In-Office Corneal Procedures

A Practical Guide

FIRST EDITION

In-Office Corneal Procedures

A Practical Guide

MARJAN FARID, MD

Professor of Ophthalmology
Director of Cornea, Cataract, and Refractive Surgery
Gavin Herbert Eye Institute
University of California, Irvine
California
United States

ELSEVIER

Elsevier
1600 John F. Kennedy Blvd.
Ste 1800
Philadelphia, PA 19103-2899

IN-OFFICE CORNEAL PROCEDURES: ISBN: 978-0-443-12589-8
A PRACTICAL GUIDE

Executive Content Strategist: Kayla Wolfe
Senior Content Development Specialist: Sneha Kashyap
Publishing Services Manager: Deepthi Unni
Project Manager: Nandhini Thanga Alagu
Design Direction: Patrick Ferguson

Printed in India

Last digit is the print number: 9   8   7   6   5   4   3   2   1

Working together
to grow libraries in
developing countries

www.elsevier.com • www.bookaid.org

This book is dedicated to my mentor, Dr. Roger F. Steinert. He taught me everything I know about corneal treatments and surgery; how to think about complex cases and investigate novel solutions, innovation, and leadership; and how to do it all with grace and humility.

CONTRIBUTORS

Natalie A. Afshari, MD, FACS
Professor
Department of Ophthalmology
Shiley Eye Institute
University of California, San Diego
San Diego, California
United States

Kanika Agarwal, MD
Ophthalmologist
Comprehensive Ophthalmology Service
Massachusetts Eye and Ear Infirmary
Boston, Massachusetts
United States;
Instructor
Department of Ophthalmology
Harvard Medical School
Boston, Massachusetts
United States

Tasnia Ahmed
..

Zaina Al-Mohtaseb, MD
Whitsett Vision Group
Cornea, Cataract, & Refractive Surgery
Director of Research
Houston, Texas
United States;
Associate Professor
Department of Ophthalmology
Baylor College of Medicine
Houston, Texas
United States

Brandon D. Ayres, MD
Instructor
Department of Ophthalmology
Sidney Kimmel Medical College Thomas
  Jefferson University
Philadelphia, Pennsylvania
United States

Alex P. Beazer, MD
Assistant Professor
Cornea
University of Washington
Seattle, Washington
United States

Cassandra C. Brooks, MD
Staff Physician
Ophthalmology
Cole Eye Institute
Cleveland, Ohio
United States

Winston Chamberlain, MD, PhD
Professor of Ophthalmology
Casey Eye Institute
Oregon Health & Science University
Portland, Oregon
United States

Lauren Chen, MD
Resident Physician
Department of Ophthalmology
UC Irvine Health
Gavin Herbert Eye Institute
University of California, Irvine
Irvine, California
United States

Jessica Blair Ciralsky, MD
Assistant Professor
Department of Ophthalmology
Weill Cornell Medical College
New York, New York
United States

Deepinder Kaur Dhaliwal, MD, L.Ac
Professor
Department of Ophthalmology
University of Pittsburgh School of Medicine
Pittsburgh, Pennsylvania
United States;
Chief of Refractive Surgery
Founder and Director, Center for Integrative
  Ophthalmology
Vice Chair, Communications and Wellness
UPMC Vision Institute
Pittsburgh, Pennsylvania
United States

Ali R. Djalilian, MD, FACS
Searls-Schenk Professor
Department of Ophthalmology and Visual
  Sciences
University of Illinois College of Medicine
Chicago, Illinois
United States

Kendall E. Donaldson, MD, MS
Professor of Ophthalmology
Bascom Palmer Eye Institute
Fort Lauderdale, Florida
United States

Marjan Farid, MD
Professor of Ophthalmology
Director of Cornea, Cataract, and Refractive
  Surgery
Gavin Herbert Eye Institute
University of California, Irvine
Irvine, California
United States

Preeya K. Gupta, MD
Managing Director
Cornea, Cataract, and Refractive Surgery
Triangle Eye Consultants
Raleigh, North Carolina
United States;
Associate Professor of Ophthalmology
Tulane University
New Orleans, Louisiana
United States

Vishal Jhanji, MD, FRCS, FRCOphth
Department of Ophthalmology
University of Pittsburgh
Pittsburgh, Pennsylvania
United States

Alexander Knezevic, MD
Professor
Ophthalmology
Cedars-Sinai Medical Center
Los Angeles, California
United States

Douglas D. Koch, MD
Professor and Allen, Mosbacher, and Law
  Chair in Ophthalmology
Department of Ophthalmology
Cullen Eye Institute
Baylor College of Medicine
Houston, Texas
United States

Amy Lin, MD
Associate Professor
Department of Ophthalmology & Visual
  Sciences
University of Utah
Salt Lake City, Utah
United States

Francis S. Mah, MD
Director, Cornea Service
Division of Ophthalmology
Scripps Clinic
La Jolla, California
United States

Parag A. Majmudar, MD
Associate Professor
Department of Ophthalmology
Rush University Medical Center
Chicago, Illinois
United States

Shivani Majmudar, MSJ, BA
Medical Student
College of Medicine
University of Illinois at Chicago
Chicago, Illinois
United States

Beeran B. Meghpara, MD
Assistant Professor
Wills Eye Hospital
Philadelphia, Pennsylvania
United States;
Assistant Professor
Department of Ophthalmology
The Sidney Kimmel Medical College
Thomas Jefferson University
Philadelphia, Pennsylvania
United States

Aman Mittal, MD
Clinical Assistant Professor
Dean McGee Eye Institute
University of Oklahoma
Oklahoma City, Oklahoma
United States

Kareem Moussa, MD
Assistant Professor
Department of Ophthalmology
UC Davis Health System
Sacramento, California
United States

Austin S. Nakatsuka, MD
Assistant Professor
University of Utah Moran Eye Center
Salt Lake City, Utah
United States

Stephen C. Pflugfelder, MD
Professor
Department of Ophthalmology
Baylor College of Medicine
Houston, Texas
United States

Margaret C. Pollard, MD
Ophthalmologist
Maine Eye Center
Portland, Maine
United States

Christopher J. Rapuano, MD
Chief, Cornea Service
Wills Eye Hospital
Philadelphia, Pennsylvania
United States;
Professor of Ophthalmology
Sidney Kimmel Medical College
Thomas Jefferson University,
Philadelphia, Pennsylvania
United States

Michelle K. Rhee, MD
Associate Clinical Professor
Department of Ophthalmology
Icahn School of Medicine at Mount Sinai
New York, New York
United States;
Medical Director
The Eye-Bank for Sight Restoration
New York, New York
United States

Eric Rosenberg, DO, MSE
Assistant Professor
Department of Ophthalmology
New York Medical College
Valhalla, New York
United States

Julie Marie Schallhorn, MD, MS
Associate Professor and Rose B. Williams
    Endowed Chair in Corneal Research
Department of Ophthalmology
University of California, San Francisco
San Francisco, California
United States

Kyoung Yul Seo, MD
Professor
Department of Ophthalmology
Yonsei University College of Medicine
Seoul, Republic of South Korea

Elizabeth Shen, MD
Ophthalmologist
Casey Eye Institute
Oregon Health & Science University
Portland, Oregon
United States

Ryan G. Smith, MD
Associate Professor
Department of Ophthalmology
School of Medicine
University of California, Irvine
Irvine, California
United States;
Cornea, Cataract, and Complex Anterior
    Segment Surgeon
Pacific Eye Institute
Upland, California
United States

Taylor W. Starnes, MD, PhD
Assistant Professor
Department of Ophthalmology and Visual
    Sciences
University of Illinois College of Medicine
Chicago, Illinois
United States

Richard Stutzman, MD
Associate Professor
Department of Ophthalmology
School of Medicine
Casey Eye Institute
Oregon Health & Science University
Portland, Oregon
United States

Miel Sundararajan, MD
Physician
Department of Ophthalmology
University of Washington
Seattle, Washington
United States

Zeba A. Syed, MD
Associate Professor
Department of Ophthalmology
Wills Eye Hospital
Philadelphia, Pennsylvania
United States

Elmer Y. Tu, BS, MD
Director, Cornea and External
    Disease Clinic
Department of Ophthalmology and Visual
    Sciences
University of Illinois College of Medicine
Chicago, Illinois
United States

Neel Vaidya, MD
Assistant Professor
Department of Ophthalmology
RUSH University
Chicago, Illinois
United States

Matthew Wade, MD
Associate Professor
Department of Ophthalmology
Gavin Herbert Eye Institute
University of California, Irvine
Irvine, California
United States

Yvonne Wang, MD
Assistant Professor
Ophthalmology and Visual Science
Yale School of Medicine
New Haven, Connecticut
United States

Kate Xie, MD
Ophthalmologist
SoCal Eye
Long Beach, California
United States

Elizabeth Yeu, MD
Partner
Virginia Eye Consultants
Norfolk, Virginia
United States;
Assistant Professor of Ophthalmology
Eastern Virginia Medical School, Norfolk
Norfolk, Virginia
United States

Corneal and ocular surface disorders are very common in all ophthalmic practices. These conditions result in loss of vision and are a significant detriment to the quality of life for our patients. Unfortunately, many of these conditions are underdiagnosed and undertreated.

All too often, beneficial techniques are not recommended or utilized because of the burden of taking the patient to the operating room. Similar to the transition of hospital-based surgery to ambulatory-based surgery, we are now seeing the transition of some procedures from the ambulatory surgery center to the clinic. This transition will reduce costs and improve efficiency and the timeliness of care. In addition, office-based care will improve the experience for the patient and medical staff. Because of the convenience, more of these beneficial procedures will be performed.

The editors and authors are to be congratulated for producing a text that contains valuable information on how to best deliver care for cornea, conjunctival, and lid disease in the office setting. Over the last several years, many innovations have occurred in the diagnosis and therapies of ocular surface disease, and many useful diagnostic techniques and treatments are outlined in detail in this book.

Patients and clinicians will both benefit from the knowledge provided by this important text.

Edward J. Holland, MD
Director of Cornea
Cincinnati Eye Institute
Professor of Ophthalmology
University of Cincinnati
Cincinnati, Ohio
United States

Dr. Marjan Farid is Professor of Clinical Ophthalmology and Director of Cornea, Refractive & Cataract Surgery at the Gavin Herbert Eye Institute, University of California-Irvine. She graduated Summa Cum Laude from UCLA with a degree in Biology and earned her medical degree at UC San Diego. Her clinical practice is divided between patient care, teaching and research. Her research interests focus on corneal surgery, specifically the use of the femtosecond laser for corneal transplantation. She is also the founder of the Severe Ocular Surface Disease Center at UCI and is a center of excellence as part of the Holland Foundation for Sight Restoration. She performs Limbal Stem Cell transplants as well as artificial corneal transplantation for the treatment of patients with severe ocular surface disease. She currently serves as the Chair of the Cornea Clinical Committee of ASCRS. Her work is published in numerous peer-reviewed journals. She has authored multiple textbook chapters and travels extensively to present her work at national and international meetings.

CONTENTS

VIDEO CONTENTS

INTRODUCTION

As office-based surgery becomes more commonplace in the medical field, ophthalmology will lead the charge. Many of our treatments are already performed within the examination lane and minor procedure room of our clinics. This case-based manual is a practical guide for how to approach these corneal procedures encountered and treated in an office setting.

As an academic corneal specialist, I am often approached by my colleagues to ask when and how to practically perform various in-office procedures (i.e., superficial keratectomy, placement of amniotic graft, conjunctivochalasis repair). Questions such as instruments required, patient positioning, and best approaches and algorithms are covered in this practical guide. We have rounded up some of the experts in the field of cornea to guide us through various corneal pathologies requiring procedural interventions and guide us through how to expediently and efficiently manage these in the office.

The target audience includes comprehensive and corneal specialists. Procedural guides that are more general and inclusive for the comprehensive ophthalmologist, such as removal of corneal foreign bodies based on type and location, removal of conjunctival calcific concretions, and procedural approaches to dry eye and Meibomian gland dysfunction, are included. Cases that are more geared to the cornea specialist, such as various approaches to a superficial keratectomy and postkeratoplasty management, are also addressed. Finally, management of those complex and urgent cases that are often encountered on a late Friday afternoon, such as impending corneal perforations, management of acute ocular surface burns, as well as how to best culture active corneal infections, are covered.

This guidebook will be an easy-to-reference and comprehensive approach to these in-office corneal and ocular surface procedures. I sincerely hope that it will be of use to our ophthalmic community as we prepare our clinics and staff to manage and treat more procedures within the office.

CHAPTER 1

Dry Eye Disease

Michelle K. Rhee ■ Francis S. Mah

Introduction

The definition of dry eye disease (DED) has evolved over decades to reflect a deeper understanding of its pathophysiology and heterogeneous clinical presentation. Most recently, the Dry Eye WorkShop (DEWS II) convened to provide follow-up on its initial global consensus report from 2007 to include the developments over the last 10 years. Today, DED is defined as "a multifactorial disease of the ocular surface characterized by a loss of homeostasis of the tear film, and accompanied by ocular symptoms, in which tear film instability and hyperosmolarity, ocular surface inflammation and damage, and neurosensory abnormalities play etiological roles."[1]

The prevalence of DED ranges from 5% to 50% globally. The most consistent risk factors for DED are older age, female sex, and Asian ethnicity.[1] Severe DED affects patient quality of life in a manner equivalent to patients with angina pectoris and hip fractures.[2] DED is chronic and widespread, leading to an enormous economic and quality of life burden. A review of expenditures of 147 participants in the Medical Expenditure Panel Survey (a subsample of the US National Health Interview Survey) found that the total number of prescriptions for DED increased markedly after the introduction of topical cyclosporine in 2003, with the cost increasing from $55 per patient per year to $299 per patient per year.[3] Another US study found the average indirect cost of DED to be approximately $11,302 per patient (and $55.4 billion to society) due to reduced productivity.[4] The annual total mean health plan costs were US $3.05 million for the topical cyclosporine cohort ($336 per patient) and $3.28 million for the punctal plug cohort ($2.24 million [$256 per patient] for initial punctal plug procedures and an additional $1.04 million [$307 per patient] for subsequent procedures during the 365-day follow-up period).[5] The overall burden of DED on the healthcare system in the US was calculated at $3.84 billion a year.[4]

Due to its variable nature, DED remains an underdiagnosed problem with a significant burden on society. As insight into DED and diagnostics improve, stepwise, early intervention through pharmacologics and procedures may control and ameliorate the disease process. As our understanding and ability to diagnose DED continues to evolve and improve, therapeutic options will grow. To date, much of the literature focuses on the pharmacologic options for managing DED. In this chapter, we offer a perspective on office procedures helpful for DED. Meibomian gland dysfunction is discussed in a separate chapter.

Diagnosis

Recently the DEWS II and the American Society of Cataract and Refractive Surgery (ASCRS) Cornea Clinical Committee[6] each produced elegant diagnostic algorithms. The DEWS II algorithm (Fig. 1.1A) includes a subjective questionnaire (Dry Eye Questionnaire or Ocular Surface Disease Index) plus one of the following homeostasis clinical markers: tear breakup time, osmolarity, or ocular surface staining with a vital dye.

The ASCRS algorithm (Fig. 1.1B) uses a modified Standard Patient Evaluation of Eye Dryness (SPEED) questionnaire, matrix metalloproteinase-9 and osmolarity testing, and clinical examination. Notably, this algorithm is specifically for the preoperative setting, and as such, the SPEED II was developed. Notably, the DEWS II flowchart does not specifically list matrix metalloproteinase-9 and osmolarity testing as essential, and it allows for other markers of homeostasis disruption.

Cases

CASE 1

A 45-year-old female with Sjögren syndrome (SS) presents with bilateral, diffuse punctate epithelial changes of the cornea despite lubricant and antiinflammatory treatment with topical cyclosporine. She has had punctal plugs inserted in both lower puncta (Fig. 1.2) with some relief in symptoms and signs, but periodically, they spontaneously explant. A next step for punctal occlusion in the office is cauterization. Suture closure of the puncta is another procedural option but is outside the scope of this chapter.

Typically, punctal plugs are the first line in tear conservation, with a variety of materials and locations, including absorbable, nonabsorbable, punctal, and intracanalicular. A large review study of lacrimal drainage system plugs showed improved signs and symptoms of DED that topical lubrication did not address, and good tolerability by patients.[7] Punctal plugs were associated with higher rates of epiphora (9%) and plug loss (40%) compared to intracanalicular plugs. However, permanent intracanalicular plugs had a higher association with canaliculitis (8%) and pyogenic granulomas; rarely, this required surgical intervention, including canaliculotomy and dacryocystorhinostomy. For this reason, punctal plugs are preferred over permanent intracanalicular plugs. Currently, studies on absorbable intracanalicular plugs are limited.

Procedure: Punctal Plug
Supplies:
- Topical anesthetic
- See Table 1.1 (Punctal Occlusion Supplies)

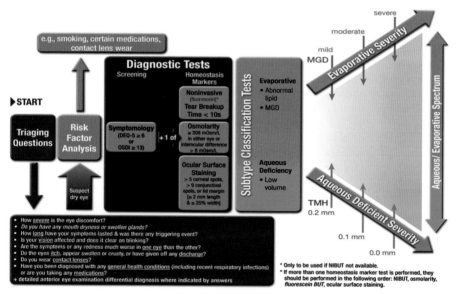

Fig 1.1 (A) DEWS II algorithm.

ASCRS PREOPERATIVE OSD ALGORITHM

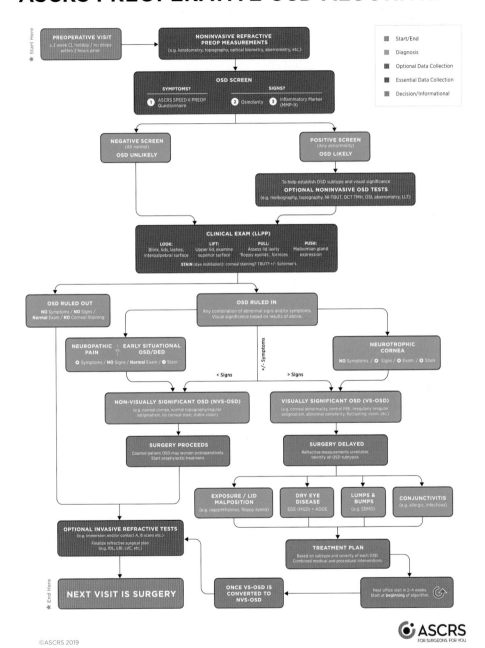

Fig 1.1 Continued (B) ASCRS algorithm. *ADDE*, Aqueous deficiency dry eye; *ASCRS*, American society of cataract and refractive surgery; *CL*, contact lens; *DED*, dry eye disease; *DEQ*, dry eye questionnaire; *EBMD*, epithelial basement membrane dystrophy; *EDE*, evaporative dry eye; *IOL*, intraocular lens; *LLT*, lipid layer thickness; *LRI*, limbal relaxing incision; *LVC*, laser vision correction; *MGD*, meibomian gland disease; *MMP9*, matrix metalloproteinase 9; *NI-TBUT*, non-invasive tear breakup time; *NVS-OSD*, non-visually significant ocular surface disease; *OCT*, ocular coherence tomography; *OSD*, ocular surface disease; *OSI*, ocular scatter index; *TBUT*, tear breakup time; *TMH*, tear meniscus height; *VS-OSD*, visually significant ocular surface disease.

©ASCRS 2019

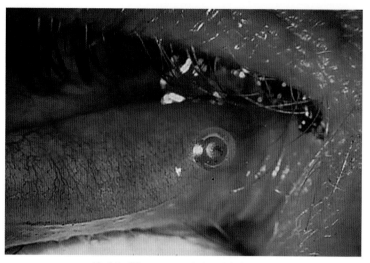

Fig 1.2   Silicone punctal plug: right inferior.

TABLE 1.1 ■ **Punctal Occlusion Supplies**

Method	Material/ Packaging	Manufacturer	Instruments
Punctal plugs (usually umbrella shaped)	• Multiple sizes • Absorbable collagen, synthetic materials • Nonabsorbable silicone, acrylic polymer • Preloaded inserter • Insert with forceps	• AlphaMed • Beaver-Visitec • EagleVision • FCI Ophthalmics • Lacrivera • Lacrimedics • Oasis • Surgical Specialties Corporation	Punctal sizer/dilator (often on the opposite end of the punctal plug inserter) Punctal plug insertion forceps
Thermal occlusion (cautery)	Single use, disposable	• Bovie • Beaver-Visitec	

Procedure: See Table 1.2 (Punctal Occlusion Technique)

Thermal occlusion via cautery is another effective in-office option for DED, especially in those patients who repeatedly have plug loss. By approaching this technique either as "superficial" or

TABLE 1.2 ■ **Punctal Occlusion Technique**

Method	Technique
Punctal plugs	• Insert at slit lamp or grossly with or without loupes. • Typically, insert both lowers; can also occlude both uppers. • Use topical anesthetic to assist in patient cooperation and comfort. • Stabilize lid tautly with finger and identify punctum. • Instruct patient to look up and temporally (away from lower punctum) as you determine size; dilate; and insert plug. • Insert plug into punctum and be ready to push the release mechanism (button on handle or squeeze device). • Use the empty plunger tip to gently maneuver the plug positioning as needed.

Thermal occlusion (cautery) modified from Holzchuh R et al.[a] and Knapp et al.[b]	• Perform under slit lamp or loupe visualization.
	• Use topical anesthetic and pledget of 4% lidocaine to punctum or infiltration of punctum with 1% lidocaine with epinephrine.
	• Stabilize lid tautly with finger and identify punctum.
	• Instruct patient to look up and temporally (away from lower punctum).
	
	For superficial cautery:
	• Tip of cautery should slightly touch the inner border of the punctum for 1–2 seconds.
	
	For deep cautery:
	• Insert cautery tip into punctum for 3 mm to include the vertical canaliculus for 1–2 seconds.
	  • Watch for whitening and closing of punctum. Repeat as needed.
	  • Postoperative antibiotic ointment or drops are given.

[a]Holzchuh R, Villa Albers MB, Osaki TH, et al. Two-year outcome of partial lacrimal punctal occlusion in the management of dry eye related to Sjögren syndrome. *Curr Eye Res.* 2011;36(6):507-512.
[b]Knapp ME, Frueh BR, Nelson CC, Musch DC. A comparison of two methods of punctal occlusion. *Am J Ophthalmol.* 1989;108(3):315-318.

"deep," the results can be nuanced to provide partial or total occlusion of the punctum. "Superficial" cautery involves superficial contact by the cautery tip to the inner border of the punctum,[8] whereas "deep" cautery requires insertion of the cautery tip into the length of the vertical canaliculus.[9] Care to avoid cautery to the external border of the punctum should be taken, as that can increase diameter.

Procedure: Thermal Occlusion of Punctum (Cautery)

Supplies:

■ Topical anesthetic
■ 4% lidocaine on pledget and/or
■ 1% lidocaine with epinephrine on 30-gauge needle for injection
■ See Table 1.1 (Punctal Occlusion Supplies)

Procedure: See Table 1.2 (Punctal Occlusion Technique)

Although punctal occlusion is an effective treatment for DED, in the setting of uncontrolled ocular surface inflammation, it can exacerbate tear inflammatory cytokines and worsen symptoms.[10] Therefore, treating with a topical steroid and/or topical chronic antiinflammatory such as cyclosporine or lifitegrast prior to punctal occlusion is generally preferred.

Other in-office procedures for DED, particularly those of neuropathic etiology, include ocular transcutaneous electrical nerve stimulation (TENS),[11] acupuncture,[12] and botulinum toxin.[13]

Discussion

SS is a systemic disease characterized by chronic inflammation of the exocrine glands, most commonly the lacrimal and salivary glands. Early diagnosis is important because it may be present alone or in conjunction with other systemic disease such as lymphoma, rheumatoid arthritis, systemic lupus erythematosus, scleroderma, and other autoimmune conditions.[14] Dry eye findings may be the first presentation of SS; 10% of predominantly aqueous-deficient dry eye has underlying SS.[15] Serologic testing (finger stick of blood to test card or phlebotomy specimen sent to laboratory) may be performed in office with the Sjö test (Bausch & Lomb), which analyzes for both traditional panels (Sjögren-specific antibody A and Sjögren-specific antibody B, antinuclear antibody, and rheumatoid factor) and novel proprietary biomarkers (salivary protein-1, carbonic anhydrase-6, and parotid secretory protein). The novel biomarkers are detected earlier in the disease.[16]

Punctal occlusion is a safe and effective in-office treatment option for DED, particularly when performed once ocular surface and lid inflammation are controlled. Historically, intracanalicular plugs for DED have not been in favor due to reports of serious adverse events. However, this experience has occurred with permanent intracanalicular plugs, where patients presented with canaliculitis and pyogenic granuloma several months to years after insertion; there is limited literature on temporary intracanalicular plugs.[7] With advances in formulation and design, temporary intracanalicular plugs may have a promising role in the treatment of DED. Currently, a self-tapering, biodegradable (about 30 days), preservative-free dexamethasone insert placed in the vertical canaliculus (Dextenza; Ocular Therapeutix Inc., Bedford, MA) is available for management of postoperative pain and inflammation.[17] Future applications of this drug delivery platform may include DED.

CASE 2

A 53-year-old male with brittle diabetes presents with visually significant punctate keratitis worse in the right eye. Despite aggressive medical management with preservative-free artificial tears and topical antiinflammatory dry eye therapies, the corneas continue to have severe keratopathy. In addition to medical therapy, in-office procedural options include the use of amniotic membrane (AM), bandage contact lens, and tarsorrhaphy.

Amniotic membrane transplantation has been used successfully for many ocular surface disorders, including as an adjunct in pterygium surgery, chemical burns, Stevens-Johnson syndrome, and persistent epithelial defects. Human AM has growth factors, collagen, fibronectin, and laminin, all of which promote regenerative healing. In addition, AM has antiinflammatory and antiscarring properties.[18] AM is available either cryopreserved or dessicated and in various sizes, shapes, and designs. For office use, two convenient and self-retained options are the cryopreserved AM attached to a conformer (Fig. 1.3) and the dessicated circular AM with a bandage contact lens overlay.

Procedure: Amniotic Membrane Transplantation for Ocular Surface Disease

Supplies: See Table 1.3 (Amniotic Membrane Supplies)

Procedure: See Box 1.1 (Amniotic Membrane Technique)

The therapeutic use of contact lenses for ocular surface disease can occur as a protective device to secure AM or on its own to provide patient comfort and heal the corneal surface. Generally, contact lenses with therapeutic indications for use have high gas permeability to allow oxygen delivery to the diseased ocular surface. Not infrequently, soft contact lenses without the therapeutic indications for use are used off-label to promote epithelialization. Prosthetic replacement of the ocular surface ecosystem treatment plays a role in the management of ocular surface disease that has failed standard therapy such as bandage contact lenses.

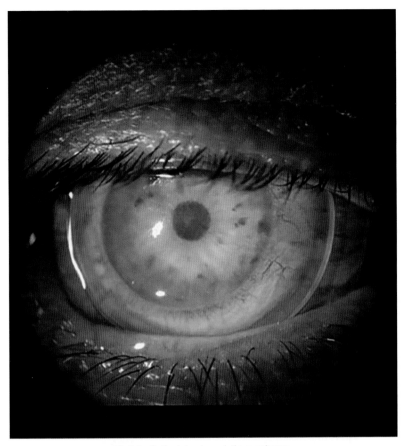

Fig 1.3   Self-retained amniotic membrane.

TABLE 1.3 ■ **Amniotic Membrane Supplies**

Method	Material/Packaging	Manufacturer	Instruments

Amniotic membrane	• Cryopreserved
	  • on polycarbonate ring conformer
	  • store at −80°C to −4°C
	  • 2-year shelf life
	  • self-retaining
	• Dessicated
	  • store at room temperature
	  • 5-year shelf life
	  • self-retaining
		• Prokera (Biotissue Inc.)
		• Ambiodisk (Katena Products Inc.)
			• Balanced salt solution bottle
			• Tegaderm
			• Eyelid speculum
			• Toothless forceps
			• Sponge spears
			• Bandage contact lens

Another in-office procedure successfully used for the management of severe punctate keratitis is the temporary suture tarsorrhaphy (Fig. 1.4) via cyanoacrylate glue,[19] botulinum toxin,[20] or suture.[21] By keeping the eyelid closed, the ocular surface is protected from exposure and evaporation of the tear film. Because of its impact on cosmesis and obscuration of vision, tarsorrhaphy is

---

BOX 1.1 ■ Amniotic Membrane Technique

Technique

For cryopreserved

- Thoroughly rinse storage solution off of device with balanced salt solution.
- Apply topical anesthetic.
- Instruct patient to keep both eyes open and to look up; this will assist in keeping the affected eye open.
- Keeping the eyelids dry facilitates the physician's fingers in fixating the eyelids apart.
- Instruct patient to look down, and insert device into superior fornix.
- Instruct patient to look straight ahead and then up so that device can settle in place.
- Inserter can assist by gently positioning lower lid to fit the device in the inferior fornix.
- Check positioning of device at slit lamp.

Optional:

- Cut Tegaderm in half and place along lateral lid to perform a "tape tarsorrhaphy" to keep device in place and retard dissolution of amniotic membrane.

To remove:

- Hold upper eyelid.
- Instruct patient to look up.
- Use forceps to grab ring along inferior fornix and remove while instructing patient to look down.

For dessicated

- Recline patient in chair.
- Apply topical anesthetic.
- Insert lid speculum.
- Dry cornea with surgical spear.
- Place amniotic membrane, basement membrane side onto epithelium, with forceps.
- Place bandage contact lens.
- Remove speculum.

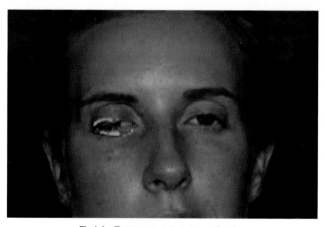

Fig 1.4   Temporary suture tarsorrhaphy.

offered when other therapy, such as topicals, punctal occlusion, AM, and/or bandage contact lens, is insufficient. Although glue, chemodenervation of the levator palpebrae, and suture tarsorrhaphy have their own advantages and disadvantages, they all work well in an office setting.

Procedure: Temporary Tarsorrhaphy for Ocular Surface Disease

Supplies: See Table 1.4 (Temporary Tarsorrhaphy Supplies)

Procedure: See Box 1.2 (Temporary Tarsorrhaphy Technique)

TABLE 1.4 ■ **Temporary Tarsorrhaphy Supplies**

Method	Material/ Packaging	Manufacturer	Instruments
Tarsorrhaphy (Temporary)	• Cyanoacrylate glue • Botulinum toxin type A • Suture	• Dermabond (Johnson and Johnson) • Botox (Allergan) • Dysport (Galderma) • Xeomin • Merz	 • Botulinum toxin • 0.9% sterile, nonpreserved saline • 1-cc syringe • 30-gauge needle • 21-gauge needle • 5-0 or 6-0 caliber silk, nylon suture, or chromic • Needle holder • Toothed forceps • Wescott scissors

---

BOX 1.2 ■ Temporary Tarsorrhaphy Technique

Technique

Cyanoacrylate glue[a]

- Instruct patient to close eyelid.
- Dry eyelid area.
- Hold eyelid closed with one hand, and apply glue directly from the applicator to the lid margin.
- Let glue dry for 60 seconds.

Note:

- Unable to visualize eye.
- Lasts up to 2 weeks.

Botulinum[b]

- Prepare botulinum according to the manufacturer's directions.
- Use half-inch 26- or 30-gauge needle to inject.
- Place needle tip near the anterior orbital roof just behind the superior orbital rim in the mid-pupillary plane. This location and use of a half-inch needle will treat the anterior-most part of the levator palpebrae (and decrease risk of superior rectus underaction and globe perforation).
- Inject 10–15 units (of Botox) aimed at the anterior-most part of the levator palpebrae.

Note:

- Expensive.
- Able to visualize eye easily.
- Complete ptosis for about 16 days and recovery of levator function at about 2 months (Kirkness et al.)[22]

Suture tarsorrhaphy[c]

- Perform grossly or with loupe visualization.
- Infiltrate eyelid skin with 1% lidocaine with epinephrine.
- Pass needle 2–3 mm inferior to the margin of lower eyelid, out through the gray line.
- Pass needle through upper eyelid gray line, out through the skin of the upper eyelid at 2–3 mm superior to the upper eyelid margin.
- Pass needle through superior eyelid skin, out through the gray line.
- Pass needle through the inferior gray line and out through the lower eyelid skin.
- Tie the suture and leave ends long.

(Continued)

BOX 1.2 ■ Temporary Tarsorrhaphy Technique—(cont'd)

- Use postoperative antibiotic ointment suture area TID × 1 week.

Note:
- Able to visualize eye.
- Lasts about 4 weeks.

[a]Donnenfeld ED, Perry HD, Nelson DB. Cyanoacrylate temporary tarsorrhaphy in the management of corneal epithelial defects. *Ophthalmic Surg.* 1991;22(10):591-593.
[b]Naik MN, Gangopadhyay N, Fernandes M, Murthy R, Honavar SG. Anterior chemodenervation of levator palpebrae superioris with botulinum toxin type-A (Botox) to induce temporary ptosis for corneal protection. *Eye.* 2008;22(9):1132-1136.
[c]Modified from Castillo GD, Remigio D. Temporary tarsorrhaphy during facial resurfacing surgery. *Arch Facial Plast Surg.* 2001;3(4):280-281.

Discussion

Fifteen percent to 35% of patients with diabetes over the age of 65 years have dry eye.[23] The mechanism of action by which diabetes causes dry eye includes neuropathy, metabolic dysfunction, and abnormal lacrimal secretions.[24] On exam, corneal sensitivity may be reduced, and dry eye complications can range from punctate keratopathy to trophic ulceration and persistent epithelial defects. When topical therapies and bandage contact lenses are inadequate, in-office procedures such as amniotic membrane transplantation and tarsorrhaphy can be highly effective in diabetics with complications of dry eye.

References

1. Craig JP, Nelson JD, Azar DT, et al. TFOS DEWS II Report executive summary. *Ocul Surf.* 2017;15(4):802–812.
2. Schiffman RM, Walt JG, Jacobsen G, et al. Utility assessment among patients with dry eye disease. *Ophthalmology.* 2003;110(7):1412–1419.
3. Galor A, Zheng DD, Arheart KL, et al. Dry eye medication use and expenditures: Data from the medical expenditure panel survey 2001 to 2006. *Cornea.* 2012;31(12):1403–1407.
4. Yu J, Asche CV, Fairchild CJ. The economic burden of dry eye disease in the United States: A decision tree analysis. *Cornea.* 2011;30(4):379–387.
5. Fiscella RG, Lee JT, Walt JG, Killian TD. Utilization characteristics of topical cyclosporine and punctal plugs in a managed care database. *Am J Manag Care.* 2008;14(3 Suppl):S107–S112.
6. Starr CE, Gupta PK, Farid M, et al. An algorithm for the preoperative diagnosis and treatment of ocular surface disorders. *J Cataract Refract Surg.* 2019;45(5):669–684.
7. Marcet M, Shtein RM, Bradley EA, et al. Safety and efficacy of lacrimal drainage system plugs for dry eye syndrome. *Ophthalmology.* 2015;122(8):1681–1687.
8. Holzchuh R, Villa Albers MB, Osaki TH, et al. Two-year outcome of partial lacrimal punctal occlusion in the management of dry eye related to Sjögren syndrome. *Curr Eye Res.* 2011;36(6):507–512.
9. Knapp ME, Frueh BR, Nelson CC, Musch DC. A comparison of two methods of punctal occlusion. *Am J Ophthalmol.* 1989;108(3):315–318.
10. Tseng SC. A practical treatment algorithm for managing ocular surface and tear disorders. *Cornea.* 2011;30(Suppl 1):S8–S14.
11. Sivanesan E, Levitt RC, Sarantopoulos CD, Patin D, Galor A. Noninvasive electrical stimulation for the treatment of chronic ocular pain and photophobia. *Neuromodulation.* 2018;21(8):727–734.
12. Dhaliwal DK, Zhou S, Samudre SS, Lo NJ, Rhee MK. Acupuncture and dry eye: Current perspectives. A double-blinded randomized controlled trial and review of the literature. *Clin Ophthalmol.* 2019;13:731–740.
13. Diel RJ, Hwang J, Kroeger ZA, et al. Photophobia and sensations of dryness in migraine patients occur independent of baseline tear volume and improve following botulinum toxin A injections. *Br J Ophthalmol.* 2019;103(8):1024–1029.

14. Liew MS, Zhang M, Kim E, Akpek EK. Prevalence and predictors of Sjögren's syndrome in a prospective cohort of patients with aqueous-deficient dry eye. *Br J Ophthalmol.* 2012;96:1498–1503.
15. Akpek EK, Klimava A, Thorne JE, et al. Evaluation of patients with dry eye for presence of underlying Sjögren syndrome. *Cornea.* 2009;28(5):493–497.
16. Bunya VY, Massaro-Giordano M, Vivino FB, et al. Prevalence of novel candidate Sjögren syndrome autoantibodies in the Penn Sjögren's International Collaborative Clinical Alliance Cohort. *Cornea.* 2019;38(12):1500–1505.
17. Brooks CC, Jabbehdari S, Gupta PK. Dexamethasone 0.4 mg sustained-release intracanalicular insert in the management of ocular inflammation and pain following ophthalmic surgery: Design, development and place in therapy. *Clin Ophthalmol.* 2020;14:89–94.
18. Suri K, Kosker M, Raber IM, et al. Sutureless amniotic membrane ProKera for ocular surface disorders: Short-term results. *Eye Contact Lens.* 2013;39(5):341–347.
19. Donnenfeld ED, Perry HD, Nelson DB. Cyanoacrylate temporary tarsorrhaphy in the management of corneal epithelial defects. *Ophthalmic Surg.* 1991;22(10):591–593.
20. Naik MN, Gangopadhyay N, Fernandes M, Murthy R, Honavar SG. Anterior chemodenervation of levator palpebrae superioris with botulinum toxin type-A (Botox) to induce temporary ptosis for corneal protection. *Eye.* 2008;22(9):1132–1136.
21. Castillo GD, Remigio D. Temporary tarsorrhaphy during facial resurfacing surgery. *Arch Facial Plast Surg.* 2001;3(4):280–281.
22. Kirkness CM, Adams GG, Dilly PN, Lee JP Botulinum toxin A-induced protective ptosis in corneal disease. *Ophthalmology.* 1988;95(4):473–480. https://doi.org/10.1016/s0161-6420(88)33163-5.
23. Manaviat MR, Rashidi M, Afkhami-Ardekani M. Prevalence of dry eye syndrome and diabetic retinopathy in type 2 diabetic patients. *BMC Ophthalmology.* 2008;8:10.
24. Inoue K, Kato S, Ohara C, et al. Ocular and systemic factors relevant to diabetic keratoepitheliopathy. *Cornea.* 2001;20(8):798–801.

CHAPTER 2

Meibomian Gland Disease

Cassandra C. Brooks ▪ Preeya K. Gupta

Introduction

Meibomian glands are important structures that create meibum, which is vital to the stability of a healthy tear film.[1] Meibum has several key functions, including acting as a physical hydrophobic barrier to foreign agents, lubricating the ocular surface to protect against irritation and decrease surface light diffraction, as well as preventing tear evaporation and subsequent surface desiccation.[2-4] Meibomian gland dysfunction (MGD) is defined as terminal duct obstruction and/or qualitative/quantitative changes in glandular secretion.[5] MGD can result in disruption of the tear film, ocular discomfort, and ocular surface disease.[6]

Meibomian gland function can be assessed at the slit lamp, specifically looking at oil quality (i.e., clear versus thickened) and oil flow (i.e., free-flowing versus obstructed).[7] Meibography is also of great value to understand the underlying anatomy of the meibomian glands.[8,9] The LipiView or LipiScan devices (Johnson & Johnson Vision) are easily integrated into clinical practice and are the most commonly available devices. It is essential for the clinician to know the degree of meibomian gland atrophy present when evaluating a patient. This information can give insight into how severe the disease stage is and also can help to set patient expectations.[10] A patient with more severe atrophy will often require multiple therapies. Meibomian gland dropout can occur with increased age, topical medication use (i.e., prostaglandin analog drugs), isotretinoin, rosacea, and Sjögren disease, all of which can be associated with chronic MGD.[9,11-16]

Case 1

A 44-year-old female who is a software engineer presents with complaints of fluctuating vision, eye fatigue, and burning. She wears soft contact lenses daily but has had increasing difficulty tolerating lens wear. She has used artificial tears intermittently and does a warm compress once daily, which provides some relief. Symptoms appear to worsen throughout the day. Past medical history is unremarkable. Slit-lamp examination of the eyelid margin reveals erythema and fine telangectasias (Fig. 2.1A). Secretions appeared thickened with poor flow. Meibography revealed mild atrophy (Fig. 2.1B).

MANAGEMENT

The goal of treatment is to improve the flow of meibomian gland secretions (MGSs) and stabilize the tear film to allow greater protection of the ocular surface and stability of vision quality.

Home Therapies

These therapies are often considered to be supportive care; however, when patients are truly symptomatic and show signs of MGD, in-office procedural treatments have been shown to be more beneficial.

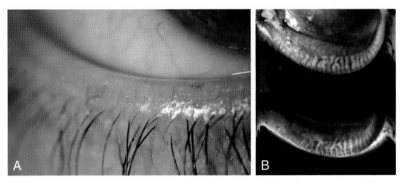

Fig. 2.1 (A) Eyelid margin with mild erythema and fine telangiectasias. (B) Meibography with mild atrophy and tortuosity.

- *Warm compresses*: Warm compresses (40.0 ± 2° C) applied for 5 minutes to the skin of closed eyelids nearly doubles the tear film lipid layer thickness.[17] Notably, room temperature (24 ± 1° C) compresses, even after 30 minutes of application, result in no change to tear film lipid layer thickness.
- *Lid hygiene*: Lid hygiene using eyelid cleanser or a gentle shampoo daily to remove debris and decrease bacterial colonization can improve clinical indices and alleviate patient symptoms.[18,19]
- *Dietary supplementation*: There is mixed evidence on the effectiveness of omega-3 essential fatty acid supplementation for the treatment of dry eye disease. Initial evidence indicated that long-term moderate daily supplementation might reduce tear osmolarity and increase tear stability in patients with dry eye disease.[20] However, recent multicentered, double-blind clinical trials suggest there are no significant differences compared to a placebo, though the study design and outcomes are frequently debated.[21,22]

In the present case, the patient has MGD with insufficient flow of meibum to support the tear film. Thermal treatments are the procedures of choice to manage patients with limited gland atrophy in the presence of MGD. There are 3 current in-office procedural thermal treatment options that can be used to relieve gland obstruction:

In-Office Procedural Options

(1) Thermal Pulsation (LipiFlow)

With US Food and Drug Administration approval in 2011, LipiFlow is a vectored thermal pulsation (VTP) device that has the longest treatment history with the most substantial data to support efficacy.[23–25] The device consists of a base console attached to a single-use sterile device with an inner and outer shell to provide 12 minutes of treatment. The shell is inserted under the eyelid and applies heat (42.5°C) to the tarsal conjunctiva of both eyelids simultaneously, while the outer portion of the device applies simultaneous precise pressure to the glands directly.

One prospective, multicenter, open-label clinical trial of 200 (400 eyes) randomized patients to a single VTP treatment (treatment group) versus twice-daily (BID) warm compresses with lid hygiene for 3 months (control group).[24] At 3 months, patients in the control group received a VTP treatment (crossover group), and the groups were monitored at 3-month intervals for 12 months for measures of MGSs and dry eye symptoms. Beginning 3 months following initial VTP treatment (month 3 in the treatment group and month 6 in the control/crossover group), patients could receive additional therapy if symptoms were inadequately controlled. At 3 months, patients in the treatment group had a statistically significant improvement in MGSs ($P < 0.0001$) and dry eye symptoms ($P = 0.0068$). At 12 months, patients in both the treatment and crossover groups had sustained improvements in both MGSs and dry eye symptoms, with only one VTP treatment in 86% and 89%, respectively, suggesting that a single treatment can lead to 12 months of sustained meibomian gland function and symptomatic relief.

A recent study demonstrated the impact of thermal pulsation on contact lens wearers with MGD and dry eye symptoms.[26] The prospective study involved 55 soft contact lens wearers with MGD and dry eye symptoms and randomized patients to a single VTP treatment or an untreated control group that received crossover VTP treatment at 3 months. MGS scores, Standard Patient Evaluation of Eye Dryness (SPEED) questionnaires, frequency of over-the-counter drop use, and hours of comfortable contact lens wear were evaluated before and after VTP treatment. VTP treatment was associated with significantly greater MGSs (12.4 vs. 1.4, $P < 0.0001$) and SPEED (-8.4 vs. -0.7, $P < 0.0001$) scores, decreased over-the-counter drop use, and a mean increase of 4 hours of comfortable contact lens wear.

Special populations including those with dry eye and MGD post–laser refractive surgery and those with Sjögren syndrome have also been shown to have benefit from LipiFlow thermal pulsation, though the benefit may not be as robust as in the typical MGD population.[27-29]

Supplies

- Topical anesthetic (i.e., tetracaine or proparacaine)
- LipiFlow Thermal Pulsation System console
- Sterile single-use LipiFlow Activator

Technique

1. Comfortably seat patient in mildly reclined exam chair
2. Remove contact lenses if applicable
3. Apply 1–2 drops of topical anesthetic to each treatment eye
4. Using a blunt spatula or spud-like instrument, gently debride the lid margin along the orifice of the meibomian glands for both the upper and lower eyelids (Fig. 2.2)
5. Attach single-use disposable LipiFlow Activators to console
6. Insert single-use disposable LipiFlow Activator to patient's eye (similar to scleral lens or surgical corneal shield) (Fig. 2.3)
7. Apply adhesive strip to device and anchor it at the bridge of the nose
8. Repeat for the other eye
9. Ask patient to gently close their eyes to ensure proper positioning
10. Begin 12-minute treatment
11. Remove single-use disposable LipiFlow Activator from patient's eyes
12. Detach and discard single-use disposable LipiFlow Activator

---

CLINICAL PEARLS

- For patients with loose or floppy eyelids:
  - "Tape tarsorrhaphy": once applicators are in place, use additional tape at the lateral canthus to secure the eyelids into the correct position for the duration of the treatment.
  - It is critical for the external compressing device to be in line with the meibomian glands; shortening the canthus with tape will not allow for the lid to slip out of the activator.
- For patients with tight eyelids or narrow fissure:
  - Placement in a tight eyelid can be challenging. The device is wider horizontally than it is vertically. The shell can be rotated 45–90 degrees and inserted into the superior fornix area while the patient is looking down. Subsequently, the shell is rotated into its normal position, and the lower lid can then be retracted to facilitate complete insertion.

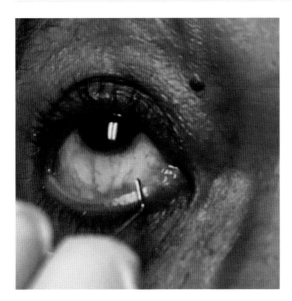

Fig. 2.2 Eyelid debridement.

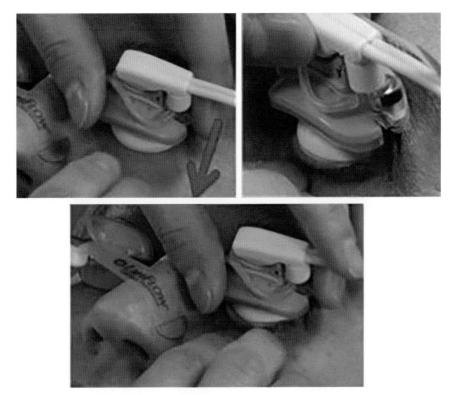

Fig. 2.3 This series of photos demonstrates insertion of the LipiFlow device.

(2) Thermal Expression (iLux)

Approved by the US Food and Drug Administration in 2017, iLux is a portable device that applies focal heat and pressure to the meibomian glands.[30] The device consists of a handheld console with a magnifier and a disposable unit that is inserted behind the eyelid being treated (Fig. 2.4A–C). The eyelid is treated in 3 areas: nasal, central, and temporal zones. All four eyelids are treated. Once the device is in place, the targeted area of meibomian glands is then warmed to 40–42°C in order to melt the meibum. Once critical temperature is achieved, the same device applies force to the express meibum from the glands. The eyelid margin and gland orifice are visualized by the magnifier, which allows for titrated application of treatment. Treatment time varies by patient.

Currently, minimal studies are available describing the efficacy of the device in various populations. However, clinical trials comparing LipiFlow and iLux are currently being undertaken.[31]

Supplies

- Topical anesthetic (i.e., tetracaine or proparacaine)
- iLux device
- Sterile single-use Smart Tip

Technique
1. Comfortably seat patient in mildly reclined exam chair
2. Remove contact lenses if necessary
3. Apply 1–2 drops of topical anesthetic to each treatment eye
4. Each eyelid will be treated in 3 segments: nasal, central, and temporal. Place inner pad in the inferior fornix adjacent to selected treatment area
5. Depress button to apply heat to desired temperature
6. Engage button to titrate expression while directly visualizing meibomian glands through the magnifier
7. Adjust heating time and compression as needed to optimize meibum expression and patient comfort

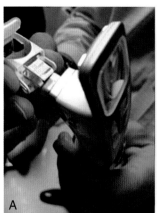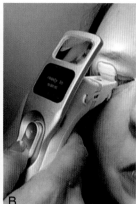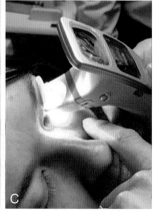

Fig. 2.4 (A) Disposable unit is attached to handheld console. (B) Place console adjacent to target treatment area and depress button. (C) Heat applied to desired temperature.

(3) Electrothermal Adhesive Thermal Treatment (TearCare)

TearCare is an external device that applies localized heat to the eyelids in order to liquefy meibum.[32] The device consists of four flexible electrothermal adhesives, and each adhesive is applied to the eyelid skin overlying the tarsal plate (Fig. 2.5). The adhesives are connected to a control unit, which delivers targeted heat between 41°C and 45°C. During the treatment, the patient is able to open their eyes and blink, thereby contributing to natural meibum expression. Following the 15-minute thermal treatment, manual expression with proprietary expression forceps is performed to complete meibum expression.

A prospective pilot study involving 24 randomized patients to a single 12-minute thermal session of TearCare treatment followed by manual expression or 4 weeks of 5-minute daily warm compresses was performed.[32] Patients were followed for 6 months. At 1 month, patients who received TearCare had improved tear breakup time (TBUT) (11.7 vs. 0.3 seconds in the warm compress group, $P < 0.0001$), MGSs, corneal and conjunctival staining, and dry eye symptoms. Improved TBUT was maintained through the 6 months. At 6 months, the treatment group was retreated and monitored for an additional 6 months.[33] The results suggest that additional treatment provides further benefit to subjective and objective parameters of dry eye, which were maintained through 12 months.

Further research comparing 15 minutes of electrothermal treatment to 12 minutes of thermal pulsation was conducted in a trial called OLYMPIA, which was completed in late 2020.[31]

Supplies

- TearCare Smart Hub
- Sterile single-use applicator adhesives
- Sterile single-use gland expression forceps

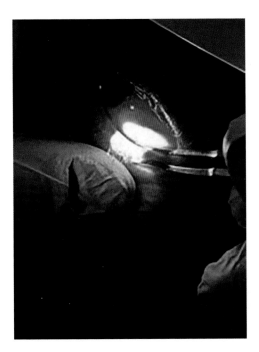

Fig. 2.5 Four flexible electrothermal adhesives each applied to the eyelid skin overlying the tarsal plate and connected to a control unit.

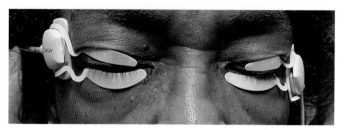

Fig. 2.6 Manual expression of meibomian glands.

Technique

1. Comfortably seat patient in exam chair
2. Remove makeup and cleanse outer eyelid skin with cleansing wipe
3. Apply one electrothermal adhesive to the skin overlying each tarsal plate
4. Attach electrothermal adhesives to controller unit
5. Engage start button to start 15-minute heating treatment
6. Remove adhesives
7. Use sterile forceps to manually express meibomian glands in all 4 lids (Fig. 2.6)

CLINICAL PEARLS

- For patients with oily skin or excessive makeup, it is essential to remove all oil and debris from skin, as this can interfere with proper adhesion of the strips to the eyelid.
- When expressing meibomian glands, have the patient look in the opposite direction to avoid corneal injury.
- Both upper and lower eyelids should be expressed (see Video 2.1).

Case 2

A 69-year-old male with a long history of dry eye presents with persistent complaints of burning, redness, and foreign body sensation. He has a history of ocular hypertension and rosacea. He is currently taking lifitegrast BID and latanoprost daily at bedtime in both eyes (QHS OU).

Slit-lamp examination of the eyelid margin reveals extensive erythema, fine telangiectasias, and keratinization of the eyelid margin (Fig. 2.7A). Secretions were thick and unable to be expressed with gentle pressure along the eyelids. External exam revealed facial rosacea. Meibography demonstrates significant gland atrophy and tortuosity (Fig. 2.7B).

MANAGEMENT

- *Topical medications:* Topical antibiotics (i.e., fluoroquinolones, macrolides) and corticosteroids can minimize eyelid bacterial colonization and inflammation associated with MGD.[34,35] Of note, a recent study that investigated 915 cases of confirmed *Staphylococcus aureus* among ocular cultures in 471 patients found an increasing incidence of methicillin-resistant *S. aureus* between 1998 and 2005, with incidences of 4.1% and 16.7%, respectively. These data suggest that more judicious use of antibiotics, as well as the potential use of antibacterials with activity against methicillin-resistant *S. aureus* in suspected cases, is warranted.[36] Interestingly, among this cohort, the most common diagnosis was blepharoconjunctivitis (78.0% in 1998 and 81.4% in 2005).

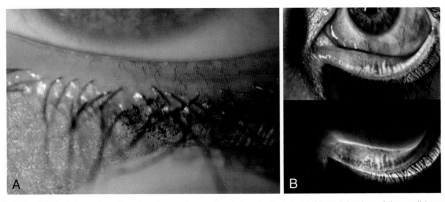

Fig. 2.7 (A) Eyelid margin with extensive erythema, fine telangiectasias, and keratinization of the eyelid margin. (B) Meibography with significant gland atrophy.

- *Oral medications*: Systemic tetracycline derivatives, such as doxycycline 20–100 mg daily or azithromycin 250–500 mg daily or 3 times per week can be utilized for their antiinflammatory and lipid-regulating properties.[37]

In-Office Procedural Options

(1) Intense Pulsed Light Therapy

Intense pulsed light (IPL) therapy has been used by dermatologists in the treatment of many skin conditions, including rosacea, for many years. Multiple prospective and retrospective trials have since recognized that IPL is an effective treatment for patients with MGD, showing that when treated with IPL, MGD patients had fewer dry eye symptoms (SPEED scores) and improved MGSs, TBUT, and corneal staining.[38–42] The treatment involves exposing the pretarsal skin to brief bursts of noncoherent polyspectrum light with wavelengths from 500 nm to 1200 nm. These wavelengths target melanin and hemoglobin in the skin and result in coagulation and ablation of fine telangiectasias along the lid margin. The mechanism of action is somewhat unclear but is believed to involve decreasing inflammatory load to the eyelid or secondary generation of heat, which softens obstructions.[43] Only patients with Fitzpatrick scale skin type <4 can be treated with IPL; patients with more pigmented skin types are at higher risk for depigmentation and should be avoided. Patients with advanced MGD or telangiectasias along the lid margin with or without rosacea or seborrheic dermatitis are ideal candidates for this procedure. However, IPL can be successfully utilized in a range of MGD severities. Patients come for 4 treatments separated by 3–5 weeks, each consisting of application of the broad-spectrum light to the lower eyelids and lateral canthal area followed by manual expression.

Supplies

- Single-use disposable IPL eye pads to protect eyes
- Ultrasound gel
- IPL unit with proprietary dry eye settings (M22; Lumenis)

Technique
1. Comfortably seat patient in exam chair
2. Remove makeup if necessary

3. Apply disposable IPL eye pads over closed eyes to prevent direct penetration of light into the eyes
4. Place ultrasound gel over desired treatment area
5. Apply light treatment to lower eyelid and lateral canthal area (recommend using dry eye settings on device; energy can range from $8 J/cm^2$ to $20 J/cm^2$)
6. Place additional ultrasound gel if needed and perform second pass with IPL
7. Remove gel
8. Apply 1 drop of topical anesthetic to each treatment eye
9. Perform manual gland expression

CLINICAL PEARLS

- Reassure patients that they will see a bright flash around the protective eye shields and that it is normal to have mild stinging from light application.
- Place a test spot on the side of the face to ensure that the settings do not induce blistering or skin irritation.
- Some patients may benefit from more than four treatments, especially in the setting of severe disease.

(2) Meibomian Gland Probing

Intraductal meibomian gland probing (MGP) is a method for removing physical barriers in order to relieve obstruction-related meibomian gland disease.[44] The technique involves introducing a wire instrument into the gland orifice and subsequently into the ductal outflow tract. Physical barriers are met with instrument resistance, and further probing can be used in an attempt to relieve those obstructions and allow the release of sequestered or retained intraductal material. A retrospective evaluation of 25 patients with MGD who underwent MGP found symptomatic relief among 96% immediately postprocedure and 100% at 4 weeks. Symptom relief averaged 11.5 months, and 80% required only 1 treatment. Further research found statistically significant changes in TBUT (5 vs. 13 seconds, $P < 0.001$), conjunctival hyperemia ($P < 0.0001$), eyelid margin vascularization ($P = 0.004$), and Ocular Surface Disease Index scores when comparing pre-MGP to 3 months post-MGP.[45] Additional investigation involving meibography pre- and post-MGP among 10 eyelids with meibography suitable for analysis found an increase in mean individual glandular area (4.87%, $P = 0.0145$).[46] This statistically significant change was observed due to increases in mean individual glandular area of 4 of the 10 eyelids, while 6 demonstrated no change. This suggests that MGP may promote growth of atrophied meibomian glands.

    Combining MGP with IPL in patients with refractory obstructive MGD has recently demonstrated a synergistic effect on SPEED, TBUT, meibum grade, and lid telangiectasia ($P < 0.5/3$).[47] Among the 45 patients (90 eyes) studied, divided into 3 treatment groups, patients in the combination treatment group did not feel the need to be retreated, compared with 35.7% and 20% in the IPL- or MGP-alone treatment groups, respectively.

Supplies

- Topical anesthetic drop (i.e., tetracaine or proparacaine) and ointment (i.e., 3.5% topical lidocaine hydrochloride jelly or 8% lidocaine with 25% jojoba wax)
- Bandage contact lens (BCL)
- Solid stainless steel probe set (76 μm in diameter with lengths of 1, 2, 4, and 6 mm) (Katena Products Inc., Denville, NJ, USA)

Technique
1. Comfortably seat patient in exam chair at slit lamp and remove makeup if necessary
2. Apply 1–2 drops of topical anesthetic to each treatment eye
3. Insert BCL
4. Apply topical anesthetic ointment to external lid margin and allow 10–15 minutes for lid to anesthetize
5. Apply additional 1 drop of topical anesthetic to treatment eye
6. Probe all meibomian gland orifices using a dart-throwing motion (hold probe in similar manner to holding a dart and make short 1- to 2-mm insertions to penetrate ducts) starting with the shortest 1 mm and using longer probes if necessary
7. Remove BCL
8. Irrigate ocular surface with copious amounts of sterile preservative-free saline
9. Use a cotton-tipped applicator to remove residual ointment and debris from eyelashes

CLINICAL PEARLS
- If patient's eyelids are still sensitive once probing has begun, place a second round of topical anesthetic ointment on lid margin.
- If there is difficulty visualizing gland orifice, red-free light, transillumination, and meibography can be used to assist.
- If you meet resistance on probing, attempt a different probe angle of entry. Resistance may be obstruction due to ductal fibrosis and can produce an audible and tactile "pop."
- A small amount of hemorrhage from the orifices is not uncommon, is self-limited, and does not require treatment.

Conclusion

Meibomian glands are essential structures that produce meibum, which is vital to stability of a healthy tear film and ocular surface. Meibomian gland function can be assessed at the slit lamp, looking at components such as oil quality and flow, or with meibography to visualize gland anatomy. Mild cases of MGD can be addressed with home therapies such as warm compresses, lid hygiene, and dietary supplements, as well as in-office procedures such as thermal pulsation (LipiFlow), thermal expression (iLux), and electrothermal adhesive thermal treatment (TearCare). Advanced MGD can be treated with topical medications, IPL therapy, and meibomian gland probing. Patients with more severe disease often require multiple therapies.

References

1. Foulks GN, Bron AJ. Meibomian gland dysfunction: a clinical scheme for description, diagnosis, classification, and grading. *Ocul Surf.* 2003;1(3):107–126.
2. Holly FJ, Lemp MA. Tear physiology and dry eyes. *Surv Ophthalmol.* 1977;22(2):69–87.
3. Mishima S, Maurice DM. The oily layer of the tear film and evaporation from the corneal surface. *Exp Eye Res.* 1961;1:39–45.
4. Tiffany JM. The lipid secretion of the meibomian glands. *Adv Lipid Res.* 1987;22:1–62.
5. Nelson JD, Shimazaki J, Benitez-del-Castillo JM, et al. The international workshop on meibomian gland dysfunction: Report of the definition and classification subcommittee. *Invest Ophthalmol Vis Sci.* 2011;52(4):1930–1937.
6. Chhadva P, Goldhardt R, Galor A. Meibomian gland disease: The role of gland dysfunction in dry eye disease. *Ophthalmology.* 2017;124(11s):S20–S26.
7. Shimazaki J, Sakata M, Tsubota K. Ocular surface changes and discomfort in patients with meibomian gland dysfunction. *Arch Ophthalmol.* 1995;113(10):1266–1270.

8. Mathers WD. Ocular evaporation in meibomian gland dysfunction and dry eye. *Ophthalmology.* 1993; 100(3):347–351.

9. Arita R, Itoh K, Inoue K, Amano S. Noncontact infrared meibography to document age-related changes of the meibomian glands in a normal population. *Ophthalmology.* 2008;115(5):911–915.

10. Arita R, Itoh K, Maeda S, et al. Proposed diagnostic criteria for obstructive meibomian gland dysfunction. *Ophthalmology.* 2009;116(11):2058–2063.e2051.

11. Mocan MC, Uzunosmanoglu E, Kocabeyoglu S, Karakaya J, Irkec M. The association of chronic topical prostaglandin analog use with meibomian gland dysfunction. *J Glaucoma.* 2016;25(9):770–774.

12. Moy A, McNamara NA, Lin MC. Effects of isotretinoin on meibomian glands. *Optom Vis Sci.* 2015; 92(9):925–930.

13. Machalinska A, Zakrzewska A, Markowska A, et al. Morphological and functional evaluation of meibomian gland dysfunction in rosacea patients. *Curr Eye Res.* 2016;41(8):1029–1034.

14. Zengin N, Tol H, Gunduz K, Okudan S, Balevi S, Endogru H. Meibomian gland dysfunction and tear film abnormalities in rosacea. *Cornea.* 1995;14(2):144–146.

15. Shimazaki J, Goto E, Ono M, Shimmura S, Tsubota K. Meibomian gland dysfunction in patients with Sjogren syndrome. *Ophthalmology.* 1998;105(8):1485–1488.

16. Sullivan DA, Dana R, Sullivan RM, et al. Meibomian gland dysfunction in primary and secondary Sjogren syndrome. *Ophthalmic Res.* 2018;59(4):193–205.

17. Olson MC, Korb DR, Greiner JV. Increase in tear film lipid layer thickness following treatment with warm compresses in patients with meibomian gland dysfunction. *Eye Contact Lens.* 2003;29(2):96–99.

18. Tanabe H, Kaido M, Kawashima M, Ishida R, Ayaki M, Tsubota K. Effect of eyelid hygiene detergent on obstructive meibomian gland dysfunction. *J Oleo Sci.* 2019;68(1):67–78.

19. Yin Y, Gong L. Reversibility of gland dropout and significance of eyelid hygiene treatment in meibomian gland dysfunction. *Cornea.* 2017;36(3):332–337.

20. Deinema LA, Vingrys AJ, Wong CY, Jackson DC, Chinnery HR, Downie LE. A randomized, double-masked, placebo-controlled clinical trial of two forms of omega-3 supplements for treating dry eye disease. *Ophthalmology.* 2017;124(1):43–52.

21. Asbell PA, Maguire MG, Pistilli M, et al. n-3 Fatty acid supplementation for the treatment of dry eye disease. *N Engl J Med.* 2018;378(18):1681–1690.

22. Oydanich M, Maguire MG, Pistilli M, et al. Effects of omega-3 supplementation on exploratory outcomes in the dry eye assessment and management study. *Ophthalmology.* 2020;127(1):136–138.

23. FDA Oks TearScience LipiFlow MGD system. https://www.reviewofophthalmology.com/article/fda-oks-tearscience-lipifl owmgd-system-29635. Published 2011. Accessed December 4, 2019.

24. Blackie CA, Coleman CA, Holland EJ. The sustained effect (12 months) of a single-dose vectored thermal pulsation procedure for meibomian gland dysfunction and evaporative dry eye. *Clin Ophthalmol.* 2016;10:1385–1396.

25. Geerling G, Baudouin C, Aragona P, et al. Emerging strategies for the diagnosis and treatment of meibomian gland dysfunction: Proceedings of the OCEAN group meeting. *Ocul Surf.* 2017;15(2):179–192.

26. Blackie CA, Coleman CA, Nichols KK, et al. A single vectored thermal pulsation treatment for meibomian gland dysfunction increases mean comfortable contact lens wearing time by approximately 4 hours per day. *Clin Ophthalmol.* 2018;12:169–183.

27. Epitropoulos AT, Goslin K, Bedi R, Blackie CA. Meibomian gland dysfunction patients with novel Sjogren's syndrome biomarkers benefit significantly from a single vectored thermal pulsation procedure: A retrospective analysis. *Clin Ophthalmol.* 2017;11:701–706.

28. Godin MR, Stinnett SS, Gupta PK. Outcomes of thermal pulsation treatment for dry eye syndrome in patients with Sjogren disease. *Cornea.* 2018;37(9):1155–1158.

29. Schallhorn CS, Schallhorn JM, Hannan S, Schallhorn SC. Effectiveness of an eyelid thermal pulsation procedure to treat recalcitrant dry eye symptoms after laser vision correction. *J Refract Surg.* 2017; 33(1):30–36.

30. US Food and Drug Administration. https://www.accessdata.fda.gov/cdrh_docs/pdf17/K172645.pdf. Accessed December 5, 2019.

31. Comparison between iLux and LipiFlow in the treatment of meibomian gland dysfunction. ClinicalTrials.gov. https://clinicaltrials.gov/ct2/show/NCT03055832. Accessed December 5, 2019.

32. Badawi D. A novel system, TearCare, for the treatment of the signs and symptoms of dry eye disease. *Clin Ophthalmol.* 2018;12:683–694.

33. Badawi D. TearCare system extension study: Evaluation of the safety, effectiveness, and durability through 12 months of a second TearCare treatment on subjects with dry eye disease. *Clin Ophthalmol.* 2019;13:189–198.
34. Dougherty JM, McCulley JP. Bacterial lipases and chronic blepharitis. *Invest Ophthalmol Vis Sci.* 1986; 27(4):486–491.
35. Lindsley K, Matsumura S, Hatef E, Akpek EK. Interventions for chronic blepharitis. *Cochrane Database Syst Rev.* 2012;2012(5):Cd005556.
36. Freidlin J, Acharya N, Lietman TM, Cevallos V, Whitcher JP, Margolis TP. Spectrum of eye disease caused by methicillin-resistant Staphylococcus aureus. *Am J Ophthalmol.* 2007;144(2):313–315.
37. Geerling G, Tauber J, Baudouin C, et al. The International Workshop on Meibomian Gland Dysfunction: Report of the subcommittee on management and treatment of meibomian gland dysfunction. *Invest Ophthalmol Vis Sci.* 2011;52(4):2050–2064.
38. Toyos R, McGill W, Briscoe D. Intense pulsed light treatment for dry eye disease due to meibomian gland dysfunction; a 3-year retrospective study. *Photomed Laser Surg.* 2015;33(1):41–46.
39. Dell SJ, Gaster RN, Barbarino SC, Cunningham DN. Prospective evaluation of intense pulsed light and meibomian gland expression efficacy on relieving signs and symptoms of dry eye disease due to meibomian gland dysfunction. *Clin Ophthalmol.* 2017;11:817–827.
40. Dell SJ. Intense pulsed light for evaporative dry eye disease. *Clin Ophthalmol.* 2017;11:1167–1173.
41. Craig JP, Chen YH, Turnbull PR. Prospective trial of intense pulsed light for the treatment of meibomian gland dysfunction. *Invest Ophthalmol Vis Sci.* 2015;56(3):1965–1970.
42. Vora GK, Gupta PK. Intense pulsed light therapy for the treatment of evaporative dry eye disease. *Curr Opin Ophthalmol.* 2015;26(4):314–318.
43. Liu R, Rong B, Tu P, et al. Analysis of cytokine levels in tears and clinical correlations after intense pulsed light treating meibomian gland dysfunction. *Am J Ophthalmol.* 2017;183:81–90.
44. Maskin SL. Intraductal meibomian gland probing relieves symptoms of obstructive meibomian gland dysfunction. *Cornea.* 2010;29(10):1145–1152.
45. Sik Sarman Z, Cucen B, Yuksel N, Cengiz A, Caglar Y. Effectiveness of intraductal meibomian gland probing for obstructive meibomian gland dysfunction. *Cornea.* 2016;35(6):721–724.
46. Maskin SL, Testa WR. Growth of meibomian gland tissue after intraductal meibomian gland probing in patients with obstructive meibomian gland dysfunction. *Br J Ophthalmol.* 2018;102(1):59–68.
47. Huang X, Qin Q, Wang L, Zheng J, Lin L, Jin X. Clinical results of intraductal meibomian gland probing combined with intense pulsed light in treating patients with refractory obstructive meibomian gland dysfunction: A randomized controlled trial. *BMC Ophthalmol.* 2019;19(1):211.

CHAPTER 3

Corneal Relaxing Incisions

Douglas D. Koch ▦ Kate Xie ▦ Marjan Farid

Introduction

Many patients undergoing cataract surgery desire good uncorrected vision. This requires accurate selection of intraocular lens (IOL) power and surgical management of astigmatism. Astigmatic refractive errors of 1–2 diopters (D) may reduce uncorrected visual acuity to the 20/30 to 20/50 level, and astigmatic errors of 2–3 D may produce uncorrected visual acuity of 20/70 to 20/100.[1] For eyes implanted with multifocal IOLs, even 0.5 D of astigmatism can reduce the distance visual acuity by 1–2 lines.[2] Using a threshold of >1.0 D, up to approximately 2/3 of patients having cataract surgery would benefit by having their astigmatism treated.[3]

Corneal relaxing incisions (CRIs) are somewhat arbitrarily categorized as "astigmatic keratotomy," or AK, if within the central 8 mm, and as "peripheral CRIs," or PCRIs, if made more peripherally. These are also often referred to as "limbal relaxing incisions," or LRIs. CRIs can be performed freehand, with a mechanical keratome, or with femtosecond laser technology.[4] With the growing popularity of femtosecond laser technology, increasing popularity of multifocal and extended depth of focus IOLs, expanding range of toric IOL implants, and technology for computer-assisted intraoperative markerless alignment, there are many excellent tools, now more than ever, to address astigmatism at the time of cataract surgery.[5] However, the ability to perform in-office manual PCRIs or LRIs remains an important skill for the ophthalmologist to maintain, especially in the setting of postsurgical astigmatism management. They may be used after implantation of a toric, multifocal, or extended-depth-of-focus lenses and after laser-assisted in situ keratomileusis (LASIK) or photorefractive keratectomy (PRK) to refine postoperative outcomes.[6]

Manual PCRIs or LRIs are created in the peripheral clear cornea by using a handheld diamond knife or a disposable steel blade knife. The incisions are created using established nomograms that vary treatment based upon the amount of astigmatism, the patient's age, and the location of the steep astigmatic meridian. They can be single or paired, and the surgical technique can vary based upon the choice of markers, blades, and nomograms. The incisions are ideally created at an 80%–90% depth with either a fixed-depth or variable-depth single-foot-plate, double-cutting diamond blade that is set based on intraoperative pachymetry readings.[7] They provide an easy and affordable method to correct corneal astigmatism.

Evaluation

PATIENT SELECTION

In general, CRIs may be considered in patients who are within 0.5 D of the targeted spherical equivalent and have refractive astigmatism of 0.50 D or more, especially if against the rule (ATR) is present and the patient desires reduced spectacle dependence.[8] An accurate history and a preoperative evaluation that includes careful examination of the patient's ocular surface and tear breakup time will help identify patients with underlying dry eye or epithelial basement membrane disease, which might exclude them from safely having PCRIs. Careful topographic screening with Placido ring and Scheimpflug imaging is recommended to rule out any ectatic corneal disorder, abnormally thin corneas, contact lens-induced corneal distortion, or irregular astigmatism. Ectatic disorders can worsen or destabilize after a relaxing incision.

PREOPERATIVE PLANNING

It is important to determine the magnitude and steep meridian of the corneal astigmatism with at least two devices, in addition to the manifest refraction, as this can be an indicator of posterior corneal astigmatism. If the amount of astigmatism on the maps is slightly asymmetric, the lengths of the paired incisions can be varied. If a large amount of asymmetry is present, a single incision may be chosen instead of paired incisions. Scheimpflug imaging is additionally helpful to evaluate corneal pachymetry and rule an ectatic disorder.

When creating the surgical plan, mild residual with-the-rule (WTR) astigmatism is desirable (at least when using monofocal implants) since most patients will drift toward ATR over their lifetime.[2]

MANUAL PCRI NOMOGRAMS

Surgeons vary in their preferred location for astigmatic incisions. Some prefer astigmatic keratotomy, typically at an 8-mm zone, whereas others primarily rely on PCRIs placed at a 9-mm or greater zone. The length and number of PCRIs are determined according to nomograms based on factors such as age, preoperative corneal astigmatism, and location of the incisions (PCRIs near the horizontal meridian induce a greater astigmatic change). We changed our existing nomogram for PCRIs based on our new posterior corneal data.[9,10] Our current PCRI nomogram in Table 3.1 is designed for use in combination with 2.2- to 2.7-mm temporal clear corneal incisions and placement of the PCRIs at the end of surgery. It is conservative in order to minimize the risk of overcorrections. In particular, for PCRIs placed along

TABLE 3.1 ■ **Nomogram for Peripheral Corneal Relaxing Incisions for Correcting Keratometric Astigmatism During Cataract Surgery[a,b]**

Preop astigmatism (D)	Age (years)	Number	Length (degree)
WTR			
1.25 to 1.75	<65	2	35[c]
	≥65	1	35
>1.75	<65	2	60
	≥65	2	45
ATR/oblique			
0.4 to 0.8	–	1	35 to 40[d]
0.81 to 1.2	–	1	45
	–	2	40
≥1.2	–	2	45

[a]Combined with temporal 2.4-mm clear corneal incision.
[b]For against-the rule astigmatism, consider doing peripheral corneal relaxing incisions (PCRIs), especially if a clear corneal incision is not centered with corneal astigmatism.
[c]One PCRI of 50 degrees if asymmetric astigmatism.
[d]Paired PCRIs of 30 degrees if symmetric astigmatism.
ATR, Against the rule, WTR, with the rule.

TABLE 3.2 ■ Nichamin Nomogram for Peripheral Corneal Relaxing Incisions

Intralimbal relaxing incision
Nomogram for modern phaco surgery
Empiric blade depth setting of 600 μm

Spherical

(up to +0.75 × 90 or +0.50 × 180)

Incision design	"Neutral" temporal clear corneal incision (i.e., 3.5 mm or less, single plane, just anterior to vascular arcade)

Against the rule

(Steep axis: 0–44 degrees/136–180 degrees)

Preop cylinder	Paired incisions in degrees of arc (if 40 degrees or less, nasal arc only)						
	30–40 yr old	41–50 yr old	51–60 yr old	61–70 yr old	71–80 yr old	81–90 yr old	91+ yr old
+0.75 to +1.25	55	50	45	40	35	35	
+1.50 to +2.00	70	65	60	55	45	40	35
+2.25 to +2.75	90	80	70	60	50	45	40
+3.00 to +3.75	90	90	85	70	60	50	45
–		optical zone = 8 mm	9 mm	9 mm	9 mm	9 mm	9 mm

Incision design	The temporal incision, if greater than 40 degrees of arc, is made by first creating a two-plane, grooved phaco incision (600 μm depth), which is then extended to the appropriate arc length at the conclusion of surgery.

With the rule

(Steep axis, 45–135 degrees)

Preop cylinder	Paired incisions in degrees of arc						
	30–40 yr old	41–50 yr old	51–60 yr old	61–70 yr old	71–80 yr old	81–90 yr old	91+ yr old
+1.00 to +1.50	50	45	40	35	30		
+1.75 to +2.25	60	55	50	45	40	35	30
+2.50 to +3.00	70	65	60	55	50	45	40
+3.25 to +3.75	80	75	70	65	60	55	45

Incision design	"Neutral" temporal clear corneal incision along with the following peripheral arcuate incisions

When placing intralimbal relaxing incisions following or concomitant with radial relaxing incisions, total arc length is decreased by 50%.

Louis D. "Skip" Nichamin, M.D. ~ Laurel Eye Clinic, Brookville, PA.

the horizontal meridian, we do not recommend exceeding 45 degrees in length. We have seen wound gape in some cases with longer incisions placed in the horizontal meridian, especially those placed nasally. Other commonly utilized PCRI nomograms include one by Nichamin (Table 3.2) and Donnenfeld (Table 3.3), which can both be found online. For PCRIs in post–refractive surgery patients, we use the nomogram described in Table 3.4.

TABLE 3.3 ■ Donnenfeld Nomogram for Corneal Relaxing Incisions

Preop cylinder	Length (limbal relaxing incision)	Length (8-mm arcuate incision)
0.50 D	1 incision, 45 degrees	1 incision, 30 degrees
0.75 D	2 incisions, 30 degrees each	2 incisions, 20 degrees each
1.50 D	2 incisions, 60 degrees each	2 incisions, 40 degrees each
3.00 D	2 incisions, 90 degrees each	2 incisions, 60 degrees each
• Use 5 degrees more for against-the-rule astigmatism • Use 5 degrees more for younger patients • Use 5 degrees less for older patients		85% depth

TABLE 3.4 ■ Nomogram for PCRIs for Corneal Relaxing Incisions for Naturally Occurring or Post Refractive Surgery

Astigmatism (D)	Age (yr)	Number	Length (degree)
WTR			
0.75–1.00	<65	2	45
	≥65	1	45
1.25–1.75	<65	2	60
	≥65	2	45
2.00 Recommend excimer laser procedure			
ATR/oblique			
0.75–1.00		2	35
1.01–1.50	<65	2	45
	≥65	2	40
1.50: Recommend excimer laser procedure			
ATR, Against the rule, WTR, with the rule.			

When adopting a nomogram for one's personal use, it is advisable to closely follow the surgical technique that was used to generate the nomogram. One can later modify this based on one's own surgical outcomes.

Case

A 31-year-old male presented to clinic with a 3-year history of blurred vision in the right eye. He had a history of myopic PRK performed 6 years previously. His uncorrected visual acuity was 20/20 in the right eye and 20/15 in the left eye. Corrected visual acuity of 20/15 was achieved in each eye with a manifest refraction of −0.25 +0.75 × 010 in the right eye and −0.50 sphere in the left eye. Examination showed a healthy ocular surface with tear breakup time of greater than 10 seconds. Dual-Scheimpflug topography showed no evidence of corneal ectasia with 0.28 D of ATR corneal astigmatism in the right eye (Fig. 3.1).

The patient underwent paired 30-degree PCRIs centered at 4 degrees in the right eye. When seen 3 months postoperatively, he reported significant improvement in his vision with no pain or discomfort. His uncorrected visual acuity was 20/15 in both eyes. Manifest refraction was plano +0.25 × 005 in the right eye. Dual-Scheimpflug topography showed 0.3 D of WTR corneal astigmatism (Fig. 3.2). The patient's vision and refraction remained stable at 6 months postoperatively.

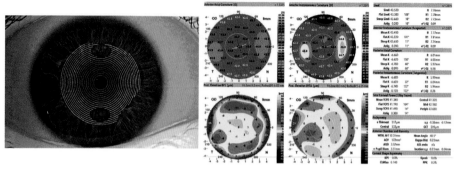

Fig. 3.1   Preoperative dual-Scheimpflug placido topography of the right eye shows good reliability with regular mires, 0.28 D of against-the-rule astigmatism, with no evidence of corneal ectasia.

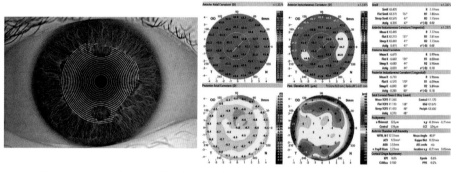

Fig. 3.2   Postoperative month-3 dual-Scheimpflug placido topography of the right eye shows good reliability with regular mires, 0.3 D of with-the-rule corneal astigmatism indicating treatment effect, with no evidence of corneal ectasia.

PROCEDURE

Manual PCRI

Supplies Needed for Manual PCRI

- Tetracaine or other anesthetic drop
- Gentian violet marker
- Eyelid speculum
- CRI blade of choice
- Fixation forceps or ring
- CRI marker of choice
- Slit lamp or operating microscope
- Handheld pachymeter (optional)
- Antibiotic drop of choice

Equipment needed for manual CRIs includes a slit lamp or microscope, an instrument to mark the incisional meridian (e.g., Sinskey hook), fixation forceps or a fixation ring, a degree marker, various zone and incision markers, a sterile marking pen or ink pad, and, depending on one's technique and the surgical indication, an ultrasonic pachymeter for intraoperative measurements. Numerous markers are available, including the Lindstrom arcuate marker (Katena Products, Denville, NJ), the Koch PCRI marker (ASICO, Inc., Chicago, IL), and the Mastel arcuate marker (Mastel Inc., Rapid City, SD) (Fig. 3.3). Some marking devices are also designed to serve as a physical guide for the diamond knife.

A large number of blade types and designs are available, which include reusable true and synthetic diamonds and other gemstones and single-use steel blades. For more central corneal incisions, an adjustable micrometer knife is desirable. For routine PCRIs, we prefer a triangular or thin trapezoidal blade with a single footplate, which allows good visibility while making the incision. With this type of blade set at 600 μm depth for incisions made at the 9-mm zone, we have found consistent results and no perforations. Microperforations can occur using 600-μm trapezoidal blades with a broad base since one can get greater depth than expected if the knife is rocked or tilted along the blade axis. Extreme care should be taken in knife selection, calibration, and maintenance to ensure reproducible cuts.

If arcuate keratotomy is being performed in an 8-mm or smaller zone, many surgeons perform pachymetry at the incision site and set the diamond blade to the desired depth, typically 80%–90% of the thinnest measurement.

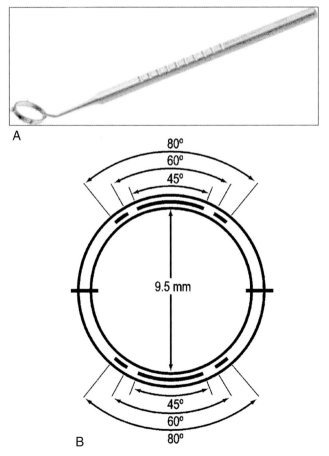

Fig. 3.3 Marker used to delineate 45-, 60-, and 80-degree incision lengths. (Koch LRI Mark; courtesy of Corza Medical ©2023.)

Manual PCRI Procedure

Accurate astigmatic surgery is highly sensitive to precise meridional alignment. Vector analysis demonstrates that a misalignment of only 15 degrees results in a 50% reduction in astigmatic correction, while a 30-degree misalignment results in no change in magnitude and induces a large shift in the astigmatic axis.[11] Errors greater than 30 degrees result in a net increase in the magnitude of the astigmatism. Swami et al.[12] demonstrated that 8% of eyes had a deviation of greater than 10 degrees when moving from an upright to a supine position; therefore, preoperative alignment marks should be obtained with the patient's head upright.

If the PCRI is performed with the patient lying down at the minor procedure room microscope of the clinic, then care needs to be taken to mark the eye prior to the patient lying supine. Various approaches can be taken to minimize alignment errors. One can make small drawings of the patient's eyes preoperatively, ensuring that they are vertically oriented at the slit lamp. Prominent conjunctival, corneal, or iris features can be used as landmarks. Landmarks at the 90- or 180-degree meridians are especially helpful. After topical anesthetic drops are administered, a Gentian violet marking pen can be used to mark the 3, 6, and 9 o'clock or 3, 6, and 12 o'clock positions while the patient looks straight ahead (Fig. 3.4). These marks may be also be made at the slit lamp using the slit lamp's orientation markers, taking care to ensure that the patient's head is not tilted.

PCRIs can be safely performed with the patient at the slit lamp. Stabilization of the head is critical, and a patient who is unable to hold a steady head position may not be the ideal candidate. Performing the incision at the slit lamp has the advantage of exact alignment on the axis without the cyclotorsion that occurs when supine. Many LRI diamond blades are available with shorter handles that are ideal for use at the slit lamp. A Gentian violet pen can be used to mark the steep axis. Most slit lamps will have the ability to align the slit beam of light to a specified

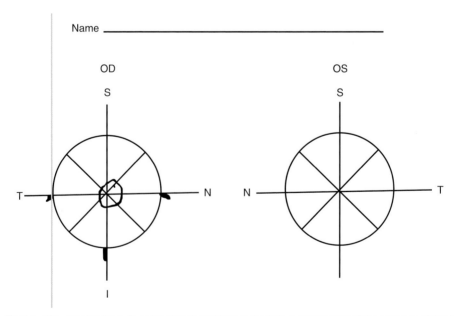

Fig. 3.4 After marking the 3, 6, and 9 o'clock positions at the limbus, assessment of the accuracy of these marks may be notated on a diagram. This diagram may be taped to the operating microscope or kept close to the surgeon to assist with intraoperative orientation. (Courtesy of Douglas Koch, MD.)

axis (Fig. 3.5). With the beam of light oriented through the visual center of the cornea and aligned to the axis, the limbus is marked (Fig. 3.6). If supine, the degree marker is aligned to the preoperative marks made at the limbus; the steep corneal meridian can be marked with a marker or hook stained with ink. The extent of the incision can be premarked by ink marks made with an instrument such as a Sinskey hook or by marks on the ring used to stabilize the globe and guide the blade. With corneal fixation forceps to grasp limbal tissue or a ring with degree marks held in one hand, the knife in the other hand is set into the cornea, pausing for 1 second. The knife is then guided slowly through the desired incision length (Fig. 3.7). A Sinskey hook, or jeweler forceps, or similar rounded-tip instrument may be used to bluntly dissect and assess the depth of the incision. Successful treatment of astigmatism can still be achieved even with a slightly irregular incision if made outside the central 9 mm.

Manual PCRI Complications

Possible complications of PCRIs include over- or undercorrection, infection, epithelial defects, perforation with hypotony, epithelial ingrowth, dry eye, and/or irregular astigmatism. Sight-threatening complications are extremely rare. It is worth noting that longer incisions may be prone to wound gape, particularly if positioned along the horizontal meridian. We recommend an upper limit of length of 45 degrees for horizontal PCRIs. Incisions may also gape if the cornea is subjected to additional stress, such as following subsequent penetrating keratoplasty. Some anecdotal evidence has suggested that longer PCRIs made in the horizontal meridian could also contribute to the development of central corneal epitheliopathy due to decreased sensation. The

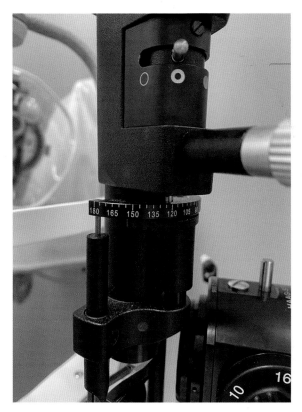

Fig. 3.5 Alignment marks on the slit lamp may be used to align the slit beam to the axis of choice. Care should be taken to align the center of the beam with the patient's visual axis and to ensure that the patient's head is not tilted.

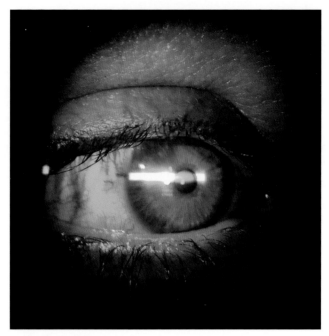

Fig. 3.6 Example of a marking made at the limbus at the slit lamp.

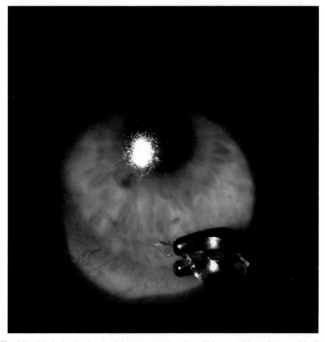

Fig. 3.7 Limbal relaxing incision created at the slit lamp with a diamond knife.

use of punctal plugs and close postoperative follow-up may help to address this before it causes damage to the corneal surface. Careful optimization of the tear film preoperatively, and extra counseling of the patient, is advised for those who require longer PCRIs in the horizontal meridian. If the PCRI inadvertently goes full thickness, resulting in a perforated and leaking wound, this should be sutured immediately (see Chapter 22 for corneal suturing at the slit lamp). These wounds once sutured will usually close and heal within a few weeks, and the suture can then be removed.

SPECIAL SITUATIONS: POSTKERATOPLASTY OR CORNEAL REFRACTIVE SURGERY

Post–Penetrating Keratoplasty Astigmatism

As many as 20% of postkeratoplasty patients have intolerable astigmatism requiring surgical intervention. Paired arcuate incisions are placed on the steep meridian either within or just central to the graft-host junction, which acts as a new functional limbus.[13] In general, one should avoid zones of less than 6 mm since they may increase irregular astigmatism. Incision lengths can range from 45 to 90 degrees and can be planned in at least three ways: (1) using a nomogram; (2) titrating intraoperatively with keratoscopy, aberrometry, or other measurements, gradually lengthening the incisions until there is a slight overcorrection;[14] or (3) using a fixed length and location for all corneas, recognizing that corneas with greater amounts of astigmatism may experience a correspondingly greater response to a given type of incision.[15] Since the result can be unpredictable due to the scarring at the graft-host junction, a conservative approach is advisable to avoid wound gape and overcorrection. Rejection has been noted after CRIs in postkeratoplasty patients, so increasing topical steroid should be considered after the procedure. Böhringer et al.[16] reported the long-term stability of manual paired arcuate corneal keratotomy in patients with high regular post–penetrating keratoplasty astigmatism. They found that arcuate corneal keratotomy is a safe and effective method to reduce high regular corneal astigmatism following penetrating keratoplasty but has limited predictability. The long-term follow-up showed an increase of keratometric astigmatism by 0.3 D per year, negating the surgical effect after 10 years, which may be explained by the slow wound healing of the cornea.

After PRK or LASIK

AK or PCRIs can also be used as an adjunct to treat residual astigmatism after PRK or LASIK. Kapadia et al.[17] studied the effectiveness of paired arcuate transverse keratotomy before and after spherical PRK treatments. Astigmatic keratotomy was performed prior to PRK in 37 eyes with 1.50 D of astigmatism. The decrease in astigmatism was significant, with a reduction from +2.40 ± 0.6 D preoperatively to +0.60 ± 0.60 D postoperatively. A second group of 86 eyes underwent AK after PRK. This group showed a significant decrease in astigmatism, +1.50 ± 0.60 D to +0.40 ± 0.40 D, 6 months postoperatively. Wang et al.[5] reported that, in a group of 33 PRK and LASIK patients treated with PCRIs, the percentage of eyes with an uncorrected visual acuity of 20/20 improved from 6% to 60%. This improvement remained stable up to 1 year. Coupling may be less predictable at higher amounts of astigmatism. When combining refractive surgery and relaxing incisions, the stability of one procedure should be ensured before performing the second procedure.

Summary

Excellent uncorrected visual acuity has become the primary goal of cataract and refractive surgery. Incisional keratotomy remains a safe and highly effective method of reducing astigmatism in cataract, post-LASIK/PRK, and corneal graft patients. Meticulous planning and technique are necessary to ensure optimal patient outcomes. Complications are rare and manageable. With experience, each surgeon will be able to develop his or her own nomograms tailored to the surgeon's equipment and technique with the goal of safely improving the vision of the patient.

References

1. Elder SS, Abrams D. *Ophthalmic Optics and Refraction. System of Ophthalmology.* St. Louis: Mosby; 1970:274–295.
2. Hayashi K, Manabe S, Yoshida M, Hayashi H. Effect of astigmatism on visual acuity in eyes with a diffractive multifocal intraocular lens. *J Cataract Refract Surg.* 2010;36:1323–1329.
3. Hoffmann PC, Heutz WW. Analysis of biometry and prevalence data for corneal astigmatism in 23239 eyes. *J Cataract Refract Surg.* 2010;36:1479–1485.
4. Wu E. Femtosecond-assisted astigmatic keratotomy. *Int Ophthalmol Clin.* 2011;51(2):77–85.
5. Wang L, Zhang S, Zhang Z, et al. Femtosecond laser penetrating corneal relaxing incisions combined with cataract surgery. *J Cataract Refract Surg.* 2016;42(7):995–1002.
6. Wang L, Swami A, Koch DD. Peripheral corneal relaxing incisions after excimer laser refractive surgery. *J Cataract Refract Surg.* 2004;30:1038–1044.
7. Rubenstein JB, Raciti M. Approaches to corneal astigmatism in cataract surgery. *Curr Opin Ophthalmol.* 2013;24:30–34.
8. Villegas EL, Alcón E, Artal P. Minimum amount of astigmatism that should be corrected. *J Cataract Refract Surg.* 2014;40:13–19.
9. Wang L, Misra M, Koch DD. Peripheral corneal relaxing incisions combined with cataract surgery. *J Cataract Refract Surg.* 2003;29:712–722.
10. Al-Mohtaseb Z, Ventura B, Wang L, eds, et al. Impact of posterior corneal astigmatism on astigmatism management during cataract surgery. In: *Curbside Consultation in Refractive and Lens-Based Surgery: 49 Clinical Questions.* Slack Books; 2014.
11. Stevens JD. Astigmatic excimer laser treatment: Theoretical effects of axis misalignment. *Eur J Implant Ref Surg.* 1994;6:310–318.
12. Swami AU, Steinert RF, Osborne WE, et al. Rotational malposition during laser in situ keratomileusis. *Am J Ophthalmol.* 2002;133:561–562.
13. Wu E. Femtosecond-assisted astigmatic keratotomy. *Int Ophthalmol Clin.* 2011;51(2):77–85.
14. Wilkins MR, Mehta JS, Larkin DF. Standardized arcuate keratotomy for postkeratoplasty astigmatism. *J Cataract Refrac Surg.* 2005;31(2):297–301.
15. Poole TR, Ficker LA. Astigmatic keratotomy for post-keratoplasty astigmatism. *J Cataract Refract Surg.* 2006;32:1175–1179.
16. Böhringer D, Dineva N, Maier P, et al. Long-term follow-up of astigmatic keratotomy for corneal astigmatism after penetrating keratoplasty. *Acta Ophthalmol.* 2016;94:e607–e611.
17. Kapadia MS, Krishna R, Shah S, Wilson SE. Arcuate transverse keratotomy remains a useful adjunct to correct astigmatism in conjunction with photorefractive keratectomy. *J Refract Surg.* 2000;16:60–68.

CHAPTER 4

Salzmann Nodular Degeneration

Marjan Farid ■ Ryan G. Smith

Introduction

Salzman nodular degeneration (SND) is a slowly progressive condition characterized by nodules noted on clinical exam of the anterior cornea. Although first described as nodular, Salzmann degeneration can also present as flat large areas of thickened subepithelial tissue (Fig. 4.1). They are generally gray-white to bluish in color. The condition was first described in 1925 as a dystrophy but since has been reclassified as a degenerative process. There are both primary and secondary forms of SND. SND has been observed with inflammatory processes such as phlyctenular disease, vernal keratoconjunctivitis, trachoma, measles, scarlet fever, and interstitial keratitis. It may also be associated with noninflammatory conditions such as epithelial membrane dystrophy, contact lens wear, and postoperatively after corneal surgery.[1] They are most often located near the limbus or in the mid-peripheral cornea. Histologically, a subepithelial nodule composed of oxytalan and other extracellular matrix was noted anterior to Bowman layer.[2] The corneal epithelium is typically thin over the overlying nodule, and violation of Bowman layer may be noted. Bowman layer may also be absent. The exact pathophysiological mechanism of nodule formation is unknown. A postulation is that Bowman layer is destroyed by enzymes, resulting in migration and proliferation of keratocytes from the posterior stroma, with resulting deposition of extracellular matrix components in nodular areas. Another theory is that there is a break in the stem cell adhesion to the cornea at the limbus that allows blood vessels to come through, resulting in exudation of a fibrous material that forms the nodule.

SND has been noted to be more common in women as well as Caucasians. It occurs bilaterally over 50% of the time. The majority of patients present either in the fifth, eighth, and ninth decades of life.[3] Associated ocular surface conditions such as meibomian gland dysfunction, chronic dry eye, contact lens wear overwear, previous ocular trauma, and history of viral infection are common.

Salzmann nodules can create visually significant irregular astigmatism and classic topographic changes. On topography, significant zones of flattening are seen in the area of the nodule. There is often an increase in higher-order aberrations from these irregular corneal surfaces. Removal of the involved nodule and surrounding subepithelial thickened areas can normalize topography and improve vision. It is important to note that SND may recur in some cases, and variable recurrence rates of 0%–31% have been reported in the literature.[3] The patient should be counseled about the risk of recurrence and the need for repeat procedures.

Case 1 Nodular Form

A 45-year-old female presents with vision changes that have been worsening over the past few months in her right eye. She has a history of contact lens use for 25 years. Her recent manifest refractions were showing changing degrees of astigmatism with a gradual decrease in best corrected visual acuity (BCVA) in that eye. She noted that she never previously required astigmatism correction in her glasses. On slit-lamp exam, a grayish-blue nodular lesion was noted superiorly (Fig. 4.2). Topographical evaluation showed obvious irregularity with a distinct flat zone

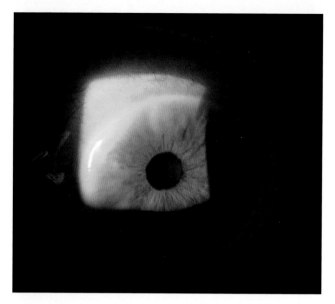

Fig. 4.1 Salzmann nodular degeneration.

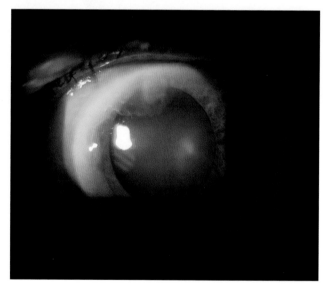

Fig. 4.2 Nodular form of Salzmann nodular degeneration (SND).

corresponding to the location of the lesion on her cornea (Fig. 4.3). The decision was made to proceed with superficial keratectomy and nodule removal.

PROCEDURE: EXCISION OF SALZMANN NODULE (SEE BOX 4.1)

The eye is prepped in the usual sterile fashion with topical betadine 0.5%. A drop of anesthetic and a drop of topical antibiotic are placed in the eye. The speculum is placed, and the patient is brought forward to the slit lamp. One prong of a jeweler forceps or a 0.12-mm forceps is used to dimple

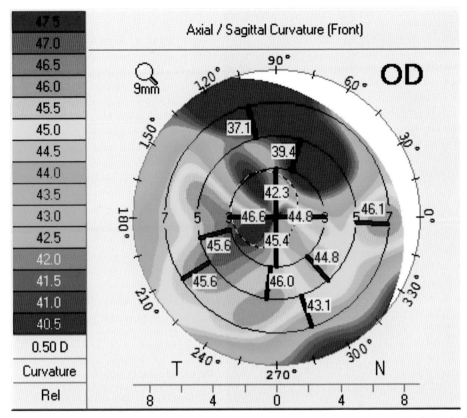

Fig. 4.3 Topography showing significant flattening and irregularity in the superior cornea corresponding to the area of Salzmann nodular degeneration (SND).

BOX 4.1 ■ Supplies

- Barraquer eye speculum
- Jeweler forceps or 0.12-mm Colibri forceps
- Povidone-iodine 5%
- Topical antibiotic drop (i.e., fluoroquinolone)
- Topical anesthetic eye drop
- no. 15 Bard Parker blade
- Bandage contact lens

---

into the cornea immediately adjacent to the nodule and find the plane under the subepithelial thickened tissue (Figs. 4.4A and 4.5A). Once the edge is identified, the nodule can often simply be grasped and smoothly peeled off without disturbing the underlying Bowman membrane (Figs. 4.4B and 4.5B). Care is taken to remove all aspects of the nodule or thickened subepithelial tissue outside the obvious nodule, as many times, there are extensions of abnormal tissue that emanate from the obvious nodule but are not immediately visualized. A gentle superficial keratectomy can be performed using a no.15 Bard Parker blade beyond the area of the observed nodule to ensure smooth transition zones into healthy epithelium, especially in the visual axis. Once all

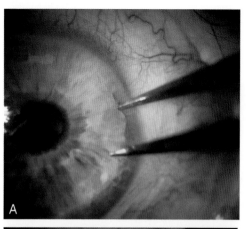

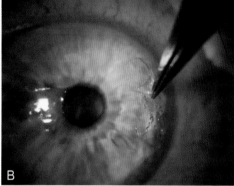

Fig. 4.4 Excision of Salzmann nodule. (A) Finding the edge and plane using one prong of the jeweler forceps. (B) Removing the nodule in one smooth sheet.

of the lesion is removed, a bandage contact lens is placed on the cornea followed by an antibiotic drop. The patient is instructed to use the antibiotic drops for 1 week or until the bandage contact lens is removed (see Video 4.1).

POSTPROCEDURE COURSE

The patient noticed some pain on postoperative day zero that was relieved with acetaminophen over the counter. Slit-lamp exam 1 week later showed full closure of the epithelial defect. Topography was done after 1 month to allow normalization and epithelial remolding to occur. This showed improvement and regularity of corneal keratometry (Fig. 4.6). The patient's BCVA went from 20/70 to 20/20.

Case 2 Diffuse Form

A 65-year-old male came in for cataract evaluation. He noted that his vision had progressively worsened over the past year and his vision was not correctable with glasses. Topography imaging for all preoperative consultations is routine for our cataract workup. In this case, a significant anterior corneal irregularity was noted on topography in his right eye. On close slit-lamp examination of the cornea, a flat, nonnodular, and less obvious area of thickened subepithelial lesion was observed with fine superficial neovascularization (Fig. 4.7). The patient had been treated in

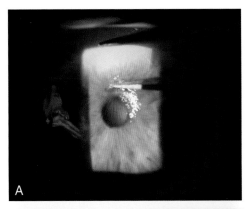

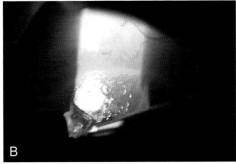

Fig. 4.5 Excision of Salzmann nodule. (A) Dimple down with one prong of the jeweler forceps to find the edge and plane of the lesion. (B) Peeling the lesion in one smooth sheet.

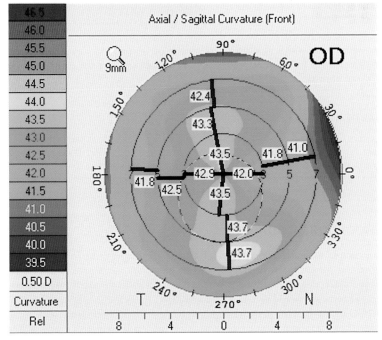

Fig. 4.6 Topography 1-month postexcision of Salzmann nodule. Now showing regularity and mild with-the-rule astigmatism.

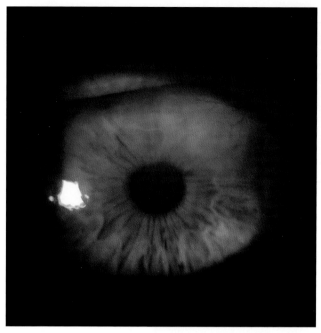

Fig. 4.7   Diffuse form of Salzmann nodular degeneration (SND).

the past for significant ocular rosacea and showed some limbal neovascularization in both eyes. Topographic evaluation of the right eye revealed significant flattening superiorly in the area of the diffuse "nodule" (Fig. 4.8). The patient wanted to reduce spectacle dependence with a presbyopic correcting intraocular lens (IOL), so the decision was made to perform a corneal excision of the Salzmann degeneration with a superficial keratometry (as discussed in Case 1) primarily and then to evaluate the patient for possible premium IOL technology once the cornea had healed and topography had normalized.

> **CLINICAL PEARLS**
>
> When performing surgical removal for diffuse SND, a larger superficial keratectomy is often necessary. Furthermore, the plane between the nodule and underlying tissue may be harder to locate. Turning the jeweler forceps such that one prong is tangential to the cornea may aid in starting the dissection and peeling process. An example of this can be seen in the supplemental surgical video.

POSTPROCEDURE COURSE

Repeat topography imaging was performed after 1 month to assess for normalization and regularity of the patient's cornea and to reassess candidacy for a premium toric monofocal or presbyopia-correcting IOL. In cases where the corneal keratometry may still be shifting, multiple measurements should be taken postoperatively to ensure stability prior to a final decision and IOL planning. Our patient's topography improved significantly with mild residual regular with-the-rule astigmatism, and the decision was made to place a monofocal toric IOL

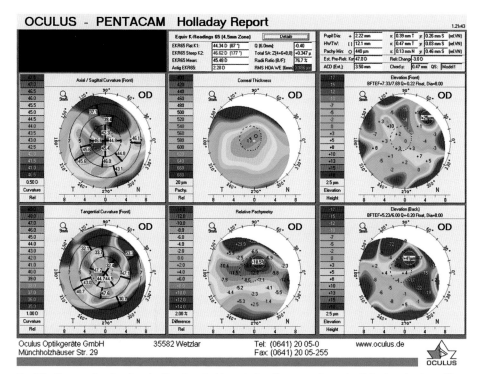

Fig. 4.8 Topography showing significant central irregularity with areas of superior flattening due to a diffuse form of Salzmann nodular degeneration (SND).

for distance correction. Following cataract surgery, the patient had 20/20 uncorrected distance visual acuity.

Conclusion

SND can cause visually significant keratometric changes and induce irregular astigmatism that greatly impacts patients' vision and quality of life. SND can manifest in nodular or diffuse form. Slit-lamp removal of these nodules can be performed at the slit lamp in the office without the need to take these patients to the operating room. Patient selection and counseling on the benefits, risks, and possibility of recurrence are paramount to achieving a successful outcome and a satisfied patient. Furthermore, removing nodules that are causing significant flattening and distortion on topography should be considered in all patients preparing for cataract extraction.

References

1. Mannis MJ, Holland EJ. *Cornea, 2-Volume Set*. 5th ed. Elsevier; 2021.
2. Obata H, Inoki T, Tsuru T. Identification of oxytalan fibers in Salzmann's nodular degeneration. *Cornea*. 2006;25(5):586–589.
3. Paranjpe V, et al. Salzmann nodular degeneration: Prevalence, impact, and management strategies. *Clin Ophthalmol*. 2019;13:1305–1314.

CHAPTER 5

Anterior Basement Dystrophy

Brandon D. Ayres

Introduction

Perhaps no other corneal dystrophy is known by more names than anterior basement membrane dystrophy (ABMD). Many people know it as map-dot-fingerprint dystrophy, some call it Cogan microcystic dystrophy, and others refer to it as epithelial basement membrane dystrophy. Call it what you may, they all refer to the same entity with the same clinical findings of corneal microcysts and map- and fingerprint-like lines in the corneal epithelial basement membrane. Most cases are considered to be a corneal degeneration secondary to trauma or involutional changes due to long-term exposure to environmental insult.

The corneal changes in ABMD cause two major symptoms in patients. The first is spontaneous and recurrent sloughing of the epithelium causing recurring corneal erosions. The second symptom is visual disturbance due to the changes in the corneal epithelium. In many cases, the changes from ABMD are in the periphery of the cornea, where they are visually insignificant; however, symptomatic patients will often have corneal changes that can be noted in the visual axis. The subtle changes in the corneal epithelium can cause irregular astigmatism and diffraction of light, causing unwanted images and blurred vision. It can often be difficult to detect ABMD on clinical exam. The dystrophy is often the cause of symptoms in patient with unexplained painless visual disturbances.[1] Careful examination of the cornea is necessary to detect the subtle changes from ABMD.

The word *dystrophy* in ABMD implies that the condition is genetic. However, to be considered a dystrophy (instead of corneal degeneration), the corneal findings need to follow some type of inheritance pattern, and many cases of ABMD are typically considered a degeneration or induced by trauma. As far back as 1976, Drs. Laibson and Krachmer noted an autosomal dominant inheritance pattern[2] in some families with ABMD. More recently, mutations in the *TGFB1* gene have been implicated in some of the familial cases of ABMD.[3] With the growing evidence of a genetic basis for ABMD in some families with ABMD, the International Committee for Classification of Corneal Dystrophies agreed that in some cases, ABMD is a true dystrophy (Category 1), but in most patients, the changes are sporadic and more likely from degenerative changes.[4]

Hematoxylin and eosin–stained slides of pathology slides will show a thickened epithelial basement membrane that migrates into the epithelial layer. The basement membrane changes can trap epithelial cells and prevent them from migrating to the superficial layer, where they are desquamated (Fig. 5.1). The trapped cells will eventually degenerate, creating cysts seen at the slit lamp.

Diagnosis

With a prevalence between 2% and 43% of the population,[5] ABMD is the most common corneal dystrophy, and it is critical to be able to correctly diagnose the condition. Making the diagnosis does not require expensive imaging equipment in the office but may require a high index of suspicion and a careful patient history and clinical exam of both corneas.

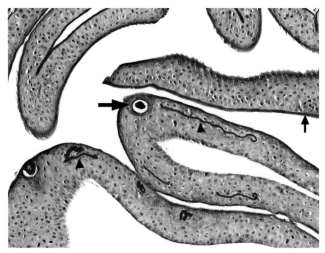

Fig. 5.1   Superficial keratectomy specimen. Folded corneal epithelium demonstrates prominently thickened basement membrane (thin arrow), epithelial reduplication with intraepithelial basement membrane formation (arrowhead), and Cogan microcysts (thick arrow) (periodic acid–Schiff stain, original magnification, ×50). Image courtesy of Tatyana Milman, MD.

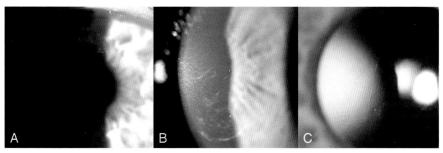

Fig. 5.2   Three of the common forms of anterior basement membrane dystrophy. (A) Microcysts. (B) Map lines. (C) Fingerprint lines.

Patients' symptoms can range from completely asymptomatic to severe blurred vision, unwanted images, and monocular diplopia. The changes in vision can be episodic and highly variable but typically progress over time. In some situations, there is a memorable event, such as a corneal abrasion or trauma, where the changes started and the vision never completely recovered. In most cases, the more symptomatic the patient the easier, it is to see the clinical findings on slit-lamp exam.

Best corrected vision may be reduced in patients with ABMD, and manifest refraction can be challenging due to irregular astigmatism. Very careful examination of the cornea will show the epithelial microcysts and map and fingerprint lines in the cornea (Fig. 5.2). Peripheral corneal changes may be less likely to cause visual complaints but should not be written off as unimportant. Peripheral corneal changes can still contribute to regular and irregular astigmatism with changes in manifest refraction over time. Patients with peripheral changes are also at increased risk of spontaneous corneal erosion or epithelial defect formation after laser vision correction and cataract surgery.

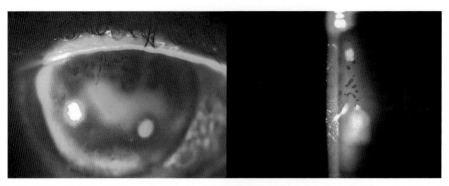

Fig. 5.3 (Right photo) Application of fluorescein will help detect the areas of corneal elevation associated with anterior basement membrane dystrophy (ABMD). In this photo, the areas of negative staining can be seen in the visual axis. (Left photo) Using the red reflex can help highlight the changes from ABMD. In this photo, several microcysts are visible in the visual axis.

When the corneal changes from ABMD appear in the visual axis, patients tend to become aware of the changes in visual quality. There are several slit-lamp techniques and diagnostic devices that can help the practitioner identify the corneal changes. One of the easiest and least expensive tests is evaluation of the cornea for negative staining. For this test, liberal amounts of fluorescein are applied to the cornea tear film. The map and fingerprint lines and microcysts of ABMD are slightly elevated. The elevation causes the fluorescein in the tear film to run off the elevated areas, leaving a dark area, or negative stain, in the corneal tear film when viewed under cobalt blue light. The negative staining simplifies detection of the cornea changes and also confirms the irregular nature of the cornea (Fig. 5.3).

A second slit-lamp technique that helps in detection of ABMD is retroillumination. With this technique, the light from the slit lamp is placed coaxial with the oculars and projected through the pupil. This will allow visualization of the red reflex. The practitioner focuses on the corneal epithelium and uses the reflected light off the retina to help highlight the changes in the corneal epithelium.

Corneal imaging such as topography and tomography are also very helpful, but nonessential, tools to help detect the presence of irregular astigmatism signifying AMBD. Looking at the Placido ring image from the topographer can highlight the irregular quality of the corneal epithelium. The location of the dystrophy is also easily seen in the Placido rings, giving a sense of the clinical significance of the corneal changes. Irregular astigmatism can also be documented by the topographer. Scheimpflug-based tomography will also show the irregular astigmatism induced by ABMD, and in some cases, the changes in the epithelium can be documented in the corneal images captured by the device. Other advanced imaging systems, such as optical coherence tomography, can also aid to visualize ABMD but, in most cases, are not necessary to make the diagnosis.

Case 1

HISTORY

An 82-year-old male was sent for evaluation of blurred vision that is worse in the right eye than the left. The patient states that he not only experiences blurred vision but also has unwanted double images when looking out of the right eye only. He has tried several changes in his glasses without success. To try and remedy the problem on his own, he has tried several types of artificial tears and lubricating gels and ointments without success.

EXAM

Vision on the right eye was 20/50 and on the left eye was 20/25, with no improvement with manifest refraction.

Slit-lamp exam showed significant blepharitis as well as map and fingerprint lines in the visual axis consistent with AMBD. Corneal topography confirmed irregular astigmatism and significant irregularity in the corneal epithelium crossing the visual axis (Fig. 5.4).

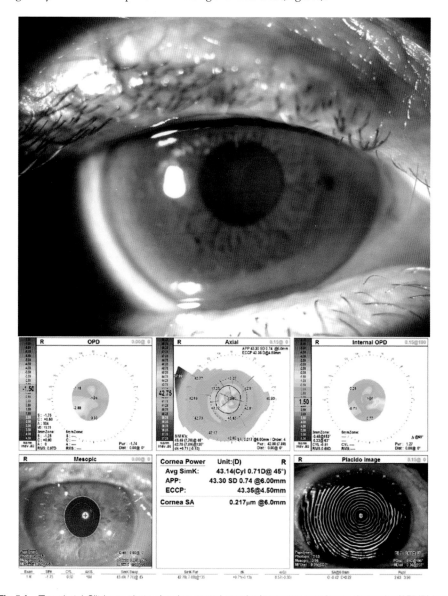

Fig. 5.4 (Top photo) Slit-lamp photo showing central anterior basement membrane dystrophy (ABMD) in a symptomatic patient. Notice how centrally located the dystrophic changes are in this patient. (Bottom photo) Placido disc topography of the same patent. Notice the irregularity of the axial topography and, even more importantly, the irregularity of the Placido image, indicating the clinical significance of the ABMD for this patient.

MEDICAL MANAGEMENT

The diagnosis of ocular surface disease coupled with ABMD was discussed with the patient. In this case, the etiology of the reduced vision was thought to be the changes from ABMD in the visual axis of the right eye. Dry eye and blepharitis were also coexistent in this patient (as is commonly the case).

Several treatment options were discussed with the patient. The most conservative in this case was to aggressively treat the ocular surface disease and see if he would experience an improvement in vision. The patient was informed that treatment would not remove the map lines from the cornea, but improvement in the tear film may give him acceptable, but not perfect, vision. If medical treatment did not alleviate his symptoms, a superficial keratectomy could be performed to remove the corneal epithelial changes. The risks and benefits of a superficial keratectomy were also discussed with the patient.

After careful consideration, the patient wanted to try topical treatment prior to agreeing to a procedure. He was started on a short course of topical steroids, preservative-free artificial tears, and a topical antiinflammatory with the goal of improving the tear film quality. He was then evaluated 3 months later with the understanding that if he experienced no improvement in vision, a superficial keratectomy could be performed.

The patient returned 3 months later for repeat evaluation. His vision had improved to 20/25 on the right eye, with minimal to no ghosting or doubling in his vision. Although he still realized that his vision was not perfect, he was satisfied enough with the result; he did not want a corneal procedure performed.

The exam still showed the changes of ABMD but with significant improvement in the tear film and quality of vision. Corneal topography was repeated, confirming an improvement in the irregular nature of the corneal shape (Fig. 5.5). With the improvement noted, medical management was continued.

DISCUSSION

This case highlights a very important aspect in the treatment of ABMD: not every case will need a surgical procedure. In many cases, patients will present with a combination of ocular surface disease and corneal changes. Treating the ocular surface has two main objectives in these cases: to improve the quality of vision and to prepare the surface for procedural intervention. Steroids, tears, and prescription dry eye medications do not remove the corneal changes seen with AMBD, but they do stabilize the precorneal tear film. In some instances, such as the case described earlier, improving the tear film will be enough to disguise some of the corneal changes and improve quality of vision to the point where patients are satisfied.

At times, the changes from ABMD are too severe and may require a superficial keratectomy to physically remove the irregular epithelium. Medical pretreatment of the ocular surface will also help prepare the cornea for a procedural intervention and speed recovery, reduce haze formation, and decrease the chances of infection.

Case 2

HISTORY

A 72-year-old male was referred for evaluation of vision in both eyes. He has noted a slow decline in his quality of vision over the past several years. He described difficulty with distance and near vision that was not improved, even with his new pair of glasses. Along with the reduced vision, he also described difficulty driving at night due to glare and multiple images. He attributed his visual decline to his cataracts and wanted cataract surgery.

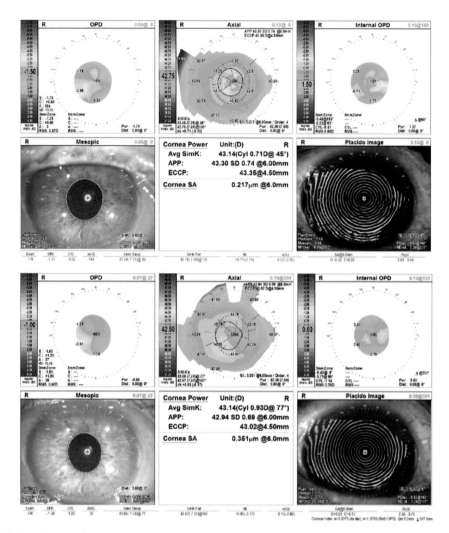

Fig. 5.5 (Top photo) Pretreatment topography showing irregular astigmatism secondary to ABMD and ocular surface disease. Note the irregularity of the mires in the Placido disc image. (Bottom photo) Topography of the same patient several months after medical treatment of the ocular surface. Note the reduction in irregular topography on the Placido disc image.

EXAM

Best corrected vision was approximately 20/40 in both eyes and did not improve with manifest refraction. A rigid gas-permeable refraction was done on both eyes, allowing the patient to read the 20/25 line in both eyes, but did not fully correct the double images.

Slit-lamp exam showed midlid changes consistent with blepharitis. The conjunctiva was quiet in both eyes, and both corneas had extensive map, dot, and fingerprint lines in the central cornea of both eyes. After application of fluorescein stain, negative staining was noted in the visual axis of both corneas. The remainder of his exam was normal outside mild nuclear sclerotic changes to both lenses. Computerized corneal topography confirmed irregular astigmatism in both eyes (Fig. 5.6).

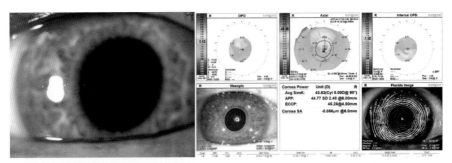

Fig. 5.6 (Right) Slit-lamp image of right eye with microcysts consistent with anterior basement membrane dystrophy (ABMD) and the corresponding topography (left) of the same eye showing marked irregular

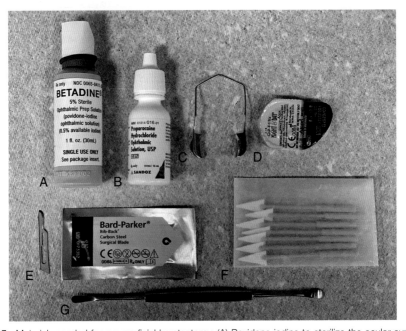

Fig. 5.7 Materials needed for a superficial keratectomy. (A) Povidone-iodine to sterilize the ocular surface. Povidone-iodine should be placed after (B) topical proparacaine or tetracaine to anesthetize the ocular surface. (C) A lid speculum can be placed to keep the eye open. Removal of the epithelium can be accomplished with a combination of (E) a surgical no. 15 or similar blade used in a sweeping motion, (F) surgical microspears and sponges, or (G) a blunted spatula. Once the epithelium is removed, a (D) bandage contact lens can be placed.

The images and topographical images were shared with the patient, and treatment options were discussed. In this particular case, with the severity of the ABMD in the visual axis, optimizing the ocular surface would likely not be enough to improve the patient's vision. Superficial keratectomy, or removal of corneal epithelium, would be necessary for full resolution of symptoms, and this procedure would likely be needed in both eyes. The risks and benefits of a superficial keratectomy were also discussed with the patient. The major risks discussed were pain and discomfort, risk of corneal infection, slow epithelial healing, corneal scar formation, and recurrence of the ABMD. After careful consideration, the patient consented to the superficial keratectomy.

PROCEDURE: SUPERFICIAL KERATECTOMY

Supplies (Fig. 5.7)
■ Topical anesthetic drop ■ Povidone-iodine drop ■ Eyelid speculum ■ Surgical microsponge/spear ■ No. 15 blade ■ Bandage contact lens (BCL)

Superficial keratectomy is one of the most straightforward in-office procedures to perform, but attention to technique is still critical. The procedure is used to remove superficial pathology in the cornea down to the Bowman layer. The keratectomy will leave a large epithelial defect, leaving the patient uncomfortable for 2 to 3 days and with blurred vision until healed. Due to the discomfort and reduced vision, the procedure is typically performed one eye at a time. Superficial keratectomy can be performed at the slit lamp with the patient seated or in a minor procedure room under a microscope. On rare occasions (usually due to patient anxiety or photophobia), the procedure can be performed in the operating room for additional anesthesia. It is some surgeons' preference to do this procedure under the excimer laser in the event that some of the corneal stroma needs to be ablated if scar tissue is present. In these cases, the procedure is called phototherapeutic keratectomy (see Chapter 6). In most cases of ABMD, a superficial keratectomy is adequate, and phototherapeutic keratectomy is not required.

Procedure

After the patient signs the surgical consent form, a drop of topical anesthetic is placed in the operative eye. Once the anesthetic has taken effect, a drop of povidone-iodine ophthalmic solution is placed in the eye, and in patients with blepharitis, it is a good idea to also use a cotton-tipped applicator to prep the eyelash margin as well. When the surgical prep is completed, the patient is positioned at the slit lamp or under the microscope for the procedure (Fig. 5.7). It is the author's preference to start the keratectomy with a dry ophthalmic sponge to debride loose epithelium. The sponge can be helpful in showing where the epithelium is more or less adherent to the underlying corneal stroma. Once the surgical sponge has been used, the no. 15 blade or spatula can be used to more smoothly remove the remaining epithelium. It is important to note that the blade is not used to cut or chisel the epithelium away; it is used in a sweeping motion to brush off the corneal epithelium, leaving the Bowman layer intact. The sweeping motion will also help to remove any subepithelial fibrosis that may have formed over time.

Once the central 8 mm of the cornea is cleared of pathology, try to leave a sharp margin of epithelium in the periphery. Minimizing epithelial tags and loose epithelium will help to speed recovery of the cornea. In most cases, epithelial removal is all that is needed to remove changes caused by ABMD; however, some surgeons will advocate the use of a diamond burr (usually 3- to 5-mm ball size) to polish the cornea under the area of epithelial removal. This is not a necessary procedure for ABMD but can be performed at the surgeon's discretion or if there is evidence of recurrent erosions (see Chapter 6).

After making sure all loose epithelium is cleaned off the surface of the eye, a BCL is placed. The BCL will help with pain management and act as a scaffold, helping the corneal epithelium heal. In most cases, the corneal epithelium will heal in 2 to 3 days, depending on the original size of the epithelial defect. Once healed, the BCL can be removed and discarded. In lieu of a BCL, a self-retaining amniotic membrane (AMT) may also be used for postprocedure epithelial healing (see Chapter 15).

Postprocedure Management

In the majority of cases, patients are started on a topical steroid 3–4 times per day starting immediately after the procedure. In many cases, a lower-potency ophthalmic steroid such as loteprednol
0.5% or fluorometholone 0.1% is enough to control the inflammation associated with the superficial keratectomy procedure. Along with the steroid, antibiotic drops are typically prescribed for
use 3–4 times per day and continued until the epithelium is healed and the BCL is removed. It is
the author's preference to also prescribe a topical nonsteroidal antiinflammatory drug (NSAID)
for use once daily if needed for pain. The NSAID is often only needed for the first few days while
the epithelium is healing. Caution must be taken when using an NSAID drop, as it can slow down
epithelial healing in patients wearing BCLs, as they have been associated with corneal melting.[6]
The problems become more likely when the NSAID is used in the absence of a topical steroid.

Patients should be reevaluated 1 day after the procedure to make sure there are no signs of
infection and to review medications. Typically, no changes to topical medications are made at this
visit. If the exam is within normal limits, the patient returns to the office about 1 week later. At
the 1-week exam, the epithelium is expected to be healed, and the BCL can be removed. Once
removed, the antibiotic and NSAID can be discontinued. The topical steroid is typically tapered
over the course of 3–4 weeks depending on surgeon preference, and the patient is seen again
approximately 1 month after the procedure. One month after the procedure, the corneal epithelium should be quite smooth and clear. A very slight haze may still be observable in the superficial corneal stroma, especially if a diamond burr has been performed. At this point, a follow-up
topography can be performed to compare to preop and to serve as a new baseline to help confirm

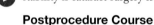

stability if cataract surgery is eventually planned (see Video 5.1).

Postprocedure Course

The patient had successful superficial keratectomies in both eyes and healed without difficulty.
One month after completion of the second eye, his exam showed no evidence of ABMD in the
visual axis and a best corrected vision of 20/20 in both eyes. Computerized topography shows
minimal regular astigmatism and crisp mires on Placido disc imaging (Fig. 5.8).

DISCUSSION

In this case, the ABMD was causing enough irregularity in the corneal epithelium that a procedural intervention was necessary. It can be tempting to blame progressive decline in the quality
of vision on the cataract and not take a close look at the cornea. If this patient had gone on to
cataract surgery without first addressing the ABMD, he likely would be unhappy with his quality
of vision even after the surgery. By correctly diagnosing and treating the ABMD, this patient was
spared unnecessary surgery, and when the cataract does become visually significant, his biometry
and intraocular lens selection will be more accurate.

It is important in patients with ABMD to also look for coexistent dry eye disease. In the case
described above, the patient was started on topical antiinflammatories prior to the procedure and
is still using them postoperatively. Treating the ocular surface is likely helpful in helping the ocular
surface to heal and keeping a healthy tear film once the ABMD has been treated with a superficial
keratectomy.

Case 3

HISTORY

A 68-year-old male presented for evaluation of reduced vision. He was told by his referring eye
care provider that he had both cataract formation as well as a corneal dystrophy and should be
seen by a corneal specialist. When questioned, the patient described not only reduced quality

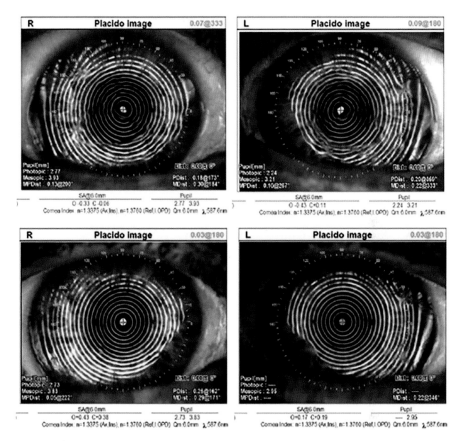

Fig. 5.8 (Top) Placido disc images of right and left eye of patient prior to superficial keratectomy. Note the extensive irregularity in the reflected images indicating irregular astigmatism. (Bottom) Placido disc images of same patient 2 months after superficial keratectomy, with marked improvement in irregular astigmatism.

of vision but also multiple images, primarily from his right eye. He had tried multiple changes in his glasses without success and was looking for a permanent solution for improved vision. The patient was also interested in trying to minimize the need for both distance and near prescriptions.

EXAM

On exam, the patient was 20/30 in the right eye and 20/25 in the left. There was minimal improvement with manifest refraction, and the patient still noted multiple images on the right side.

Slit-lamp exam showed mild moderate blepharitis of the upper and lower lids on both eyes. The conjunctiva was white. Examination of the right cornea showed significant ABMD in the visual axis with both positive and negative staining. The left eye had a normal corneal epithelium. The remainder of the anterior segment was within normal limits with the exception of 2+ nuclear sclerotic and cortical changes to both lenses (Fig. 5.9). Examination of the retina was within normal limits. Computerized corneal topography showed moderate irregular astigmatism, as well as distortion of the Placido disc mires. Biometry revealed approximately 2.5 diopters of astigmatism, resulting in the need for placement of a T5 toric intraocular lens (IOL). (Fig. 5.10).

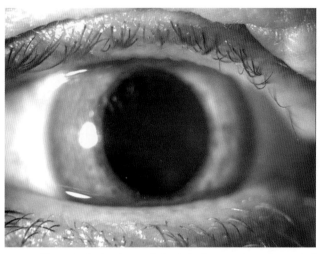

Fig. 5.9 Slit-lamp exam. The radar is showing central anterior basement membrane dystrophy as well as nuclear and cortical lens changes. Note how the ABMD changes are in the center of the cornea, leading to symptoms of multiple images.

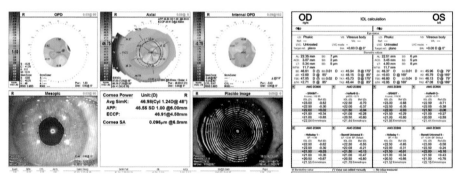

Fig. 5.10 (Left) Computerized corneal topography showing distortions in the Placido disc image and irregular astigmatism in the visual axis attributed to the anterior basement membrane dystrophy. (Right) Biometry shows approximately 2.5 diopters of astigmatism requiring a toric intraocular lens (IOL) for correction.

After examination, the patient was given the diagnosis of ABMD as well as visually significant cataracts in both eyes. The overall reduction in vision was likely secondary to the cataract formation in the multiple images coming from the corneal dystrophy. After a thorough discussion of the risks and benefits of both cataract surgery and superficial keratectomy, the patient decided to have a superficial keratectomy on the right eye followed by cataract surgery once the right cornea stabilized, using a trifocal lens implant.

The superficial keratectomy was performed as described previously in this chapter. The patient tolerated the procedure well and was followed closely for approximately 6–8 weeks with serial topography until the keratometric measurements appeared stable. One stable, biometry was repeated, revealing little to no astigmatism, and a spherical trifocal lens implant was selected for use (Fig. 5.11).

The patient underwent successful cataract surgery in both eyes with placement of a spherical trifocal implant. By postoperative month one, uncorrected distance vision had improved to 20/20 in both eyes and J1 reading vision at near and intermediate.

Measurement 1 — OD right, IOL calc

LS: Phakic | VS: Vitreous body
Ref: --- | VA: ---
LVC mode: - | LVC mode:
Target ref.: plano | SIA: +0.00 D @ 0°

AL: 22.35 mm SD: 7 µm
ACD: 3.07 mm SD: 2 µm
LT: 5.34 mm SD: 5 µm
WTW: 11.7 mm
SE: 46.81 D (!) SD:0.01 D K1: 45.54 D @ 175°
ΔK: +2.60 D @ 85° K2: 48.15 D @ 85°
TSE: 47.05 D (!) SD:0.02 D TK1: 45.73 D @ 175°
ΔTK: +2.71 D @ 85° TK2: 48.44 D @ 85°

AMO ZCB00 – SRK®/T – A const: 119.30		AMO ZCB00 – Hoffer® Q – pACD: +5.71	
IOL (D)	Ref (D)	IOL (D)	Ref (D)
+23.00	-0.62	+22.50	-0.70
+22.50	-0.30	+22.00	-0.37
+22.00	+0.02	+21.50	-0.04
+21.50	+0.34	+21.00	+0.28
+21.00	+0.65	+20.50	+0.60
+22.04 Emmetropia		+21.44 Emmetropia	

AMO ZCB00 – Holladay 1 – SF: +1.93		AMO ZCB00 – Barrett Universal II – LF: +2.04 DF: Default	
IOL (D)	Ref (D)	IOL (D)	Ref (D)
+22.50	-0.62	+22.50	-0.55
+22.00	-0.30	+22.00	-0.21
+21.50	+0.03	+21.50	+0.13
+21.00	+0.35	+21.00	+0.47
+20.50	+0.67	+20.50	+0.80
+21.55 Emmetropia		+21.70 Emmetropia	

Measurement 2 — OD right, IOL calc

LS: Phakic | VS: Vitreous body
Ref: --- | VA: ---
LVC mode: Untreated | LVC mode: -
Target ref.: plano | SIA: +0.00 D @ 0°

AL: 22.35 mm SD: 6 µm
ACD: 3.11 mm SD: 7 µm
LT: 5.26 mm SD: 11 µm
WTW: 11.6 mm
SE: 46.28 D SD:0.02 D K1: 45.88 D @ 92°
ΔK: +0.82 D @ 2° K2: 46.70 D @ 2°
TSE: 46.41 D SD:0.06 D TK1: 45.96 D @ 86°
ΔTK: +0.90 D @ 176° TK2: 46.86 D @ 176°

Alcon SN60WF – SRK®/T – A const: 119.00		Alcon SN60WF – Hoffer® Q – pACD: +5.64	
IOL (D)	Ref (D)	IOL (D)	Ref (D)
+23.00	-0.54	+23.00	-0.66
+22.50	-0.21	+22.50	-0.32
+22.00	+0.12	+22.00	+0.01
+21.50	+0.45	+21.50	+0.33
+21.00	+0.77	+21.00	+0.66
+22.18 Emmetropia		+22.01 Emmetropia	

Alcon SN60WF – Holladay 1 – SF: +1.84		Alcon SN60WF – Barrett Universal II – LF: +1.88 DF: +5.0	
IOL (D)	Ref (D)	IOL (D)	Ref (D)
+23.00	-0.65	+23.00	-0.61
+22.50	-0.32	+22.50	-0.25
+22.00	+0.01	+22.00	+0.09
+21.50	+0.34	+21.50	+0.44
+21.00	+0.67	+21.00	+0.78
+22.02 Emmetropia		+22.14 Emmetropia	

Measurement 3 — OD right, IOL calc

LS: Phakic | VS: Vitreous body
Ref: --- | VA: ---
LVC mode: Untreated | LVC mode: -
Target ref.: plano | SIA: +0.00 D @ 0°

AL: 22.37 mm SD: 4 µm
ACD: 3.10 mm SD: 4 µm
LT: 5.29 mm SD: 7 µm
WTW: 11.6 mm
SE: 46.92 D SD:0.01 D K1: 46.80 D @ 68°
ΔK: +0.24 D @ 158° K2: 47.03 D @ 158°
TSE: 47.10 D SD:0.02 D TK1: 46.92 D @ 62°
ΔTK: +0.36 D @ 152° TK2: 47.28 D @ 152°

Alcon SN60WF – SRK®/T – A const: 119.00		Alcon SN60WF – Hoffer® Q – pACD: +5.64	
IOL (D)	Ref (D)	IOL (D)	Ref (D)
+22.50	-0.69	+22.00	-0.62
+22.00	-0.37	+21.50	-0.29
+21.50	-0.04	+21.00	+0.04
+21.00	+0.28	+20.50	+0.36
+20.50	+0.60	+20.00	+0.68
+21.44 Emmetropia		+21.06 Emmetropia	

Alcon SN60WF – Holladay 1 – SF: +1.84		Alcon SN60WF – Barrett Universal II – LF: +1.88 DF: +5.0	
IOL (D)	Ref (D)	IOL (D)	Ref (D)
+22.00	-0.56	+22.00	-0.57
+21.50	-0.23	+21.50	-0.23
+21.00	+0.09	+21.00	+0.13
+20.50	+0.42	+20.50	+0.47
+20.00	+0.73	+20.00	+0.81
+21.14 Emmetropia		+21.19 Emmetropia	

Fig. 5.11 Three consecutive biometry measurements showing the change in levels of astigmatism with healing of the cornea after a superficial keratectomy. Stability is often achieved at 6 to 8 weeks but may take longer in some patients. It is advisable to wait until 2 measurements taken a few weeks apart give similar results.

DISCUSSION

This case highlights the importance of a careful corneal exam and the impact it can have on biometry. Without the help of corneal topography and careful clinical exam, a toric IOL could have been incorrectly selected for this patient. This certainly would have led to a suboptimal result, leading to an unhappy patient and possibly an IOL exchange. It is critical to recognize and treat visually significant ABMD in patients to deliver optimal results with cataract surgery. Just as critical is to follow patients postprocedure until keratometry has stabilized. Typically, it will take 6 to 8 weeks for stabilization, but in some cases, it can be significantly longer.

Conclusion

ABMD is one of the most common dystrophies/degenerations of the cornea, and every eye care professional will see it in their practice. The changes can be very subtle and difficult to detect on exam but can cause very bothersome symptoms for patients. With a detailed history and careful slit lamp exam, the corneal changes from ABMD were documented for both presence and clinical significance.

Treatment for ABMD starts with evaluation and management of the ocular surface. In mild cases of ABMD, improvement in the tear film can translate into reduced symptoms, preventing the patient from needing surgical intervention. In more severe cases with irregular astigmatism and visual symptoms, procedural treatment is indicated. The primary surgical treatment for ABMD is superficial keratectomy, a simple and effective treatment option to erase the central corneal changes seen in dystrophy. With the proper postoperative care, the cornea can be restored to its healthy state, giving good vision for years to come or for improved results after cataract surgery.

References

1. Reed JW, Jacoby BG, Weaver RG. Corneal epithelial basement membrane dystrophy: an overlooked cause of painless visual disturbances. *Ann Ophthalmol.* 1992;24(12):471–474.
2. Laibson PR, Krachmer JH. Familial occurrence of dot (microcystic), map, fingerprint dystrophy of the cornea. *Invest Ophthalmol.* 1975;14(5):397–399.
3. Boutboul S, Black GC, Moore JE, et al. A subset of patients with epithelial basement membrane corneal dystrophy have mutations in TGFBI/BIGH3. *Hum Mutat.* 2006;27(6):553–557. https://doi.org/10.1002/humu.20331.
4. Weiss JS, Møller HU, Aldave AJ, et al. The IC3D classification of the corneal dystrophies. *Cornea.* 2008;27(Suppl 2):S1–S83. https://doi.org/10.1097/ICO.0b013e31817780fb.
5. Werblin TP, Hirst LW, Stark WJ, et al. Prevalence of map-dot-fingerprint changes in the cornea. *Br J Ophthalmol.* 1981;65(6):401–409.
6. Rigas B, Huang W. Honkanen R, et al. NSAID-induced corneal melt: Clinical importance, pathogenesis, and risk mitigation. *Surv Ophthalmol.* 2020;65(1):1–11. https://doi.org/10.1016/j.survophthal.2019.07.001.

CHAPTER 6

Recurrent Corneal Erosions

Kanika Agarwal ▪ Elizabeth Yeu

Introduction

Recurrent corneal erosion syndrome (RCES) is a fairly common disorder that can be fairly frustrating for both the clinician and the patient. Forty-five percent to 64% of patients have a prior history of trauma, and 19%–29% present with epithelial basement membrane dystrophy (EBMD).[1] Onset usually occurs around age 30–40, and there has been a higher prevalence in patients with dry eye syndrome, diabetes mellitus, blepharitis, and ocular rosacea.[1] Past ocular history may be unremarkable, but additional risk factors include ocular trauma such as prior corneal abrasion with a fingernail, ocular surgery, and corneal epithelial and stromal dystrophies such as Reis Buckler, Thiel-Behnke, lattice, and granular and macular dystrophies.[1] Patients typically present with pain upon awakening, tearing, photophobia, eye redness, and decreased vision. Onset of symptoms can occur at any time after an inciting event if applicable.

Diagnosis involves slit-lamp examination with direct illumination to identify irregular corneal epithelium, small cysts, epithelial defects, map lines or fingerprint patterns, or negative staining. There may be scarring where prior repeated episodes have occurred. Diagnostic testing modalities, including confocal microscopy and optical coherence tomography, have also been utilized if the diagnosis remains unclear.[2,3] Patients can also be assessed at the slit lamp for subclinical RCES by using a cotton swab or Weck-Cel spear at areas of loose epithelium to determine if these areas slough off easily, confirming the diagnosis.[4]

Initially, patients are treated with aggressive topical and systemic regimens. However, if these conservative measures are refractory or patients have frequent symptomatic recurrences, more aggressive intervention should be pursued.

Medical Management

Initial management of recurrent erosions includes an aggressive topical regimen including hypertonic saline, preservative-free artificial tears, oral tetracyclines such as 50 mg doxycycline twice daily, punctal occlusion, and bandage contact lens. In up to 43% of patients, these measures alone will offer patients symptomatic relief.[5] However, if recurrences become frequent or symptoms are unable to be adequately controlled, consider one of the procedural interventions described below depending on the clinical presentation and location of erosions.

Case 1

A 52-year-old hyperopic male with EBMD was symptomatic from recurrent erosions involving his central visual axis, which was refractory to conservative medical management. After repeated and more frequent episodes, he opted for more aggressive treatment. The decision was made to proceed with epithelial debridement and diamond burr polishing of the Bowman membrane. See Fig. 6.1A–D.

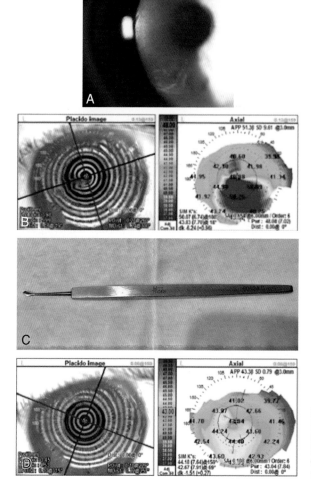

Fig. 6.1 (A and B) EBMD preepithelial debridement and diamond burr polishing of Bowman membrane. (C) Blunt spatula used to debride epithelium. (D) Postepithelial debridement with diamond burr.

PROCEDURE: EPITHELIAL DEBRIDEMENT AND DIAMOND BURR POLISHING OF BOWMAN MEMBRANE

Supplies
▪ Eyelid speculum ▪ No. 15 blade or spatula ▪ Weck-Cel spears ▪ Diamond burr ▪ Bandage contact lens

Procedure

The eye is prepped in the usual sterile fashion with topical betadine 0.5% or pretreated with a drop of antibiotic. Topical anesthetic drops are instilled in the eye, and an eyelid speculum is placed.

The areas of loose epithelium are identified by light debridement with a Weck-Cel spear or a no. 15 blade and scraped off. The underlying basement membrane is then polished with a fine-grit diamond burr mounted on a battery-powered Algerbrush low-torque motor for 10–15 seconds. A drop of topical antibiotic is given, and then a bandage contact lens is placed. A drop each of a nonsteroidal antiinflammatory drug and steroid can be applied afterward to help with inflammation and pain (See Video 6.1).

DISCUSSION

The success rate of treating recurrent erosions with conservative medical management alone is up to 75%, but patients can have recurrences.[1] Superficial keratectomy with diamond burr polishing prevents recurrent erosions by both removing the abnormal basement membrane to allow a smooth surface for reepithelialization and stimulating a reactive fibrosis to allow for stronger adhesion of corneal epithelium. Epithelial debridement and diamond burr polishing have a recurrence rate of 6% versus epithelial debridement alone, which has a recurrence rate of 15%–18%.[5] The documented success rate (defined as resolution of recurrent erosions at 18 months follow-up) had been as high as 80%–96% in patients treated with diamond burr polishing of the Bowman membrane. The only drawback of this method is surgically induced subepithelial haze, which occurred in 9.4% of eyes after 1 month. However, the haze was not visually significant.[6]

Case 2

A 35-year-old female with a prior corneal abrasion secondary to a fingernail injury 5 years ago presented with recurrent erosions refractory to conservative medical therapy. The affected area was in the superior peripheral cornea and spanned an area of 1 mm vertically and 2.5 mm horizontally. The patient decided to proceed with stromal micropuncture of the affected area.

PROCEDURE: STROMAL MICROPUNCTURE

Supplies
■ 5/8-inch 25-gauge needle attached to a 1-mL syringe ■ Eyelid speculum (if necessary) ■ Bandage contact lens ■ Slit lamp

Procedure

Topical anesthetic drops are administered to the affected eye. The patient is positioned at the slit lamp, and an eyelid speculum is placed if deemed necessary. The 25-gauge needle tip is bent near the needle hub by using the plastic needle cover or other instrument such as a needle driver, ensuring the needle tip is not dulled. The surgeon aims the needle tip 90 degrees to the corneal surface to gently indent the epithelium to create micropunctures that feel loose on contact. Enough pressure is gauged by feeling resistance against the stroma (usually around 5%–10% stromal depth). Punctures are made less than 1 mm apart. The procedure can be performed with fluorescein and cobalt blue light to identify intrastromal, which appear as triangular, versus subepithelial bubbles, which are rounder. Instrastromal bubbles confirm that the needle tip has penetrated the stroma enough to allow for better adhesion of epithelium. The number of micropunctures is determined by the area that requires treatment, and they are typically placed close enough together to minimize risk of recurrent erosion between spots. A bandage contact lens is applied, and topical antibiotics and steroids are given (see Video 6.2).

DISCUSSION

Stromal micropuncture aims to improve epithelial adherence to the underlying anterior stroma by inducing scar tissue formation with penetration of the Bowman membrane by the needle. It is best to perform this on patients with peripheral corneal pathology, as scarring could be visually significant if present on the visual axis. The advantages of performing stromal micropuncture are the low costs associated with performing the procedure and the ability to perform right at the slit lamp compared to superficial keratectomy with or without a diamond burr or phototherapeutic keratectomy (PTK). Although a history of trauma has not been demonstrated to have a higher rate of success compared to other etiologies, stromal micropuncture can offer a variable success rate from 63%–85%.[7]

Case 3

A 33-year-old male presents 15 years after having laser-assisted in situ keratomileusis (LASIK) in both eyes with decreased vision at counting fingers and recurrent corneal erosions in his right eye. He is found to have granular dystrophy that was confirmed by genetic testing and thought to have been activated by his LASIK procedure. He was offered treatment options of corneal transplantation versus PTK with epithelial debridement. He opted for PTK, with resolution of his symptoms and a visual acuity without correction at 20/25 at postop month 1. See Fig. 6.2A–C.

PROCEDURE: PTK WITH EPITHELIAL DEBRIDEMENT

Supplies

- Eyelid speculum
- Spatula
- PTK laser (AMO vs. Allegretto)
  - The Allegretto laser performs PTK with an estimate of 15.3 microns of tissue ablated per diopter.[8]
    - Refraction set to target for the depth necessary. For RCES in a naive cornea, a depth of 5–10 microns is sufficient.
  - AMO Visx excimer laser parameters:
    - 6- to 6.5-mm treatment zone
    - 193-nm UV-C beam at a fluence of 160 mJ/cm^2 with a repetition rate of 2 Hz
    - Transition zone, 1 mm
    - 5–10 microns of tissue removal after removal of epithelium (15–30 pulses)
- Diamond burr
- Weck-Cel spears
- Mitomycin C
- Bandage contact lens

Procedure

Topical anesthetic drops are administered to the affected eye. The eye is prepped and draped in the usual sterile fashion, and the laser microscope is positioned into place. An eyelid speculum is placed and seated temporally. A spatula is used to remove the diseased corneal epithelium and superficial lesions. The laser is turned on for the determined diopter/pulses (dependent on the type of laser) applicable to the patient. The epithelial edges are inspected and inverted toward the corneal center. The underlying Bowman layer and corneal stroma are polished with a diamond-dusted burr in the periphery for three passes. This is crucial for lesions in the

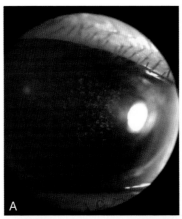

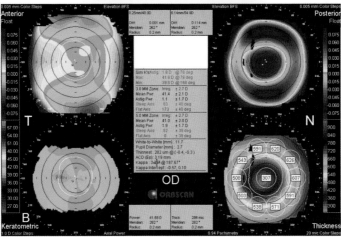

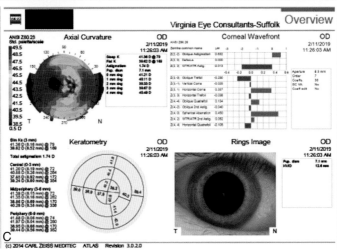

Fig. 6.2 (A) Slit lamp photo. (B) Orbscan. (C) Atlas: granular dystrophy pre-PTK.

periphery that cannot be reached by the laser. Mitomycin C 0.02% to 0.04% for 6 to 12 seconds can be used, as the patient is a post-LASIK patient, and to prevent haze formation. The cornea is then copiously irrigated with 1.5 bottles of balanced salt solution. A drop of antibiotics and a bandage contact lens are placed. The bandage contact lens is used for 2 months and exchanged every 1–2 weeks.

Transepithelial PTK can also be performed where the epithelium is not removed completely. A variety of methods exist:

1. The epithelium is loosened but not removed entirely and is preserved as a hinged flap. PTK is then performed over the exposed Bowman membrane and the epithelial flap replaced.[9]

2. The laser is passed through intact epithelium. In order to do this, the laser ablation depth has to be adjusted to aim for anterior stroma/Bowman based on the patient's pachymetry and accounting for epithelial thickness, which is usually around 45 microns.[10] Another method consists of applying 2 pulses × 40 pulses for an ablation depth of 18–20 microns with postoperative use of autologous serum eyedrops.[11] Faster recovery time and decreased postoperative pain are advantages of this technique. However, epithelial surface irregularities may be translated to the underlying Bowman membrane and anterior stroma.[9]

3. "Wet" transepithelial PTK involves a 50-micron ablation removing epithelial tissue of the surrounding affected erosion area without stromal ablation. The second step of ablation is done up to a depth of 10 microns to flatten the corneal surface. The tear fluid acts as a "masking agent" in the zone of the epithelial defect/erosion site, whereas the epithelium is the "natural masking agent" adjacent to this area of pathology. This way, the epithelium is removed evenly, allowing an even ablation of Bowman and anterior stroma so that the ablation extends beyond the affected area to even the boundaries between the affected and unaffected anterior surface. This method may be more effective when a nonhealing epithelial defect from an erosion is present.[12]

DISCUSSION

PTK has a high rate of success—as high as 88%—in reducing the recurrence of recurrent erosions, especially in those related to trauma[13] and corneal dystrophies.[14] The goal of PTK is to remove enough of the Bowman layer to allow for formation of new hemidesmosomes and to strengthen the adhesion of the basal epithelial cells to the underlying tissue via anchoring fibrils, which can take 6–8 weeks.[15] The ablation depth can vary between 5–10 microns of Bowman layer after epithelium removal, but some have found that removal of 10 microns results in fewer occurrences.[16] Although rare, those that do have a recurrence are retreated with PTK and found to not have a recurrence after the second treatment.[17] Overall, refractive error does not change after treatment with PTK if done conservatively.[10] However, there is a larger risk for refractive change can if the number of pulses is >50 and/or more than 50–100 microns of tissue are ablated.[14,18]

References

1. Miller DD, Hasan SA, Simmons NL, Stewart MW. Recurrent corneal erosion: A comprehensive review. *Clin Ophthalmol.* 2019;13:325–335. https://doi.org/10.2147/OPTH.S157430.
2. Diez-Feijóo E, Durán JA. Optical coherence tomography findings in recurrent corneal erosion syndrome. *Cornea.* 2015;34(3):290–295.
3. Rosenberg ME, Tervo TM, Petroll WM, Vesaluoma MH. In vivo confocal microscopy of patients with corneal recurrent erosion syndrome or epithelial basement membrane dystrophy. *Ophthalmology.* 2000;107(3):565–573.

4. Ryan G, Lee GA, Maccheron L. Epithelial debridement with diamond burr superficial keratectomy for the treatment of recurrent corneal erosion. *Clin Experiment Ophthalmol.* 2013;41(6):621–622. https://doi.org/10.1111/ceo.12052.

5. Ewald M, Hammersmith KM. Review of diagnosis and management of recurrent erosion syndrome. *Curr Opin Ophthalmol.* 2009;20(4):287–291. https://doi.org/10.1097/ICU.0b013e32832c9716.

6. Vo RC, Chen JL, Sanchez PJ, Yu F, Aldave AJ. Long-term outcomes of epithelial debridement and diamond burr polishing for corneal epithelial irregularity and recurrent corneal erosion. *Cornea.* 2015;34(10):1259–1265. https://doi.org/10.1097/ICO.0000000000000554.

7. Avni Zauberman N, Artornsombudh P, Elbaz U, Goldich Y, Rootman DS, Chan CC. Anterior stromal puncture for the treatment of recurrent corneal erosion syndrome: patient clinical features and outcomes. *Am J Ophthalmol.* 2014;157(2):273–279. https://doi.org/10.1016/j.ajo.2013.10.005. e1.

8. El Bahrawy M, Alió JL. Excimer laser 6(th) generation: state of the art and refractive surgical outcomes. *Eye Vis (Lond).* 2015;2:6. https://doi.org/10.1186/s40662-015-0015-5.

9. Miller DD, Hasan SA, Simmons NL, Stewart MW. Recurrent corneal erosion: a comprehensive review. *Clin Ophthalmol.* 2019;13:325–335. https://doi.org/10.2147/OPTH.S157430.

10. Rapuano CJ. A stepwise approach to laser PTK. Review of Ophthalmology. Published September 6, 2012. Accessed May 30, 2020. https://www.reviewofophthalmology.com/article/a-stepwise-approach-to-laser-ptk.

11. Holzer MP, Auffarth GU, Specht H, Kruse FE. Combination of transepithelial phototherapeutic keratectomy and autologous serum eyedrops for treatment of recurrent corneal erosions. *J Cataract Refract Surg.* 2005;31(8):1603–1606. https://doi.org/10.1016/j.jcrs.2005.01.014.

12. Churashov SV, Kudryashova EV, Kulikov AN, Boiko EV, Chernysh VF, Maltsev DS. "Wet" transepithelial phototherapeutic keratectomy in the management of persistent epithelial defects in the graft. *Clin Ophthalmol.* 2018;12:895–901. https://doi.org/10.2147/OPTH.S161018.

13. Lee W-S, Lam C, Manche EE. Phototherapeutic keratectomy for epithelial basement membrane dystrophy. *Clin Ophthalmol.* 2016;11:15–22. https://doi.org/10.2147/OPTH.S122870.

14. Cavanaugh TB, Lind DM, Cutarelli PE, et al. Phototherapeutic keratectomy for recurrent erosion syndrome in anterior basement membrane dystrophy. *Ophthalmology.* 1999;106(5):971–976. https://doi.org/10.1016/S0161-6420(99)00540-0.

15. Maini R. Phototherapeutic keratectomy re-treatment for recurrent corneal erosion syndrome. *Br J Ophthalmol.* 2002;86(3):270–272. https://doi.org/10.1136/bjo.86.3.270.

16. Phototherapeutic keratectomy. American Academy of Ophthalmology. Published January 8, 2014. Accessed February 14, 2020. https://www.aao.org/current-insight/phototherapeutic-keratectomy-3.

17. Dedes W, Faes L, Schipper I, Bachmann LM, Thiel MA. Phototherapeutic keratectomy (PTK) for treatment of recurrent corneal erosion: correlation between etiology and prognosis – prospective longitudinal study. *Graefes Arch Clin Exp Ophthalmol.* 2015;253(10):1745–1749. https://doi.org/10.1007/s00417-015-2990-6.

18. Garg S., McColgin A.Z., Steinert R.F. Phototherapeutic Keratectomy. American Academy of Ophthalmology. Published January 8, 2014. Accessed May 9, 2020. https://www.aao.org/current-insight/phototherapeutic-keratectomy-3.

CHAPTER 7

Band Keratopathy

Alexander Knezevic ▪ Marjan Farid

Introduction

Band keratopathy is a chronic degenerative disease that may present in both calcific and non-calcific forms. Calcific band keratopathy is characterized by gray or white calcium opacities on the corneal surface. It was first described by Dixon in 1848 to start peripherally and then progress slowly along the interpalpebral zone.[1] While it is typically slowly progressive, there are case reports of rapid progression over a few weeks to months.[2,3] It can be seen primarily or secondary to chronic inflammation and systemic or hereditary disease. Chronic ocular conditions like uveitis, prolonged corneal edema, or chemical burns can result in calcific band keratopathy.[4] Hypercalcemia secondary to systemic disease such as chronic renal failure, vitamin D toxicity, or hyperparathyroidism may also cause band keratopathy.[5,6]

The primary mineral deposited is calcium hydroxyapatite. Histopathologically, basophilic calcific particles are seen at the level of the Bowman layer.[7] The exact mechanism of deposition is debated, but it has been hypothesized to be due to pH changes, increased calcium concentration, and increased evaporation of tears.[8]

Band keratopathy can be surprisingly asymptomatic in the earlier stages of disease. As the deposits start peripherally, many patients will not notice any changes until the visual axis is impacted. As the disease progresses, there can be decreased visual acuity, glare, and pain if there is a break in the corneal epithelium.

In a setting where the contributing factor is unknown, a workup should be pursued. This should include serum calcium, phosphorus, vitamin D, uric acid, blood urea nitrogen (BUN), and creatinine. The physician can also consider serum parathyroid hormone and angiotensin-converting enzyme levels. Recognition of an underlying medical condition is important both due to other possible comorbidities and improvement in band keratopathy after calcium levels normalize.[9]

In visually significant or symptomatic band keratopathy, therapy is directed at removal of the calcium deposits. A preferred initial therapy is disodium ethylenediaminetetraacetic acid (EDTA).[10,11] The chelation treatment requires epithelium to be removed first, followed by 1.7% (0.05 molar) EDTA applied directly to the calcific areas. Alternative therapies that have been described include using a Neodymium:yttrium-aluminum-garnet (Nd:YAG) laser,[12] diamond burr or no. 15 blade,[10] excimer laser,[12] and amniotic membrane (AM) transplantation.[13] Another novel approach has used dipotassium-EDTA as a chelating agent.[14]

Case 1

A 20-year-old presents with hand motion vision in an eye with a history of multiple previous surgeries for retinal detachment. He was recently counting fingers and reports a recent decline in vision with increased haziness and "whitening" of his cornea (Fig. 7.1).

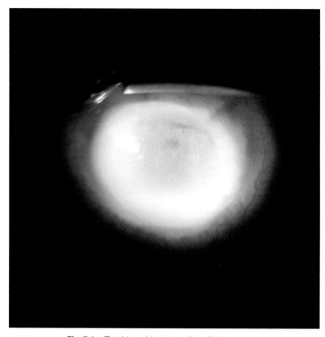

Fig. 7.1   Total band keratopathy of the cornea.

PROCEDURE: EDTA CHELATION

See Box 7.1 *for supplies.*

BOX 7.1 ■ Supplies

- Barraquer eyelid speculum
- Jeweler forceps
- Povidone-iodine 5%
- Ofloxacin ophthalmic solution 0.3% (or equivalent antibiotic eye drop)
- Proparacaine hydrochloride 0.5% (or equivalent anesthetic eye drop)
- No. 15 Bard Parker blade or No. 57 blade
- Corneal shield
- 1.7% disodium ethylenediaminetetraacetic acid (EDTA)
- Bandage contact lens

Procedure

A drop of proparacaine hydrochloride 0.5% is placed in the eye. The lids and lashes are prepped with povidone-iodine in typical fashion for an ocular procedure, including a drop in the fornix. An antibiotic drop is placed in the eye. The speculum is placed, and the patient is brought forward to the slit lamp. Superficial keratectomy is performed using a No. 15 Bard Parker or No. 57 blade over the entire area of band keratopathy. The patient is laid supine with the speculum still in place. An EDTA-soaked corneal shield is placed on the central cornea (Fig. 7.2) for approximately 5–10 minutes to allow chelation of calcium to occur. Gross visualization of the cornea is done

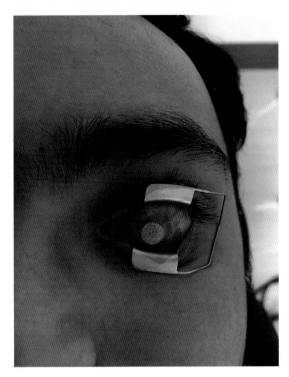

Fig. 7.2 Ethylenediaminetetraacetic acid (EDTA)–soaked sponge placed on the cornea to allow chelation.

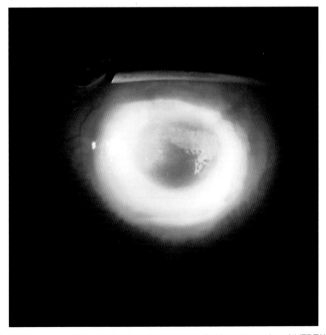

Fig. 7.3   Partial clearance of the calcification after ethylenediaminetetraacetic acid (EDTA) chelation.

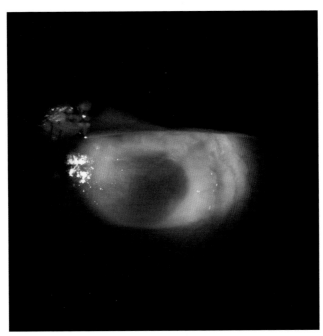

Fig. 7.4 Restoration of a clear corneal visual axis after ethylenediaminetetraacetic acid (EDTA) chelation and removal of final calcific plaques with forceps.

every 10 minutes to assess the degree of chelation and clearing of the calcification. The patient is brought back forward to the slit lamp to check for residual calcium (Fig. 7.3). With a jeweler forceps and the No. 15 Bard Parker blade, additional scraping or removal of plaques can be performed if necessary. The procedure is repeated until the central corneal calcification has dissolved and cleared the visual axis (Fig. 7.4). A bandage contact lens is placed on the cornea to facilitate reepithelialization, and the patient is instructed to use antibiotic drops and preservative-free artificial tears until the lens is removed in 5–7 days.

Conclusion

When calcification of the cornea becomes visually significant or is causing chronic pain and foreign body sensation, a superficial keratectomy with a chelating agent will successfully decrease the calcium burden on the cornea. The goal may be either to fully eliminate all calcium (especially in the central axis) to clear the vision, or it may be to debulk areas of calcific roughness to improve pain. This procedure can be safely accomplished as an in-office procedure. Long-term monitoring should be done, as recurrence of the calcification is common.

References

1. Dixon J. Dixon's guide to the practical study of diseases of the eye. *Br Foreign Med Chir Rev.* 1866;38:560.
2. Lemp MA, Ralph RA. Rapid development of band keratopathy in dry eyes. *Am J Ophthalmol.* 1977;83:657–659. https://doi.org/10.1016/0002-9394(77)90131-3.
3. Moisseiev E, et al. Acute calcific band keratopathy: Case report and literature review. *J Cataract Refract Surg.* 2013;39:292–294. https://doi.org/10.1016/j.jcrs.2012.12.020.
4. Mannis MJ, Holland EJ. *Cornea E-Book.* Elsevier Health Sciences; 2016.

5. Porter R, Crombie AL. Corneal and conjunctival calcification in chronic renal failure. *Br J Ophthalmol.* 1973;57:339–343. https://doi.org/10.1136/bjo.57.5.339.
6. Porter R, Crombie AL. Corneal calcification as a presenting and diagnostic sign in hyperparathyroidism. *Br J Ophthalmol.* 1973;57:665–668. https://doi.org/10.1136/bjo.57.9.665.
7. Cursino JW, Fine BS. A histologic study of calcific and noncalcific band keratopathies. *Am J Ophthalmol.* 1976;82:395–404. https://doi.org/10.1016/0002-9394(76)90488-8.
8. O'Connor GR. Calcific band keratopathy. *Trans Am Ophthalmol Soc.* 1972;70:58–81.
9. Johnston RL, Stanford MR, Verma S, Green WT, Graham EM. Resolution of calcific band keratopathy after lowering elevated serum calcium in a patient with sarcoidosis. *Br J Ophthalmol.* 1995;79:1050. https://doi.org/10.1136/bjo.79.11.1050.
10. Wood TO, Walker GG. Treatment of band keratopathy. *Am J Ophthalmol.* 1975;80:550.
11. Bokosky JE, Meyer RF, Sugar A. Surgical treatment of calcific band keratopathy. *Ophthalmic Surg.* 1985;16:645–647.
12. O'Brart DP, et al. Treatment of band keratopathy by excimer laser phototherapeutic keratecomy: Surgical techniques and long term follow up. *Br J Ophthalmol.* 1993;77:702–708. https://doi.org/10.1136/bjo.77.11.702.
13. Im SK, Lee KH, Yoon KC. Combined ethylenediaminetetraacetic acid chelation, phototherapeutic keratectomy and amniotic membrane transplantation for treatment of band keratopathy. *Korean J Ophthalmol.* 2010;24:73–77. https://doi.org/10.3341/kjo.2010.24.2.73.
14. Lee ME, Ouano DP, Shapiro B, Fong A, Coroneo MT. "Off-the-shelf" K2-EDTA for calcific band keratopathy. *Cornea.* 2018;37:916–918. https://doi.org/10.1097/ICO.0000000000001558.

CHAPTER 8

Epithelial Ingrowth Under a LASIK Flap

Zeba A. Syed ▪ Beeran B. Meghpara ▪ Christopher J. Rapuano

Introduction

The construction of a laser-assisted in situ keratomileusis (LASIK) flap results in a potential space between the underlying corneal stroma and overlying flap. A possible complication resulting from the creation of this space is the entry of epithelial cells, a process called epithelial ingrowth. Many risk factors have been identified for epithelial ingrowth after LASIK; flap lifting for enhancement is a well-documented predisposing factor. The decision to pursue treatment for epithelial ingrowth is guided largely by patient symptoms and health of the overlying flap, as a significant proportion of cases of epithelial ingrowth are mild and asymptomatic. Various office-based techniques exist to treat epithelial ingrowth, and often the initial approach is flap lifting with mechanical debridement of both the stromal surface and underside of the flap. Flap lifting and debridement can be performed either alone or combined with suture placement, adhesives such as hydrogel sealant or fibrin glue, or adjuvant therapy including alcohol, mitomycin C, or phototherapeutic keratectomy (PTK). Neodymium:yttrium-aluminum-garnet (Nd:YAG) laser treatment has also been employed in the management of epithelial ingrowth. In this chapter, we review this spectrum of procedural options for epithelial ingrowth by using a case-based approach. We discuss the instruments required for each technique, the risks associated with these treatments, and outcomes. Success rates have varied across these different techniques in case reports and case series, and large-scale studies are needed to compare these treatments systematically.

Epithelial ingrowth involves the migration of corneal epithelium into the flap interface (Fig. 8.1). The incidence of epithelial ingrowth after primary LASIK has been reported to range from 0% to 3.9%,[1–4] but postmortem histopathologic investigations have identified a rate of 50%.[5] Epithelial ingrowth typically develops within a month after primary treatment or flap lifting for LASIK enhancement.[4]

Two general processes underlie the mechanism of post-LASIK epithelial ingrowth. First, the introduction of corneal epithelial cells during initial flap construction results in the deposition of epithelial clusters a distance away from the flap edge. These cells typically exhibit low proliferative activity secondary to their decreased access to the ocular surface and its nourishment. Furthermore, this colony of implanted cells is not connected to the limbal stem cells. Second, poor flap adhesion may permit the invasion of epithelial cells into the flap-stroma interface. Proliferation of these cells may result in the development of a fistula and progressive epithelial ingrowth.[6] Over time, the stroma overlying and underlying these epithelial cells can undergo remodeling, resulting in keratolysis.

Risk Factors

Although the overall risk of epithelial ingrowth after primary LASIK is low, this risk increases in several situations. For example, when the LASIK flap is lifted for enhancement, the rate of epithelial ingrowth is 10% to 20%.[7–9] In addition, flap lifts that take place 3 or more years after

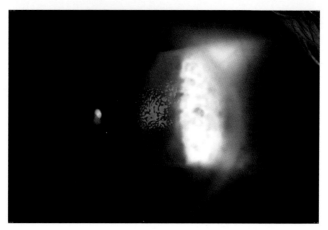

Fig. 8.1   Anterior segment photograph demonstrating epithelial ingrowth.

initial treatment are associated with a greater risk of epithelial ingrowth compared to flap lifts performed earlier.[1] The technique for initial flap construction affects the risk of epithelial ingrowth after retreatment due to the resulting geometry of the flap edge. Femtosecond flaps are associated with a lower risk of epithelial ingrowth following flap lifting compared to those created using a microkeratome (1.4% versus 8.3%).[7] Furthermore, using the femtosecond laser to create inverted side-cut angle flaps may further decrease the risk of epithelial ingrowth.[10]

Epithelial injury during LASIK may also increase the risk of epithelial ingrowth.[11,12] Large epithelial defects inadvertently created during LASIK may be associated with increased flap edema and poorer flap adhesion, resulting in an increased risk of epithelial ingrowth.[4] The use of a Pinelli spatula or a similar device to release the flap edge prior to flap-lift retreatment may reduce the chances of epithelial ingrowth compared to forceps due to the increased epithelial trauma associated with the latter.[13]

Other risk factors for epithelial ingrowth that have been documented in the literature include traumatic flap dislocation,[14,15] epithelial basement membrane dystrophy (EBMD),[12] and hyperopic LASIK compared to myopic LASIK.[3]

Clinical Features

The clinical presentation associated with epithelial ingrowth ranges from an asymptomatic and incidental finding to severe vision loss and flap melt. In addition to visible nests of epithelial cells in the flap-stroma interface, other slit-lamp findings associated with epithelial ingrowth include (1) fluorescein pooling at the flap periphery due to partial lifting of the flap secondary to a sheet of underlying epithelial cells, (2) a fibrotic demarcation line along the advancing edge of epithelial cells, and (3) keratolysis of the flap, most commonly at the flap edge, with resulting flap edge irregularity (Fig. 8.2).[4]

Although clinical evaluation with slit-lamp examination is the primary method to detect epithelial ingrowth, other tools may be employed to identify and monitor the condition. These include anterior segment optical coherence tomography, which can identify small epithelial nests that may be subtle on slit-lamp evaluation. Alternatively, corneal topography can identify ocular surface irregularities induced by epithelial ingrowth. Finally, corneal densitometry can also be employed to objectively measure the severity of epithelial ingrowth and document progression.[16]

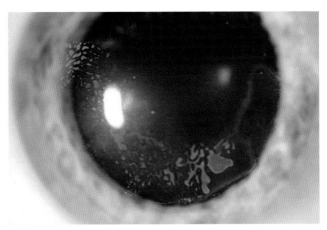

Fig. 8.2 Anterior segment photograph demonstrating epithelial ingrowth that resulted in flap melt and resulting flap edge irregularity.

Treatment Indications

The decision to pursue treatment of epithelial ingrowth is primarily dictated by the patient's symptoms, although other characteristics such as location, severity, health of the overlying flap, and associated flap dislocation or dehiscence also factor into the assessment. Up to 64% of eyes with post-LASIK epithelial ingrowth do not warrant intervention.[17] For example, cases of nonprogressive epithelial ingrowth located within 1–2 mm of the flap edge and which do not distort flap anatomy typically do not require treatment.

In general, epithelial ingrowth necessitates surgical intervention for one of five reasons: (1) the ingrowth may encroach into the visual axis, affecting the patient's visual acuity; (2) the epithelial ingrowth may trigger glare symptoms due to its proximity to the pupil; (3) the epithelial ingrowth may result in keratolysis or flap melt, requiring urgent intervention; (4) by elevating the flap in a focal region, the epithelial ingrowth may induce irregular (or less commonly regular) astigmatism, causing visual aberrations and affecting quality of vision; and (5) the ingrowth may result in epithelial irregularity, causing ocular surface symptoms such as foreign body sensation.

Case 1

A 50-year-old female presented for evaluation of decreased vision. She underwent cataract surgery in the left eye 3 years prior to presentation, and residual refractive error was treated with LASIK 2 months later. Two years later, she underwent a LASIK enhancement, which was complicated by significant epithelial ingrowth. She was treated with a flap lift and mechanical debridement but had recurrent ingrowth. The patient reported symptoms of progressively worsening vision and light sensitivity in her left eye.

On initial evaluation, she had an uncorrected visual acuity of 20/25 in the right eye and 20/200 in the left eye. Her best corrected visual acuity (BCVA) in the left eye was 20/40 with a manifest refraction of −0.75 +1.75 × 180. Slit-lamp examination of the left eye demonstrated a LASIK flap with a superior hinge and epithelial ingrowth extending from the superonasal flap edge approximately 3.5 mm toward the visual axis (Fig. 8.3). The LASIK flap edges were noted to be ragged around the area of ingrowth. Topography demonstrated irregular astigmatism with central steepening (Fig. 8.4). The patient was scheduled for *mechanical debridement of the epithelial ingrowth with flap suture placement* (see Video 8.1).

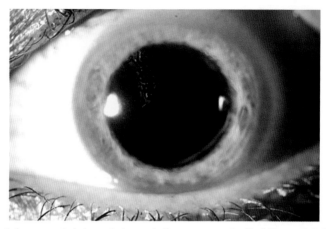

Fig. 8.3 Anterior segment photograph demonstrating superonasal epithelial ingrowth in the left eye.

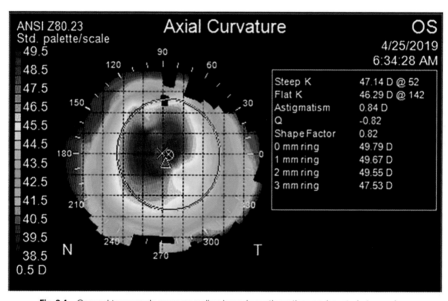

Fig. 8.4 Corneal topography map revealing irregular astigmatism and central steepening.

PROCEDURE: MECHANICAL DEBRIDEMENT OF EPITHELIAL INGROWTH WITH FLAP SUTURE PLACEMENT (BOX 8.1)

An eyelid speculum was placed for exposure. A Sclerotome blade no. 57 was used to debride epithelium around the circumference of the flap edge, extending approximately 1 mm both centrally and peripherally from the flap edge. Weck-Cel spears were also used to remove epithelial debris. A Sinskey hook was then used to elevate the flap edges. Nontoothed forceps were employed to gently elevate the flap. Once the flap was completely free from the stromal bed, the Sclerotome blade no. 57 was used to scrape epithelial cells off the stromal bed and the underside of the flap. Special care was taken to make sure all the epithelium was removed from the very edge of the flap.

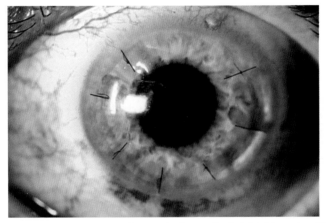

Fig. 8.5 Postoperative anterior segment photograph after mechanical debridement and flap suturing.

The flap was then floated into the correct position using balanced salt solution and a LASIK flap cannula. Seven 10-0 nylon sutures were placed symmetrically around the edge of the flap to tightly reapproximate the flap edges to the stroma, taking care to not create flap striae. Vannas scissors were used to trim the suture tails prior to rotating the knots away from the flap. A Bandage contact lens was placed on the cornea at the end of the case.

On postoperative day one, the patient had a visual acuity in the left eye of counting fingers at 5 feet. The flap was in good position with all sutures intact (Fig. 8.5). About 6 weeks after the procedure, half of the flap sutures were removed. One month later, the remaining sutures were removed. At her most recent follow-up visit 7 months after surgery, the patient had an uncorrected visual acuity of 20/40 in the left eye. No recurrent epithelial ingrowth was noted at that visit (Fig. 8.6). On topography, the central steepening associated with the prior area of epithelial ingrowth had flattened (Fig. 8.7).

DISCUSSION

One option for the treatment of epithelial ingrowth is simple debridement of the interface epithelium. The patient is reclined in a supine position, and a sterile drape is placed over the eye. A wire lid speculum is inserted in the fornices for exposure.

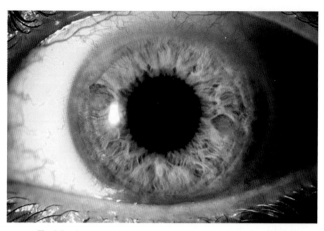

Fig. 8.6 Anterior segment photograph after suture removal.

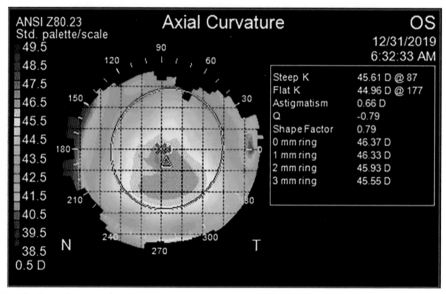

Fig. 8.7 Corneal topography map performed 7 months after treatment revealing improvement in irregular astigmatism and flattening in the area of prior epithelial ingrowth.

Although there is no consensus over the necessity of this step, many surgeons prefer to remove the epithelium surrounding the circumference of the flap edge (approximately 1 mm on either side of the flap edge) prior to lifting the flap. This step theoretically reduces the risk of ingrowth while the flap heals by temporarily eliminating adjacent epithelial cells. Epithelium can be removed with a number of instruments such as a Sclerotome blade no. 57. Other options include a Maloney spatula, Beaver blade, or crescent blade.

Following surface epithelial removal from the flap edge, the surgeon separates the LASIK flap from the underlying stroma using a blunt hook such as a Sinskey hook. Other instruments available to separate the LASIK flap include a LASIK flap manipulator, Katzen LASIK flap unzipper, MacRae LASIK flap spatula, or Pinelli spatula.

Once the peripheral LASIK flap has been separated from the underlying stroma, the flap can be lifted using various instruments. Any set of nontoothed forceps, such as tying forceps, can be used to elevate the flap. Other instruments available to elevate the flap include Hersh LASIK retreatment forceps or LASIK corneal flap forceps.

After the flap is lifted, the epithelium from the stromal bed and the underside of the flap needs to be scraped off. The instrument used to remove the surface epithelium around the flap periphery can also be used for this step, such as a Sclerotome blade no. 57. Alternatively, cellulose sponges such as Weck-Cel spears can be used to polish the stromal bed and underside of the flap. Special care must be taken to remove all the epithelium from the edges of the flap, as it is often quite adherent in that location.

As a final step after mechanical debridement, the flap should be repositioned with copious irrigation using balanced saline solution. Similar to the primary LASIK procedure, the repositioned flap should be brushed lightly with a moistened sponge to achieve optimal flap edge apposition. Finally, most surgeons will elect to place a bandage soft contact lens over the surface of the cornea to enhance flap adhesion and reduce the chances of flap dislocation. The bandage soft contact lens typically remains in place until the epithelium completely heals, or about 1 week. A typical postoperative drop regimen includes an antibiotic and steroid, each four times daily for the first week (or as long as the bandage contact lens remains in place). Thereafter, the antibiotic is discontinued, and the steroid is tapered weekly over the course of about a month.

The incidence of recurrence of epithelial ingrowth after flap interface debridement alone is documented to be as high as 44%, although clinically significant recurrence is reported to be approximately 23%.[4] Many surgeons opt to combine debridement with a technique to more tightly secure the flap to the stromal bed, as described below.

Combined With Flap Suturing

Tightly suturing the LASIK flap to cause apposition of the flap to the stromal bed can be done with the goal of reducing the risk of recurrent epithelial ingrowth. After mechanical debridement as described above, the flap is tightly sutured into place using 10-0 nylon sutures. Typically, a total of 5 to 12 interrupted sutures, depending on the amount of the flap that required elevation, are placed symmetrically around the area that was previously lifted. Care is taken to avoid the creation of flap striae. A Bandage contact lens is usually applied at the conclusion of the surgery and removed after a week. Patients should be counseled that, due to the tightness of the sutures, vision does not immediately recover. Rather, improvement may not occur until after all sutures are removed. Typically, half of the sutures are removed 4 to 6 weeks after the surgery. The remaining half of the sutures are usually removed 4 to 6 weeks later.

The success rate of this approach has been reported to be higher than mechanical debridement alone. In one study comparing mechanical debridement alone and mechanical debridement with flap suturing, debridement alone resulted in significantly better immediate postoperative visual outcomes but higher epithelial ingrowth recurrence rates.[18] Long-term visual acuity results were similar between the two groups.[18] The rate of clinically significant recurrence of epithelial ingrowth following mechanical debridement with flap suturing has been reported to range from 0% to 22%.[2,17,19]

Combined With Hydrogel Sealant or Fibrin Glue

As an alternative to suture placement, which requires more frequent follow-ups for suture removal, some practitioners have opted to use tissue adhesives to secure the flap edge after removal of epithelial ingrowth. Additionally, some surgeons believe that the use of adhesives avoids the possible striae and irregular astigmatism that may be associated with tight suture placement. After the flap is irrigated and repositioned as described above, the edge is dried, and an adhesive is applied around the circumference of the flap edge.

The hydrogel ReSure sealant has been used for this purpose. Although there are no rigorous trials comparing the use of hydrogel sealant to flap sutures, case series using sealant have shown promising results. The two reports using this technique, totaling three eyes, demonstrated a 0% rate of clinically significant recurrent epithelial ingrowth.[20,21]

A substitute for sealant is the use of fibrin glue. Similar to hydrogel sealant, once the flap is irrigated into position, the margins are dried off prior to placement of fibrin glue. Tisseel has been studied for this indication. The rate of recurrence of epithelial ingrowth after mechanical debridement followed by fibrin glue placement has ranged from 0% to 7.7% across several studies.[22-24] Fibrin glue, furthermore, may have inhibitory properties that reduce the migration of ocular surface epithelial cells.[25]

Combined With Alcohol or Mitomycin C

Due to its ability to delaminate corneal epithelium, alcohol has been considered an adjunct to mechanical debridement in the management of epithelial ingrowth. Various protocols have been used, and these approaches differ in (1) the form of alcohol used, (2) the concentration of alcohol employed, (3) the length of time alcohol is applied, and (4) whether alcohol is applied to the flap and stromal surfaces prior to or after debridement.

The mechanical debridement step is performed as described above. However, a corneal sponge soaked in alcohol is placed between the stromal and LASIK flap surfaces for between 10 and 30 seconds. Several forms and concentrations of alcohol may be employed, and reports have used ethanol (between 10% and 50%) and 70% isopropyl alcohol.

Outcomes after the adjunctive use of alcohol have varied, with studies demonstrating between a 0% and 36% recurrence rate of epithelial ingrowth.[26,27] Overall, there is no definitive evidence supporting the use of alcohol in the management of epithelial ingrowth. Reports of flap melt among patients treated in this manner reinforce that the use of this agent in the flap-stroma interface should be considered cautiously.[28] Furthermore, diffuse lamellar keratitis has also been reported after the use of higher concentrations (>50%) of ethanol at the flap-stroma interface.[29]

In addition to alcohol, mitomycin C has been suggested as an option to reduce the recurrence of epithelial ingrowth. One study combined mechanical debridement with the sequential application of both alcohol and mitomycin C 0.02% to the stromal bed and underside of the flap. Clinically significant epithelial ingrowth did not recur in any of the four eyes treated in this manner during this study.[30] While such cases exist, there are no robust data to support the use of mitomycin C in the management of epithelial ingrowth. The potential toxicity associated with mitomycin C, possibly leading to scleromalacia, corneal melt, limbal stem cell deficiency, and punctal stenosis, warrant extreme caution in its use to treat epithelial ingrowth.[31]

Case 2

A 45-year-old male presented for evaluation of decreased vision and glare symptoms. He had a history of LASIK treatment 12 years prior to presentation. He suffered from trauma with a wire to the right eye 2 years prior to presentation, and he was noted to have epithelial ingrowth after this injury. One year prior to presentation, he was treated with flap relifting and mechanical debridement. However, the epithelial ingrowth recurred.

On initial evaluation, he had an uncorrected distance visual acuity of 20/60 in the right eye and 20/20 in the left eye. His best corrected visual acuity in the right eye was 20/40 with a manifest refraction of −2.50 +2.00 × 155. Slit-lamp examination of the right eye demonstrated a LASIK flap with a superior hinge. At the 9:00 flap edge, epithelial ingrowth was noted to extend approximately 4 mm toward the visual axis. The central edge of epithelial ingrowth featured a moderately dense fibrotic demarcation line. Examination of the left eye revealed a LASIK flap without any epithelial ingrowth. Given the level of fibrosis, the patient was scheduled for *mechanical debridement combined with phototherapeutic keractectomy (PTK)a.*

BOX 8.2 ■ Supplies

Eyelid speculum
Sclerotome blade no. 57
Weck-Cel spears
Sinskey hook
Nontoothed forceps
Excimer laser
LASIK flap cannula on a BSS syringe
Bandage contact lens

PROCEDURE: MECHANICAL DEBRIDEMENT COMBINED WITH PHOTOTHERAPEUTIC KERATECTOMY (BOX 8.2)

An eyelid speculum was inserted to optimize exposure. A Sclerotome blade no. 57 was used to scrape the epithelium around the flap edge, extending approximately 1 mm both centrally and peripherally. Weck-Cel spears were utilized to clear up residual epithelial debris. A Sinskey hook was then employed to elevate the flap margin, and nontoothed forceps were used to gently grasp and elevate the flap. The Sclerotome blade no. 57 was again used to scrape epithelial cells off the stromal bed and the underside of the flap. Next, using an excimer laser PTK set at a 6.5-mm-diameter treatment zone, approximately 7 μm of tissue was ablated centrally from both the stromal surface and flap underside. The flap was then floated into position using balanced salt solution on a LASIK flap cannula. A Bandage contact lens was placed on the cornea at the end of the case.

On postoperative day one, the patient had a visual acuity in the right eye of 20/50. The flap was in a good position, and no fibrosis was noted clinically. By postoperative month one, the patient's uncorrected visual acuity was 20/30, and the best corrected visual acuity was 20/20 with a manifest refraction of −1.00 +1.50 × 155. At the most recent follow-up visit 6 months after the procedure, no recurrent epithelial ingrowth was noted.

DISCUSSION

Excimer laser PTK has been used to maximize the removal of all remaining epithelial cells after mechanical debridement. Furthermore, the laser may ablate areas of fibrosis or other scar-related pathology that may promote further epithelial cell invasion. Smoother surfaces between the stromal bed and flap may optimize adhesion, and successful attachment is required to prevent future epithelial cell migration.

The depth of treatment is set to remove between 7 μm and 10 μm from both the stromal and flap surfaces.[32] This treatment depth is preferred because it minimizes refractive changes from the treatment yet still ablates a few layers of cells. There is no consensus on treatment protocol, and one study recommended using two 7-mm treatment zones plus transition zones of 0.5 mm on both stromal and flap surfaces.[32] One caveat to this approach is that it primarily treats the central zone, reducing local astigmatism and accomplishing better adhesion between the stromal bed and flap centrally; peripheral ingrowth is not targeted by this therapy. The rate of recurrence of significant epithelial ingrowth after debridement with PTK was 20% in this study.[32] Significant changes in refractive error, typically a hyperopic shift, can occur depending on the depth of treatment.

A usual postoperative drop regimen includes an antibiotic and steroid, each four times daily for the first week after surgery. Subsequently, the antibiotic is discontinued, and the steroid is tapered weekly over the course of about a month.

Case 3

A 59-year-old female presented for evaluation of progressively decreasing vision. She underwent LASIK in both eyes 10 years prior to presentation. One year after her original surgery, the patient underwent bilateral LASIK enhancements with flap relifting. She later developed epithelial ingrowth in her right eye that was treated with repeat flap lifting and mechanical debridement 6 months prior to presentation. Three months prior to presentation, the left LASIK flap was also lifted with mechanical debridement to treat epithelial ingrowth. However, this latter procedure was complicated by inadvertent flap amputation. The flap was repositioned, and a bandage contact lens was placed for mechanical support.

On initial evaluation, the patient had an uncorrected visual acuity of 20/30 in the right eye and 20/40 in the left eye. Her best corrected visual acuity in the right eye was 20/20 with a manifest refraction of −1.50 +1.00 × 090. Her left eye vision could not be improved with refraction. Slit-lamp examination of the right eye demonstrated a LASIK flap with a superior hinge and a small degree of peripheral epithelial ingrowth at 1:00 and 9:00. Examination of the left eye revealed a free LASIK flap and a moderate degree of epithelial ingrowth at the superior paracentral region encroaching on the visual axis (Fig. 8.8). To avoid mechanically disrupting the already traumatized LASIK flap, the patient was scheduled for *Nd:YAG laser treatment of the epithelial ingrowth*.

PROCEDURE: ND:YAG LASER TREATMENT (BOX 8.3)

The patient was positioned at the Nd:YAG laser, and an Abraham capsulotomy lens was placed over the left eye to stabilize the globe. Power settings were adjusted between 0.7 mJ and 0.9 mJ, and a spot size of 8 μm was used. Approximately 20 shots were performed and aimed at the plane of epithelial ingrowth. The goal of the individual laser sessions was to create a set of confluent gas bubbles at the LASIK interface (Fig. 8.9).

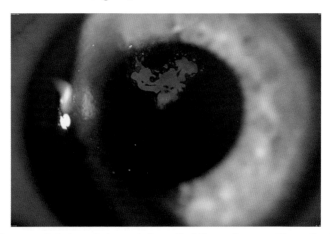

Fig. 8.8   Anterior segment photograph demonstrating epithelial ingrowth encroaching on the visual axis.

BOX 8.3 ■ Supplies

Nd:YAG laser
Abraham capsulotomy lens

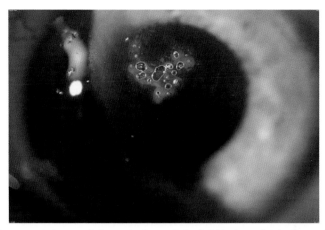

Fig. 8.9 Anterior segment photograph demonstrating cavitation bubbles immediately after neodymium:yttrium-aluminum-garnet (Nd:YAG) laser treatment for epithelial ingrowth.

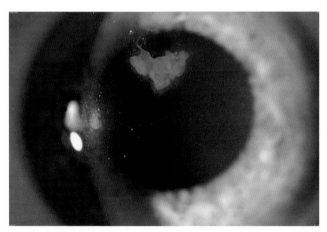

Fig. 8.10 Anterior segment photograph demonstrating improvement in epithelial ingrowth 1 month after neodymium:yttrium-aluminum-garnet (Nd:YAG) laser treatment.

One month after this treatment, the area of epithelial ingrowth had shrunken (Fig. 8.10). A second session of Nd:YAG laser was performed. A month after the second treatment, further improvement of the residual epithelial ingrowth was noted (Fig. 8.11). A third and final treatment was completed at that time. Approximately 18 months after the final treatment, the epithelial ingrowth was noted to be very faint (Fig. 8.12). The patient's best corrected visual acuity was 20/20 in the left eye with a manifest refraction of −1.75 +1.25 × 155.

DISCUSSION

Another option for managing epithelial ingrowth is Nd:YAG laser treatment. This option is particularly attractive in situations where the surgeon would like to avoid lifting the LASIK flap. The laser employs infrared light at a wavelength of 1064 nm and is used in ophthalmology to treat posterior capsular opacification, to create peripheral iridotomies, and for vitreolysis. However, its application in corneal surgery is less well defined.

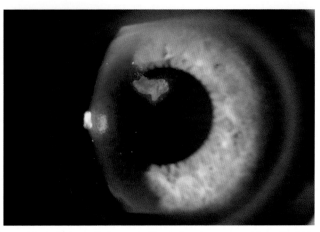

Fig. 8.11 Anterior segment photograph demonstrating further improvement in epithelial ingrowth 1 month after second neodymium:yttrium-aluminum-garnet (Nd:YAG) laser treatment.

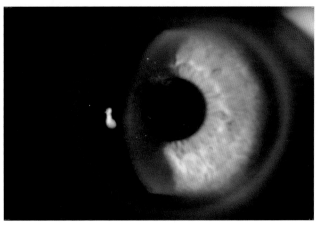

Fig. 8.12 Anterior segment photograph demonstrating faint residual epithelial ingrowth 18 months after third neodymium:yttrium-aluminum-garnet (Nd:YAG) laser treatment.

Different protocols can be used to treat epithelial ingrowth with the Nd:YAG laser. One approach involves using an Abraham capsulotomy lens to stabilize the globe, while the Nd:YAG laser is used to create confluent vacuoles along the track of epithelial ingrowth.[33] Spot size may vary depending on the focal area of epithelial ingrowth being treated, and 8 μm is often used. A power of 0.6 mJ to 0.9 mJ is typically sufficient to cause disruption of the epithelial ingrowth cells. The shots should be placed so that the resulting cavitation bubbles coalesce, with each subsequent laser placement at the periphery of the bubble created by the prior shot. In this manner, the entire region of ingrowth can be treated.[33]

Some surgeons will limit the number of shots to approximately 20 per session to avoid corneal melt. In one report, after 65 shots of 0.6 mJ energy, localized melt was noted at the flap periphery.[34] As a result, it may be reasonable to consider fewer laser shots during one session and to repeat sessions 1 or 2 weeks apart. Furthermore, Nd:YAG may result in unintentional new fistulas at the flap edges and new areas of ingrowth.[35] The postoperative treatment regimen usually includes a topical steroid three to four times daily for a week.

Although no large-scale comparative analyses have been performed using Nd:YAG to treat epithelial ingrowth, existing reports show promising results with 0% recurrence rates across several studies, but it typically requires multiple sessions.[33,36,37]

Conclusion

While epithelial ingrowth is a relatively rare complication after primary LASIK, the risk increases considerably after flap lift for retreatment and traumatic flap dehiscence. Many options exist to treat epithelial ingrowth. Mechanical debridement alone may be considered, but data suggest that debridement combined with suture placement may provide improved results. Alternative options include mechanical debridement with hydrogel sealant or fibrin glue, mechanical debridement with alcohol or mitomycin C, mechanical debridement with PTK, or Nd:YAG laser. Although case reports and case studies exist for these options, large-scale randomized studies comparing various approaches are needed to guide clinicians on the appropriate course of action in different scenarios.

References

1. Caster AI, Friess DW, Schwendeman FJ. Incidence of epithelial ingrowth in primary and retreatment laser in situ keratomileusis. *J Cataract Refract Surg*. 2010;36:97–101.
2. Guell JL, Verdaguer P, Mateu-Figueras G, et al. Epithelial ingrowth after LASIK: Visual and refractive results after cleaning the interface and suturing the lenticule. *Cornea*. 2014;33:1046–1050.
3. Mohamed TA, Hoffman RS, Fine IH, Packer M. Post-laser assisted in situ keratomileusis epithelial ingrowth and its relation to pretreatment refractive error. *Cornea*. 2011;30:550–552.
4. Wang MY, Maloney RK. Epithelial ingrowth after laser in situ keratomileusis. *Am J Ophthalmol*. 2000;129:746–751.
5. Kramer TR, Chuckpaiwong V, Dawson DG, L'Hernault N, Grossniklaus HE, Edelhauser HF. Pathologic findings in postmortem corneas after successful laser in situ keratomileusis. *Cornea*. 2005;24:92–102.
6. Ting DSJ, Srinivasan S, Danjoux JP. Epithelial ingrowth following laser in situ keratomileusis (LASIK): Prevalence, risk factors, management and visual outcomes. *BMJ Open Ophthalmol*. 2018;3:e000133.
7. Letko E, Price MO, Price Jr. FW. Influence of original flap creation method on incidence of epithelial ingrowth after LASIK retreatment. *J Refract Surg*. 2009;25:1039–1041.
8. Ortega-Usobiaga J, Llovet-Osuna F, Katz T, et al. Comparison of 5468 retreatments after laser in situ keratomileusis by lifting the flap or performing photorefractive keratectomy on the flap. *Arch Soc Esp Oftalmol*. 2018;93:60–68.
9. Schallhorn SC, Venter JA, Hannan SJ, Hettinger KA, Teenan D. Flap lift and photorefractive keratectomy enhancements after primary laser in situ keratomileusis using a wavefront-guided ablation profile: refractive and visual outcomes. *J Cataract Refract Surg*. 2015;41:2501–2512.
10. Jhanji V, Chan TC, Li WY, et al. Conventional versus inverted side-cut flaps for femtosecond laser-assisted LASIK: Laboratory and clinical evaluation. *J Refract Surg*. 2017;33:96–103.
11. Asano-Kato N, Toda I, Hori-Komai Y, Takano Y, Tsubota K. Epithelial ingrowth after laser in situ keratomileusis: clinical features and possible mechanisms. *Am J Ophthalmol*. 2002;134:801–807.
12. Jabbur NS, Chicani CF, Kuo IC, O'Brien TP. Risk factors in interface epithelialization after laser in situ keratomileusis. *J Refract Surg*. 2004;20:343–348.
13. Chan CC, Boxer Wachler BS. Comparison of the effects of LASIK retreatment techniques on epithelial ingrowth rates. *Ophthalmology*. 2007;114:640–642.
14. Holt DG, Sikder S, Mifflin MD. Surgical management of traumatic LASIK flap dislocation with macrostriae and epithelial ingrowth 14 years postoperatively. *J Cataract Refract Surg*. 2012;38:357–361.
15. Xiao J, Jiang C, Zhang M, Jiang H, Li S, Zhang Y. When case report became case series: 45 cases of late traumatic flap complications after laser-assisted in situ keratomileusis and review of Chinese literature. *Br J Ophthalmol*. 2014;98:1282–1286.

16. Adran D, Vaillancourt L, Harissi-Dagher M, et al. Corneal densitometry as a tool to measure epithelial ingrowth after laser in situ keratomileusis. *Cornea.* 2017;36:406–410.

17. Rapuano CJ. Management of epithelial ingrowth after laser in situ keratomileusis on a tertiary care cornea service. *Cornea.* 2010;29:307–313.

18. Yesilirmak N, Chhadva P, Cabot F, Galor A, Yoo SH. Post-laser in situ keratomileusis epithelial ingrowth: treatment, recurrence, and long-term results. *Cornea.* 2018;37:1517–1521.

19. Rojas MC, Lumba JD, Manche EE. Treatment of epithelial ingrowth after laser in situ keratomileusis with mechanical debridement and flap suturing. *Arch Ophthalmol.* 2004;122:997–1001.

20. Ramsook SS, Hersh PS. Use of a hydrogel sealant in epithelial ingrowth removal after laser in situ keratomileusis. *J Cataract Refract Surg.* 2015;41:2768–2771.

21. Yesilirmak N, Diakonis VF, Battle JF, Yoo SH. Application of a hydrogel ocular sealant to avoid recurrence of epithelial ingrowth after LASIK enhancement. *J Refract Surg.* 2015;31:275–277.

22. Anderson NJ, Hardten DR. Fibrin glue for the prevention of epithelial ingrowth after laser in situ keratomileusis. *J Cataract Refract Surg.* 2003;29:1425–1429.

23. Hardten DR, Fahmy MM, Vora GK, Berdahl JP, Kim T. Fibrin adhesive in conjunction with epithelial ingrowth removal after laser in situ keratomileusis: Long-term results. *J Cataract Refract Surg.* 2015;41:1400–1405.

24. Yeh DL, Bushley DM, Kim T. Treatment of traumatic LASIK flap dislocation and epithelial ingrowth with fibrin glue. *Am J Ophthalmol.* 2006;141:960–962.

25. Yeung AM, Faraj LA, McIntosh OD, Dhillon VK, Dua HS. Fibrin glue inhibits migration of ocular surface epithelial cells. *Eye (Lond).* 2016;30:1389–1394.

26. Haw WW, Manche EE. Treatment of progressive or recurrent epithelial ingrowth with ethanol following laser in situ keratomileusis. *J Refract Surg.* 2001;17:63–68.

27. Lahners WJ, Hardten DR, Lindstrom RL. Alcohol and mechanical scraping for epithelial ingrowth following laser in situ keratomileusis. *J Refract Surg.* 2005;21:148–151.

28. Vroman DT, Karp CL. Complication from use of alcohol to treat epithelial ingrowth after laser-assisted in situ keratomileusis. *Arch Ophthalmol.* 2001;119:1378–1379.

29. Kim P, Briganti EM, Sutton GL, Lawless MA, Rogers CM, Hodge C. Laser in situ keratomileusis for refractive error after cataract surgery. *J Cataract Refract Surg.* 2005;31:979–986.

30. Wilde C, Messina M, Dua HS. Management of recurrent epithelial ingrowth following laser in situ keratomileusis with mechanical debridement, alcohol, mitomycin-C, and fibrin glue. *J Cataract Refract Surg.* 2017;43:980–984.

31. Khong JJ, Muecke J. Complications of mitomycin C therapy in 100 eyes with ocular surface neoplasia. *Br J Ophthalmol.* 2006;90:819–822.

32. Fagerholm P, Molander N, Podskochy A, Sundelin S. Epithelial ingrowth after LASIK treatment with scraping and phototherapeutic keratectomy. *Acta Ophthalmol Scand.* 2004;82:707–713.

33. Mohammed OA, Mounir A, Hassan AA, Alsmman AH, Mostafa EM. Nd:YAG laser for epithelial ingrowth after laser in situ keratomileusis. *Int Ophthalmol.* 2019;39:1225–1230.

34. Kucukevcilioglu M, Hurmeric V. Localized flap melt after Nd-YAG laser treatment in recurrent post-LASIK epithelial ingrowth. *Arq Bras Oftalmol.* 2015;78:250–251.

35. Lapid-Gortzak R, Hughes JM, Nieuwendaal CP, Mourits MP, van der Meulen IJ. LASIK flap breakthrough in Nd:YAG laser treatment of epithelial ingrowth. *J Refract Surg.* 2015;31:342–345.

36. Ayala MJ, Alio JL, Mulet ME, De La Hoz F. Treatment of laser in situ keratomileusis interface epithelial ingrowth with neodymium:yytrium-aluminum-garnet laser. *Am J Ophthalmol.* 2008;145:630–634.

37. Kim JM, Goel M, Pathak A. Epithelial ingrowth-Nd:YAG laser approach. *Clin Exp Ophthalmol.* 2014;42:389–390.

CHAPTER 9

LASIK Flap Striae

Aman Mittal ■ Beeran B. Meghpara

Introduction

Laser-assisted in situ keratomileusis (LASIK) requires creating an anterior corneal flap with either a microkeratome blade or femtosecond laser and precisely aligning the flap back into position after excimer laser ablation. A potential flap-related complication is the development of postoperative flap striae. Postoperative flap striae can limit visual acuity depending on the size and location of the striae. The decision to pursue treatment is guided largely by patient symptoms, as a proportion of flap striae are mild and asymptomatic. Various office-based treatments exist to treat flap striae. Often, the initial approach is flap lifting, stretching, and repositioning. Flap repositioning can be performed either alone or in combination with flap hydration, heating, suturing, or even flap removal. Flap striae seen immediately after surgery can be treated with refloating and repositioning of the flap. In this chapter, we review the treatment options for LASIK flap striae using a case-based approach, including techniques, instruments required, and outcomes.

Clinical Features

Flap striae are generally apparent within 24 hours after LASIK and can be divided into two categories: microstriae and macrostriae.[1,2] Microstriae are fine, randomly oriented wrinkles in the anterior cornea that can produce a negative-staining pattern after application of fluorescein dye due to disruption of the overlying tear film.[3] Microstriae are subtle, and slit-lamp retroillumination or broad oblique illumination is used to help visualization. Microstriae are often too small to be seen on corneal topography and generally have a minimal effect on visual acuity, as they can be masked by the overlying epithelium.[2]

Macrostriae, or folds, are larger parallel, or near-parallel, lines that are straight ("washboard") or somewhat "wavy," often involving the full thickness of the flap. Examination of the flap edge can reveal a widened gutter or partial flap dislocation. Fluorescein dye will demonstrate negative staining over the macrostriae and pooling in the gutter.[3] Macrostriae are more readily apparent on slit-lamp examination and are often visually significant.[2] Retroillumination can help with visualization and flap striae have been documented with anterior segment optical coherence tomography imaging.[4,5]

Vision changes associated with flap striae include loss of best corrected visual acuity (BCVA) as well as ghosting of images, monocular diplopia, increased glare or halos, and decreased contrast sensitivity. Flap striae have been reported to induce visually streaks of light perpendicular to the striae in a similar fashion to a Maddox rod.[6]

Epidemiology

LASIK flaps were originally created mechanically with a microkeratome; more recently, this has been done with the femtosecond laser. Femtosecond laser flaps are associated with a lower complication risk, including epithelial ingrowth, buttonholes, free flaps, and flap striae. The incidence of postoperative flap striae ranges of 0.1%–12.8% with microkeratome flaps and 0%–10.4% with femtosecond-created flaps.

Horizontal striae are more common with nasal-hinged flaps, and vertical striae are more common with superior-hinged flaps.[7] Although the overall risk of flap striae after LASIK is low, this risk increases in several situations, including lesser surgeon experience; preoperative brimonidine use; intraoperative flap misalignment, desiccation and contracture during LASIK; flap "tenting," especially with larger treatments; thinner flaps; larger-diameter flaps; minimal trauma such as eye rubbing; and postoperative epithelial defect.[8–12] Flap striae can also be caused by trauma that results in partial flap dislocation, which can occur years after the initial surgery.[13,14]

Management

Early diagnosis of flap striae, ideally within 24 hours of surgery, is crucial as treatment becomes more difficult once the flap epithelium, Bowman layer, and stroma have begun to remodel.[7] The decision to pursue treatment of flap striae is primarily dictated by the patient's symptoms, although other characteristics such as chronicity, severity, health of the overlying flap, and associated epithelial ingrowth also factor into the assessment. Medical treatment for visually significant flap striae is correction with spectacles or contact lenses. Spectacles, however, are unlikely to address all symptoms, as they do not correct optical higher-order aberrations and irregular astigmatism. A hard contact lens, such as a rigid gas-permeable or scleral lens, however, can correct these aberrations. The RK4 reverse-geometry contact lens was described as treatment in a case of bilateral visually significant flap striae that initially underwent flap lifting, refloating, and stretching twice. Despite the initial treatments, the patient still had decreased best corrected visual acuity, which ultimately improved to 20/20 in each eye with the use of the rigid contact lens.[15]

Procedural management of flap striae begins with lifting and refloating the flap. Lifting the flap and replacing it into proper position is often sufficient to treat the striae, especially if done early in the postoperative phase. In this technique, the flap edge is lifted using a Sinskey hook. Once the peripheral LASIK flap has been separated from the underlying stroma, the flap can be lifted using various instruments, including any nontoothed forceps or a long blunt hook found on the Seibel IntraLase flap lifter. Prior to lifting, the flap edge can be marked prior to the procedure to ensure that the flap is repositioned correctly, with the markings misaligned, following lifting and refloating.[4] If flap striae are noted immediately postoperatively, an alternative treatment is stretching the flap at the slit lamp using a dry cotton-tip applicator. Gentle pressure is applied perpendicular to the striae until the flap appears symmetric and the striae have resolved. This technique has been reported as a comparable alternative to flap lift and refloat for striae noted immediately postoperatively. Benefits of this technique include decreased requirement for additional anesthesia, decreased manipulation of the flap, and improved optics for the surgeon at the slit lamp.[16] Massaging the flap has also been described as an early treatment for flap striae at the slit lamp. In this technique, pressure is applied to the central flap by using a smooth, flat instrument, followed by concentric massaging of the flap expanding peripherally. In a series of 25 eyes, 20 eyes had uncorrected visual acuity (UCVA) improvement to 20/20 following up to three serial flap massages, with only one refractory case requiring flap lift.[17]

Flap repositioning can be performed either alone or in combination with adjuvant techniques, including flap hydration, stretching, compression, heating, suturing, or epithelial removal. The use of hypotonic balanced salt solution or deionized water to hydrate the flap has been described. Hydrating the flap allows expansion, aiding in the removal of striae or folds in the flap.[1,18] The flap is then repositioned over the stromal bed. Prior to placing the flap in its final position, two dry cellulose sponges or cotton-tip applicators can be used to stretch the flap by applying force perpendicular to the orientation of the striae.

For longstanding flap striae (>4 weeks), epithelial and stromal collagen remodeling can take place; treatment using the aforementioned techniques may be less effective, and additional measures may be needed.

Case 1

A 36-year-old female presented for a second opinion 1 month following bilateral LASIK surgery. She complained of blurry vision and photophobia in her right eye. The patient reported that there was difficulty with flap creation during the surgery but could not provide any additional details. She reported significant pain the night of surgery in the affected right eye, and a Bandage contact lens (BCL) had been placed on the eye by her surgeon at the postoperative day 1 visit.

On initial presentation to us, the patient had an UCVA of 20/100 in the right eye and 20/20 in the left eye. Her best corrected vision acuity (BCVA) in the right eye was 20/50 with a manifest refraction of +1.50 + 0.75 × 120. Slit-lamp examination of the right eye revealed a LASIK flap with a nasal hinge with vertical and horizontal striae most prominent nasally and extending into the visual axis (Fig. 9.1). Topography demonstrated irregular astigmatism with nasal steepening (Fig.9.2). The patient was scheduled for *repair of visually significant LASIK flap striae* (See Video 9.1). ▶

PROCEDURE: FLAP LIFT AND REFLOAT WITH FLAP SUTURING (BOX 9.1)

After topical anesthetic was instilled, an eyelid speculum was placed for exposure. A Sclerotome blade no. 57 was used to debride the epithelium overlying the striae. A Sinskey hook was then used to lift the flap edge along the entire circumference of the flap. Next, a nontoothed forceps was used to gently lift and reflect the flap nasally. An area of epithelial ingrowth was noted, and the blade no. 57 was used to scrape the epithelial cells off both the stromal bed and underside of the flap. Debridement of the corneal epithelium was extended approximately 1 mm beyond the flap edge to reduce risk of repeat epithelial ingrowth. The flap was floated back into position using balanced salt solution on a 27-gauge canula. Two dry Weck-Cel spears were used to stretch the flap perpendicularly to the orientation of the striae. Given the chronicity of the striae, the decision was made to suture the flap back down using several interrupted 10-0 nylon

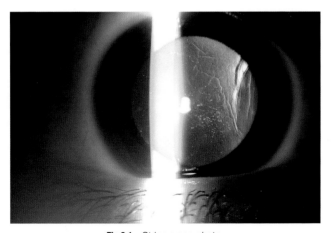

Fig 9.1 Striae preop photo.

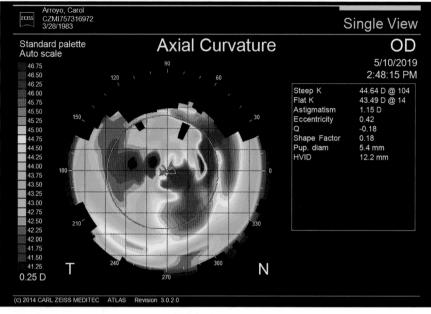

Fig 9.2 Preop axial.

BOX 9.1 ■ Equipment Utilized for Flap Lifting and Re-suturing

Topical anesthetic eye drop
Eyelid speculum and drape
Sclerotome blade no. 57
Weck-Cel spears
Sinskey hook
Nontoothed forceps
Bonn 0.12-mm forceps
27-gauge cannula on a BSS syringe
Needle driver and 10-0 nylon suture
Vannas scissors
Bandage contact lens

---

sutures. The sutures were tied tight enough to put the flap on stretch but not too tightly so as to prevent inducing new striae in the opposite meridian. The knots were carefully buried away from the flap. At the end of the case, there were no visible striae, and a Bandage contact lens was placed on the cornea.

For several weeks after the procedure, the patient expectedly had poor vision, as the tight sutures induced significant refractive error. Six weeks after the surgery, half of the sutures were removed. After another 6 weeks, the remaining sutures were removed. At her final follow-up, approximately 4 months after surgery, her UCVA was 20/25 with resolution of the striae on slit-lamp examination (Fig. 9.3). Corneal topography demonstrated a more regular area of central flattening typically seen in myopic laser vision correction (Fig. 9.4).

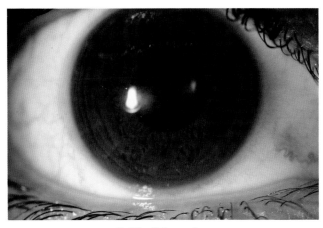

Fig 9.3   Striae postop.

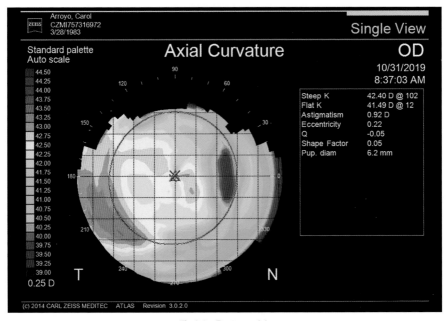

Fig 9.4   Postop axial.

DISCUSSION

The corneal epithelium can remodel to fill in the valleys and thin out over the peaks of long-standing flap striae, making treatment more challenging. Some surgeons advocate removal of the epithelium to aid in flattening of the striae, as this allows relaxation of the stroma and Bowman layer.[1,19] A typical postoperative drop regimen includes topical antibiotic and steroid drops, each four times daily for the first week (or as long as the Bandage contact lens remains in place). Thereafter, the antibiotic is discontinued, and the steroid is tapered over the course of 2 to 4 weeks. Disadvantages of debridement include increased patient discomfort during the recovery period, longer visual recovery, and increased risk of infectious keratitis and haze formation.[19]

Hyperthermic treatment of LASIK flaps has also been described to successfully treat chronic flap striae. In this technique, a heated spatula is applied to the LASIK flap to relax and stretch collagen fibers.[20] A platinum spatula is immersed in a sterile 65°C water bath for 30 seconds and then used to massage the flap suspended in air with forceps. The spatula is again placed in the heated water bath to reheat for 30 seconds, and the massage is repeated. This procedure is done until the striae have resolved on visual inspection, approximately 5–10 minutes in total. In a series of 36 eyes that underwent hyperthermic treatment of flap striae, all patients had reduction of striae and improvement of symptoms with stable to improved best corrected visual acuity (BCVA).[21]

If the combination of flap lifting, hydration, stretching, and heat are unable to flatten striae, additional radial tension can be applied with 10-0 nylon sutures placed at the flap edge. The sutures are oriented perpendicular to the meridian of the striae and are tied tight enough to flatten the striae but not so tight as to induce striae in the opposite meridian. Slipknots are used to titrate suture tension, and the tails are buried away from the flap. A Bandage contact lens is usually applied at the conclusion of the surgery and removed after a week. Patients should be counseled that due to the tightness of the sutures, vision does not immediately recover. Rather, improvement may not occur until after all sutures are removed. Jackson et al. reported a series of 7 eyes that underwent suturing for chronic flap striae, with a mean interval of 12 months following LASIK. Most of these eyes had failed flap lift and reposition previously. Six eyes ultimately had BCVA of 20/20 or better, and one eye had mild recurrence of striae with BCVA of 20/32.[22] A running suture technique has also been described where the flap is sequentially lifted and sutured 120 degrees at a time. The suture is then adjusted to ensure maximal tension perpendicular to the striae and the knot buried. The suture can be removed a minimum of 3 weeks later.[23]

Phototherapeutic keratectomy (PTK) is another technique that has been described as a treatment for chronic macrostriae. In a procedure pioneered by Steinert et al., transepithelial PTK is used to treat the epithelium and anterior stroma such that the peaks of the striae are ablated with the epithelium acting as a masking agent in the valleys. PTK is performed with a broad-beam excimer laser, using an optical zone of 6.5 mm. The treatment is monitored until the epithelial fluorescence recedes between striae, signifying that the stroma had been reached (usually after 180–220 pulses). At this point, artificial tears are used as a masking agent, and PTK is resumed to reduce the height of the striae and ablate the peaks in the stromal bed (usually 80–100 pulses). In the series by Ashrafzadeh et al., mean BCVA improved from 20/32 to 20/22 following PTK, and mean UCVA improved from 20/48 to 20/33. One patient developed mild anterior stromal haze with decreased BCVA.[24]

Depending on the severity of striae and response to other treatments, flap amputation can be used as a last resort to address refractory flap striae. The free cap can be sutured back into place, verifying the original orientation, or excised completely allowing reepithelialization of the stromal bed.[25] In this case, subsequent laser vision correction such as photorefractive keratectomy can be performed to address the hyperopic shift and improve the final visual outcome if residual stromal thickness allows.

Conclusion

While flap striae are a well-described complication after LASIK, no consensus has been reached on the optimal treatment. Early recognition of this condition is important, as treatment is more successful the earlier it is performed and can be as noninvasive as flap stretching at the slit lamp. Flap lifting, stretching, and repositioning alone can be considered if treatment is performed relatively early; however, as striae become more longstanding, additional procedures such as flap hydration, compression, heating, suturing, PTK, and partial or complete severing of the flap hinge may be necessary. Although case reports and case studies exist for each of these options, large-scale randomized studies comparing various approaches are needed to guide clinicians on the appropriate course of action in different scenarios.

References

1. Probst LE, Machat J. Removal of flap striae following laser in situ keratomileusis. *J Cataract Refract Surg.* 1998;24(2):153–155.
2. Steinert RF, Ashrafzadeh A, Hersh PS. Results of phototherapeutic keratectomy in the management of flap striae after LASIK. *Ophthalmology.* 2004;111(4):740–746.
3. Rabinowitz YS, Rasheed K. Fluorescein test for the detection of striae in the corneal flap after laser in situ keratomileusis. *Am J Ophthalmol.* 1999;127:717–718.
4. Von Kulajta P, Stark WJ, O'Brien TP. Management of flap striae. *Int J Ophthalmol Clin.* 2000;40(3):87–92.
5. Cho KJ, Chung PS. Optical coherence tomography images of epithelial ingrowth and flap striae in traumatic complication of laser-assisted in situ keratomileusis cornea. *Med Lasers.* 2016;5(1):47–49.
6. Choi CJ, Melki SA. Maddox rod effect to confirm the visual significance of laser in situ keratomileusis flap striae. *J Cataract Refract Surg.* 2011;37(10):1748–1750.
7. Hernandez-Matamoros J, Iradier MT, Moreno E. Treating folds and striae after laser in situ keratomileusis. *J Cataract Refract Surg.* 2001;27(3):350–352.
8. Charman WN. Mismatch between flap and stromal areas after laser in situ keratomileusis as source of flap striae. *J Cataract Refract Surg.* 2002;28:2146–2152.
9. Walter KA, Gilbert DD. The adverse effect of perioperative brimonidine tartrate 0.2% on flap adherence and enhancement rates in laser in situ keratomileusis patients. *Ophthalmology.* 2001;108(8):1434–1438.
10. Muñoz G, Albarrán-Diego C, Sakla HF, Javaloy J. Increased risk for flap dislocation with perioperative brimonidine use in femtosecond laser in situ keratomileusis. *J Cataract Refract Surg.* 2009;35(8):1338–1342.
11. Galvis V, Tello A, Guerra AR, Rey JJ, Camacho PA. Risk factors and visual results in cases of LASIK flap repositioning due to folds or dislocation: Case series and literature review. *Int J Ophthalmol.* 2014;34(1):19–26.
12. Gimbel HV, Basti S, Kaye GB, Ferensowicz M. Experience during the learning curve of laser in situ keratomileusis. *J Cataract Refract Surg.* 1996;22(5):542–550.
13. Ursea R, Feng MT. Traumatic flap striae 6 years after LASIK: Case report and literature review. *J Refract Surg.* 2010;26(11):899–905.
14. Sinha R, Shekhar H, Tinwala S, Gangar A, Titiyal JS. Late post-traumatic flap dislocation and macrostriae after laser in situ keratomileusis. *Oman J Ophthalmol.* 2014;7(1):25.
15. Lin JC, Rapuano CJ, Cohen EJ. RK4 lens fitting for a flap striae in a LASIK patient. *Eye Contact Lens.* 2003;29(2):76–78.
16. Solomon R, Donnenfeld ED, Perry HD, Doshi S, Biser S. Slitlamp stretching of the corneal flap after laser in situ keratomileusis to reduce corneal striae. *J Cataract Refract Surg.* 2000;29(7):1292–1296.
17. Fox ML, Harmer E. Therapeutic flap massage for microstriae after laser in situ keratomileusis. *J Cataract Refract Surg.* 2004;30(2):369–373.
18. Muñoz G, Alió JL, Pérez-Santonja JJ, Attia WH. Successful treatment of severe wrinkled corneal flap after laser in situ keratomileusis with deionized water. *Am J Ophthalmol.* 2000;129(1):91–92.
19. Kuo IC, Ou R, Hwang DG. Flap haze after epithelial debridement and flap hydration for treatment of post–laser in situ keratomileusis striae. *Cornea.* 2001;20(3):339–341.
20. Goldblatt WS, Finger PT, Perry HD, Stroh EM, Weiser DS, Donnenfeld ED. Hyperthermic treatment of rabbit corneas. *Invest Ophthalmol Vis Sci.* 1989;30(8):1778-1783.
21. Donnenfeld ED, Perry HD, Doshi SJ, Biser SA, Solomon R. Hyperthermic treatment of post-LASIK corneal striae. *J Cataract Refract Surg.* 2004;30(3):620–625.
22. Jackson DW, Hamill MB, Koch DD. Laser in situ keratomileusis flap suturing to treat recalcitrant flap striae. *J Cataract Refract Surg.* 2003;29(2):264–269.

23. Mackool RJ, Monsanto VR. Sequential lift and suture technique for post-LASIK corneal striae. *J Cataract Refract Surg.* 2003;29(4):785–787.
24. Ashrafzadeh A, Steinert RF. Results of phototherapeutic keratectomy in the management of flap striae after LASIK before and after developing a standardized protocol: Long-term follow-up in an expanded patient population. *Ophthalmology.* 2007;114:1118–1123.
25. Lam DS, Leung AT, Wu JT, et al. Management of severe flap wrinkling or dislodgment after laser in situ keratomileusis. *J Cataract Refract Surg.* 1999;25(11):1441–1447.

CHAPTER 10

Corneal Foreign Bodies

Elizabeth Shen ▓ Richard Stutzman ▓ Winston Chamberlain

Introduction

Eye injuries are the most common eye-related emergency department visits in the United States. Many occupational eye injuries are caused by projectile corneal foreign bodies that are preventable with protective eyewear. Retained corneal foreign bodies may result in infection, inflammation, long-term scarring, and vision loss and must be evaluated by an eye professional. Ophthalmologists should be familiar with the clinical sequelae of common inorganic and organic particles, as the nature of the foreign body guides management. Most metallic foreign bodies and organic particles cause robust ocular inflammation, while other inorganic substances, such as glass or graphite, may remain inert. It is crucial to perform a complete ophthalmic examination and rule out a perforating ocular injury. Anterior segment imaging can help characterize the location, depth, and type of foreign body. Many nonperforating corneal foreign bodies may be removed at the slit lamp under topical anesthesia (Video 10.1). Corneal scarring, irregular astigmatism, and neovascularization are long-term sequelae that may necessitate further treatment if visually significant.

Incidence and Epidemiology

Eye injury is the most common reason for eye-related emergency department visits in the United States.[1] A population-based study of eye-related emergency visits between 2006 and 2011 found 4 million patients were treated for eye injuries, representing 36.3% of all ophthalmic-related emergency department visits.[1] Foreign body injuries account for approximately 67% of injuries at work and 31% of injuries at home.[2] These injuries can result in a deterioration of vision secondary to infection and scarring.

The incidence of eye injury reported in the literature varies based on data sources and study population. Moreover, one limitation of these population studies is that they exclude visits directly seen by ophthalmologists and optometrists. Nash and Margo reported a rate of 447 per 100,000 in 1993. Of these, 72.6 per 100,000 (and of which 92% were male) were diagnosed with a foreign body on the external eye.[3] A later study reported 315 eye injuries per population of 100,000 in 2000, of which 45% were caused by a foreign body.[2] Channa et al.'s more recent study reported a 24% decline between 2006 and 2011 in the incidence of eye injuries from 280 to 212 per 100,000.[1] The mean age of these patients was 32 years, and 66% were male. The leading mechanism, accounting for 30% of all eye injuries, was accidental entry of a projected foreign body to the eye and/or adnexa. The second most common mechanism of injury (18%) was from being struck by an object or person.

There appears to be a gradual decline in the incidence of eye injuries, and this has been attributed to policy and behavior interventions, such as eye protection in the workplace and the increase in use of seatbelts.[1] Understanding the burden of care for eye injuries is important to identify preventative strategies and find ways to provide more cost-effective care.

Prevention and Diagnosis

PREVENTION

Many eye injuries are preventable with eyewear protection, and despite workplace requirements for protective eyewear, failure to comply is common. Workers may neglect to wear eye protection due to a lack of education on the seriousness and potential consequences of eye injuries. One study from Melbourne, Australia, showed that as many as 45% of patients suffering from a corneal foreign body were wearing protective eyewear at the time of injury.[4] Safety education or workshops in the workplace and increased enforcement by management may increase compliance with proper equipment. However, there are also cases in which injury occurred in spite of eye protection.[5] Certain eye protection devices may not provide adequate barriers, and normal wear and tear may render them ineffective.

The United States Eye Injury Registry (useir.org) was created in 1988 in response to the lack of national eye injury epidemiological data.[6] However, this resource is unfamiliar to most practicing ophthalmologists and optometrists. Healthcare providers are encouraged to participate in this registry to improve data collection on incidence and treatment outcomes and to develop public health strategies for prevention.

Inorganic Material

Metallic particles are one of the most commonly encountered foreign bodies made of inorganic material. These injuries are often a result of high-speed grinding tools and metal-on-metal hammering common in construction and the metal industry.[4,5,7] Iron foreign bodies notoriously produce a "rust ring" that can cause inflammation and edema (Fig. 10.1).[8,9] Copper, if retained, may diffuse into the adjacent corneal layers, producing a reddish-brown hue. It is imperative to rule out intraocular iron or copper. These intraocular foreign bodies can cause siderosis (iron) or chalcosis (copper), resulting in extensive ocular damage, including retina and retinal pigment epithelial

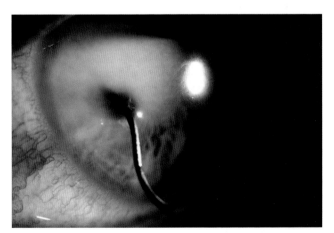

Fig. 10.1　A corneal rust ring typically forms as a reaction to iron deposits in the cornea and itself can cause a robust inflammatory reaction. (EyeRounds.org. The University of Iowa. https://webeye.ophth.uiowa.edu/eyeforum/atlas/pages/Penetrating-ocular-trauma/index.htm. Last accessed November 24, 2023.)

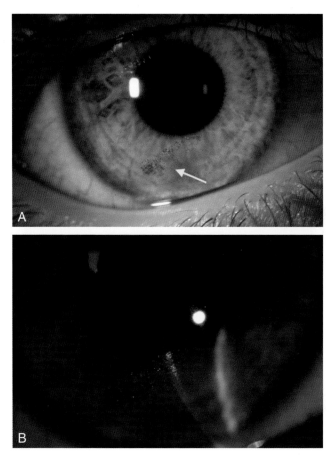

Fig. 10.2 (A) Pencil graphite is a relatively inert metallic substance that can remain in the cornea without inciting an inflammatory response. (B) Pencil graphite particles from (A) viewed with an angled slit beam.

atrophy.[10,11] Other findings in chalcosis include deposits in the Descemet membrane, iris discoloration, greenish aqueous particles, "sunflower" cataract, reddish-brown vitreous opacities, and metallic flecks on the retina.[12] The extent of intraocular damage depends on the copper or iron content of the metal alloy. Zinc and aluminum are less toxic than iron or copper but may also incite inflammation.

Inert substances, including glass, sand, plastic, graphite (i.e., pencil tip trauma), and fiberglass, are well tolerated and can remain in the cornea for prolonged periods without inciting an inflammatory response (Fig. 10.2A–B).[13–16] In these cases, removal of the foreign body is not always required. Corneal edema that ensues could be related to mechanical irritation or epithelial breakdown rather than an inflammatory response to the particles.[14] If the inert foreign body resides in the central visual axis or induces significant astigmatism, treatment options include removal or use of rigid gas-permeable lenses.[17]

Organic Material

Organic material often consists of vegetative matter or insect injuries. Plant substances, such as tree sap, can cause severe toxic reactions when contacting the ocular surface. Well-known offenders include the pencil tree (*Euphorbia tirucalli*), manchineel tree (*Hippomane mancinella)*, and dieffenbachia plant species (*Araceae* family), which can cause acute keratoconjunctivitis, epithelial defects, and stromal infiltration.[8] Aggressive irrigation of the ocular surface should be performed in addition to removal of any foreign bodies. Vegetative matter in the eye for any prolonged duration puts it at risk for fungal keratitis and should be suspected in cases that fail to resolve or worsen despite antibacterial therapy.

Coral foreign bodies have also been reported, especially in patients with exposure to aquariums and fish tanks. Even in the absence of a coral foreign body, palytoxins from the coral inhibit sodium-potassium ATPase pumps on cell membranes, causing severe anterior segment inflammation and even stromal melt.[18,19]

Insect injuries consisting of bee and wasp stings are less common but have been reported (Fig. 10.3A). These can result in significant conjunctival injection and chemosis, as well as corneal edema and stroma infiltrates.[8,20] Stingers should be removed if possible and as early as possible.

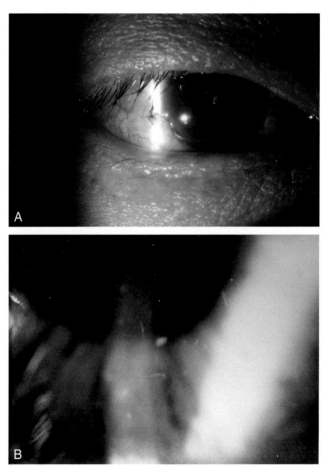

Fig. 10.3 Insect injuries. (A) Slit-lamp photo of bee stinger embedded in the cornea. (Courtesy of Lung-Kun Yeh, MD, PhD.) (B) Tarantula hairs (courtesy of Vernon C. Parmley, MD) lodged in the cornea are difficult to remove due to their barbed endings, known as urticating setae.

However, retained stingers may remain inert since it is the venom injected that is responsible for the acute inflammatory reaction.[21]

More challenging are caterpillar and tarantula hairs, which are urticating, or barbed, hairs that embed deeply into tissue and are extremely difficult to remove (Fig. 10.3B).[22-26] The inflammatory reaction that ensues in the eye includes conjunctival chemosis, lid edema, linear corneal abrasions, and corneal edema.[26] The name for this reaction, ophthalmia nodosum, was first coined in 1883 and is most common in Europe and North Africa.[27] Multiple hairs are often found; however, removal of all hair may not be necessary, as this may result in further disruption of tissue. Published case reports have shown good resolution despite retained hairs.[26,27]

Clinical Evaluation of Corneal Foreign Bodies

1. **History:** Determine the mechanism of injury and the possibility of an intraocular foreign body, particularly if there is a history of a high-speed metallic foreign body. Inquire whether the patient was wearing protective eyewear and if the injury occurred as a result of an occupational hazard.
2. **External ophthalmic examination:** Test visual acuity, intraocular pressure (not directly over the foreign body and after verifying that the globe is not ruptured), extraocular motility, and pupils.
3. **Slit-Lamp Examination**: Assess the conjunctiva, cornea, anterior chamber (AC), and iris, paying special attention to the location, size, and depth of the foreign body.
   a. *Ocular Adnexa:* Look for multiple foreign bodies in the conjunctiva and fornices. Evert the upper eyelid to rule out foreign bodies embedded in the palpebral conjunctiva.
   b. *Cornea*: Varying illumination techniques should be utilized, including a high-magnification angled narrow slit beam to evaluate depth of the foreign body. Additionally, sclerotic scatter, broad illumination, and retroillumination with reflection of light off fundus in eye with dilated pupil can help identify the location and distribution of finer particles. Assess for signs of previous surgical intervention, including previous penetrating or partial keratoplasty.
   c. *Anterior segment*: Look for evidence of perforating injury, such as a peaked pupil, capsular violation, iris tears, transillumination defects, hyphema, or AC shallowing. Perform gonioscopy prior to dilation to evaluate for any foreign bodies in the AC angles. If the foreign body extends to the AC or if there are signs of a perforating injury, globe exploration and foreign body removal in the operating room are advised.
   d. *Fundus*: A dilated fundus exam to look for an intraocular foreign body or retinal or vitreous hemorrhage is part of the complete eye exam.
4. **Ultrasound and Orbital Imaging:** If there is not an adequate view of the posterior fundus, consider gentle B-scan ultrasonography, including high-resolution ultrasound biomicroscopy, to visualize features of the anterior segment or occult foreign bodies that may be behind the iris or embedded in the lens. If one suspects intraocular involvement, a computed tomography scan of the orbit should be obtained. Avoid an MRI scan if there is a question of a metallic foreign body.

Anterior Segment Imaging of Corneal Foreign Bodies

Anterior segment optical coherence tomography (OCT) is a useful noninvasive, noncontact tool to further characterize and verify the location, size, and depth of the foreign body. Spectral-domain OCT has superior speed and resolution to the slower time domain OCT used in the earliest models. An important consideration in anterior segment imaging is the wavelength; shorter wavelength light in the 830- to 840-nm range gives higher resolution in the cornea. Longer-wavelength (~1310-nm) light penetrates deeper into the sclera and iris but has coarser resolution, and the best operating wavelength will depend on what portions of the eye need to be imaged.[28]

Metal appears hyperreflective with a shadowing effect. Glass, sand, and plastic, or polymethyl methacrylate, are hyporeflective with hyperreflective borders.[29] Pencil graphite also presents with a hyperreflective anterior border followed by a shadowing effect posteriorly.[30] Wood and plant materials exhibit variable reflectivity, depending on the concentration of the material.[31,32]

In vivo confocal microscopy is a noninvasive imaging and diagnostic tool that provides optical sections via contact applanation that is able to resolve the corneal surface epithelium, stromal keratocytes, collagen fibers, and nerves and the endothelial cell layer. This imaging modality has been used to detect iron deposits,[33] caterpillar hairs,[34] and bee stings.[35] Confocal microscopy has the advantage of providing much higher resolution in situations where embedded particles are microscopic or inflammatory reactions are subclinical.

In cases where an inert foreign body in the visual axis persists without an inflammatory response, corneal topography and tomography may be beneficial for evaluating astigmatism induced by the material.

Case 1

A 19-year-old healthy male presented with foreign body sensation and eye redness in the right eye several days after a fleck from a copper stop valve hit the eye (Fig. 10.4A–B). Visual acuity was 20/250 uncorrected. On exam, the patient had a 1-mm copper foreign body at 7 o'clock in the midperipheral cornea that was fully epithelialized. The foreign body was lodged at an approximate 50% stromal depth. The AC was deep with 3+ AC cell. A dilated fundus exam was normal. An anterior segment OCT was performed, confirming the depth and nature of the foreign body (Fig. 10.4C). The patient consented to foreign body removal at the slit lamp.

PROCEDURE

1. Gather supplies needed for metallic foreign body removal (Box 10.1).
2. Administer a topical anesthetic (i.e., 0.5% proparacaine hydrochloride).
3. Ensure the patient is comfortably and securely positioned at the slit lamp.
4. Consider instillation of topical 1%–5% povidone-iodine solution if the foreign body is not to be cultured.
5. Determine what instrument will be most suitable for the foreign body removal. For round metallic foreign bodies embedded in the stroma, a 25-, 27-, or 30-gauge needle (with or without a syringe) is effective for dislodging the metal. For irregular foreign bodies that have a protruding aspect, jeweler forceps may be used to grasp and remove the foreign body. In the event of inadvertent penetration or discovery of a Seidel-positive wound, use of a tissue adhesive and/or therapeutic bandage contact lens can be used to tamponade the leak. Surgical repair may be necessary if these measures fail to seal the leak.
6. Rust rings formed from iron foreign bodies should be removed as much as possible without perforating the cornea. This can be done either with a 25-, 27-, or 30-gauge needle or with

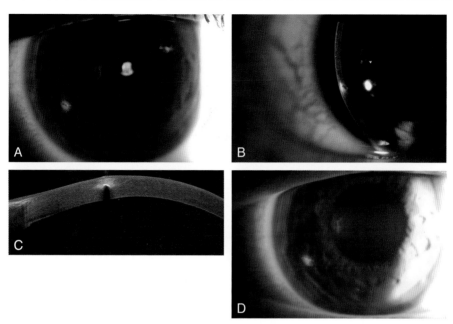

Fig. 10.4 Copper foreign body from blast injury. (A) Copper foreign body embedded in the midperipheral cornea one week after the initial injury. (B) Use of a thin angled slit beam at high magnification, highlighting at least 50% depth of the embedded copper foreign body. (C) Anterior segment optical coherence tomography (OCT) of the copper foreign body appears hyperreflective with a shadowing effect. (D) Residual corneal opacity 4 days after the copper foreign body was removed at the slit lamp.

BOX 10.1 ■ Corneal Metallic Foreign Body Removal Supplies (Fig. 10.5A–I)

- Topical anesthetic (e.g., 0.5% proparacaine hydrochloride)
- 1%–5% povidone-iodine solution
- 25-, 27-, or 30-gauge needle
- Jeweler forceps
- Topical antibiotic

Optional:
- Ophthalmic burr
- Bandage contact lens
- Tissue adhesive
- Topical cycloplegic (e.g., 1% atropine sulfate)
- Topical antibiotic (eg., 0.3% ofloxacin solution)

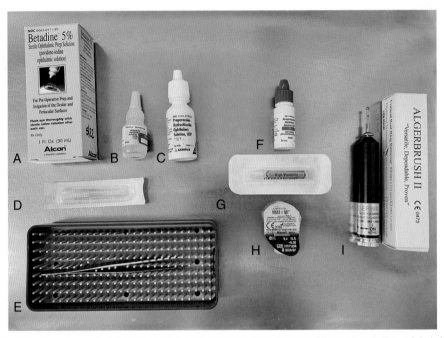

Fig. 10.5 Supplies needed for office-based corneal foreign body removal: (A) povidone-iodine ophthalmic solution, (B) topical antibiotic (e.g., 0.3% ofloxacin solution), (C) topical anesthetic, (D) 25-, 27-, or 30-gauge needle, and (E) jeweler forceps. Optional supplies: (F) topical cycloplegic (e.g., 1% atropine sulfate), (G) tissue adhesive, (H) bandage contact lens, and (I) ophthalmic diamond burr.

an ophthalmic burr (Alger brush). A residual rust ring that extends deep into the stroma may be left, as these often migrate superficially with time, making removal at a later time easier and safer. Aggressive tissue disruption from the burr should be avoided, as it can lead to increased scar formation and corneal dellen.

7. Measure and document the epithelial defect remaining, as well as the amount of inflammation noted in the AC. Be sure to note the presence of an infiltrate, especially if there is delayed presentation.

8. A topical antibiotic should be prescribed until the epithelial defect is healed or infiltrate is resolved. Consideration of a topical cycloplegic is helpful in improving patient comfort during the healing period and reducing the risk of posterior synechia in the setting of an AC reaction. If there is significant AC inflammation and no evidence of infectious keratitis, a topical corticosteroid may be considered. The patient should be monitored closely in the event that an infection develops.

DISCUSSION

The patient tolerated the procedure well and was prescribed 1 drop topical 0.3% ofloxacin four times daily, atropine 1% twice daily, and prednisolone acetate 1% 4 times daily. He followed up 3 days later with a resolved epithelial defect, no infiltrate, and a corneal opacity (Fig. 10.4D).

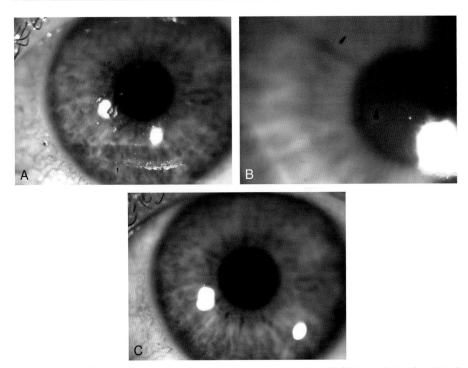

Fig. 10.6 (A) and (B) Caterpillar hairs lodged in the cornea and conjunctiva. (C) Slit-lamp photo taken 1 week after the caterpillar hairs were removed. (Courtesy of Naveen K. Rao, MD.)

Not all anterior segment foreign bodies can be removed in the clinic. An experienced ophthalmic surgeon and, in particular, a cornea specialist may need to remove foreign bodies under local or general anesthesia in order to reduce complications related to patient pain, spread of infection, and perforation and to adequately restore the integrity of a compromised globe.

Case 2

A 25-year-old female presented with a persistent foreign body sensation, tearing, and redness in the eye 2 days after a caterpillar hit her eye. She was standing on a friend's porch when her friend's mother spotted a caterpillar crawling on the balcony railing and swatted it away with her hand. The caterpillar inadvertently hit the patient directly in the left eye. On presentation, visual acuity was 20/20; slit-lamp examination showed four hairs in the cornea and one in the conjunctiva (Fig. 10.6A–B).

PROCEDURE

1. Gather supplies needed for the removal of corneal urticating hair (Box 10.2).
2. Perform steps 2–4 from the above section.

BOX 10.2 ■ Corneal Urticating Hair Removal Supplies

- Topical anesthetic (i.e., proparacaine)
- 1%–5% povidone-iodine solution
- No. 15 or no. 69 blade
- 27- or 30-gauge needle
- Jeweler forceps
- Topical antibiotic

Optional:

- Bandage contact lens
- Topical cycloplegic

---

3. Do not attempt to pull the hair directly because the one-way barb at the end of the shaft will lodge the hair deeper into the cornea.
4. Use a no. 11 or no. 69 blade to debride the epithelium overlying the hair.
5. Use a 27- or 30-gauge needle to rotate each hair within its track such that the barbed tip points anteriorly and the base points posteriorly. This allows for smoother removal of the barbed end.
6. Use jeweler forceps to grasp and remove the hair.
7. Perform steps 4–6 repeatedly until all foreign bodies are removed if possible.

DISCUSSION

The patient tolerated the procedure well and was prescribed 1 drop topical 0.3% gatifloxacin 4 times daily, 1 drop 1% cyclopentolate twice daily, and 1 drop 1% prednisolone acetate 4 times daily. She also had a bandage contact lens placed. She followed up 1 week later with resolved epithelial defects and a visual acuity of 20/20 (Fig. 10.6C).

Conclusion

Corneal foreign bodies are commonly a result of eye injury, which comprises a significant percentage of ophthalmic emergency department visits each year in the United States. Many eye injuries occurring in an occupational setting are preventable with protective eyewear. Given possible clinical sequelae of corneal foreign bodies (even after removal), ophthalmologists should be involved early in evaluation and treatment. Corneal foreign bodies can introduce infections or incite minimal to robust inflammatory responses, depending on the substance, and can also result in long-term sequelae such as visually significant astigmatism, scarring, neovascularization, and loss of vision. Anterior segment imaging is a useful adjunctive tool in the clinical evaluation of corneal foreign bodies.

References

1. Channa R, Zafar SN, Canner JK, Haring RS, Schneider EB, Friedman DS. Epidemiology of eye-related emergency department visits. *JAMA Ophthalmol.* 2016;134(3):312–319.
2. McGwin Jr G, Owsley C. Incidence of emergency department-treated eye injury in the United States. *Arch Ophthalmol.* 2005;123(5):662–666.
3. Nash EA, Margo CE. Patterns of emergency department visits for disorders of the eye and ocular adnexa. *Arch Ophthalmol.* 1998;116(9):1222–1226.

4. Ramakrishnan T, Constantinou M, Jhanji V, Vajpayee RB. Corneal metallic foreign body injuries due to suboptimal ocular protection. *Arch Environ Occup Health.* 2012;67(1):48–50.
5. Jones NP, Griffith GA. Eye injuries at work: A prospective population-based survey within the chemical industry. *Eye (Lond).* 1992;6(Pt 4):381–385.
6. US Eye Injury Registry. https://useir.org. Last accessed November 21, 2023.
7. Welch LS, Hunting KL, Mawudeku A. Injury surveillance in construction: Eye injuries. *Appl Occup Environ Hyg.* 2001;16(7):755–762.
8. External Disease and Cornea. *Basic and Clinical Science Course, Section 8.* San Francisco, CA: American Academy of Ophthalmology; 2017–2018.
9. Zuckerman BD, Lieberman TW. Corneal rust ring. Etiology and histology. *Arch Ophthalmol.* 1960;63:254–265.
10. Sneed SR, Weingeist TA. Management of siderosis bulbi due to a retained iron-containing intraocular foreign body. *Ophthalmology.* 1990;97(3):375–379.
11. Weiss MJ, Hofeldt AJ, Behrens M, Fisher K. Ocular siderosis: Diagnosis and management. *Retina.* 1997;17(2):105–108.
12. Neumann R, Belkin M, Loewenthal E, Gorodetsky R. A long-term follow-up of metallic intraocular foreign bodies, employing diagnostic x-ray spectrometry. *Arch Ophthalmol.* 1992;110(9):1269–1272.
13. Hersch PS, Zagelbaum BM, Kenyon KR, Shingelto BJ. Management of anterior segment trauma. In: Tasman W, Jaeger E, eds. *Duane's Ophthalmology.* Philadelphia: Lippincott Williams and Wilkins; 1995:1–19.
14. McDonald PR, Ashodian MJ. Retained glass foreign bodies in the anterior chamber. *Am J Ophthalm.* 1959;48:747–750.
15. Mostafavi D, Olumba K, Shrier EM. Fiberglass intraocular foreign body with no initial ocular symptoms. *Retin Cases Brief Rep.* 2014;8(1):10–12.
16. Philip SS, John D, John SS. Asymptomatic intracorneal graphite deposits following graphite pencil injury. *Case Rep Ophthalmol Med.* 2012;2012:720201.
17. Estrada LN, Rosenstiel CE. RGP lens treats irregular astigmatism from intracorneal glass. *Eye Contact Lens.* 2003;29(3):193–194.
18. Farooq AV, Gibbons AG, Council MD, et al. Corneal toxicity associated with aquarium coral palytoxin. *Am J Ophthalmol.* 2017;174:119–125.
19. Keamy J, Umlas J, Lee Y. Red coral keratitis. *Cornea.* 2000;19(6):859–860.
20. Lin PH, Wang NK, Hwang YS, Ma DH, Yeh LK. Bee sting of the cornea and conjunctiva: Management and outcomes. *Cornea.* 2011;30(4):392–394.
21. Mackler BF, Kreil G. Honey bee venom melittin: Correlation of nonspecific inflammatory activities with amino acid sequences. *Inflammation.* 1977;2:55–65.
22. Horng CT, Chou PI, Liang JB. Caterpillar setae in the deep cornea and anterior chamber. *Am J Ophthalmol.* 2000;129:384–385.
23. Corkey JA. Ophthalmia nodosa due to caterpillar hairs. *Br J Ophthalmol.* 1955;39:301–306.
24. Gundersen T, Heath P, Garron LK. Ophthalmia nodosa. *Trans Am Ophthalmol Soc.* 1950;48:151–169.
25. Bernardino CR, Rapuano C. Ophthalmia nodosa caused by casual handling of a tarantula. *CLAO J.* 2000;26:111–112.
26. Doshi PY, Usgaonkar U, Kamat P. A Hairy affair: Ophthalmia nodosa due to caterpillar hairs. *Ocul Immunol Inflamm.* 2018;26(1):136–141.
27. Portero A, Carreño E, Galarreta D, Herreras JM. Corneal inflammation from pine processionary caterpillar hairs. *Cornea.* 2013;32(2):161–164.
28. Baenninger PB, Li Y, Nanji AA, Tang M, et al. Anterior segment optical coherence tomography. In: Krachmer J, Mannis M, Holland E, eds. *Cornea.* 4th ed. Elsevier; 2015.
29. Al-Ghadeer HA, Al-Assiri A. Identification and localization of multiple intrastromal foreign bodies with anterior segment optical coherence tomography and ocular Pentacam. *Int Ophthalmol.* 2014;34(2):355–358.
30. Vijitha VS, Kapoor AG, Mohammed M, Roy A. Corneal graphite deposit on anterior segment optical coherence tomography. *Indian J Ophthalmol.* 2019;67(7):1178.

31. Armarnik S, Mimouni M, Goldenberg D, et al. Characterization of deeply embedded corneal foreign bodies with anterior segment optical coherence tomography. *Graefes Arch Clin Exp Ophthalmol.* 2019;257(6):1247–1252.

32. Mahmoud A, Messaoud R, Abid F, Ksiaa I, Bouzayene M, Khairallah M. Anterior segment optical coherence tomography and retained vegetal intraocular foreign body masquerading as chronic anterior uveitis. *J Ophthalmic Inflamm Infect.* 2017;7(1):13.

33. Witherspoon SR, Hogan RN, Petroll WM, Mootha VV. Slit-lamp, confocal, and light microscopic findings of corneal siderosis. *Cornea.* 2007;26(10):1270–1272.

34. Wong BW, Lai JS, Law RW, Lam DS. In vivo confocal microscopy of corneal insect foreign body. *Cornea.* 2003;22(1):56–58.

35. Yuen KS, Lai JS, Law RW, Lam DS. Confocal microscopy in bee sting corneal injury. *Eye (Lond).* 2003;17(7):845–847.

CHAPTER **11**

Conjunctival Concretions and Cysts

Eric Rosenberg ▦ Tasnia Ahmed ▦ Jessica Blair Ciralsky

Conjunctival Concretions

Conjunctival concretions are yellow-whitish deposits found in the palpebral conjunctiva and fornix, more commonly in the inferior palpebral conjunctiva and fornix. They are typically small, <1 mm, and discrete, although they can become confluent. They have a gelatinous paste-like consistency, and for this reason, most patients are asymptomatic. Symptoms may develop if the concretions erode through the conjunctival epithelium, and they may include foreign body sensation, irritation, and tearing.[1,2]

EPIDEMIOLOGY

Concretions are frequently incidental findings. The prevalence, therefore, is difficult to estimate. In a paper by Haici et al., 500 consecutive patients were examined. They had a mean age of 46.8 years (13–103), with 190 patients being male and 310 female. Although 39.6% (198 patients) of surveyed patients had concretions, only 6% were symptomatic. There was no statistical difference in location or laterality (upper vs lower lids, right vs left eyes).[3] A second article from the Plymouth Royal Eye Infirmary studied 100 consecutive patients in the casualty department. Similarly, concretions were found in 42% of studied patients. Only 3 patients (7%) were symptomatic from the concretions.[4]

DEVELOPMENT AND PATHOGENESIS

The main risk factor for the development of concretions is normal aging. However, chronic inflammation may predispose patients to the development of concretions. Several inflammatory conditions have been associated with concretions, including trachomatous degeneration, atopic keratoconjunctivitis, meibomian gland dysfunction, prolonged contact lens wear, and long-term use of certain topical medications such as sulfadiazine.[1,2,5]

Several groups have proposed theories about how concretions form. Chang et al. suggest that concretions form when the conjunctival epithelium becomes hyperplastic with glandular transformation and invaginates into the substantia propria, forming the pseudogland of Henle in response to a chronic inflammatory process. This recess opening becomes obstructed by shed epithelial cells and secretory material, and as the process continues, the epithelial lining attenuates to a single cell layer. The accumulated material may (1) extrude through the epithelium and cause a foreign body sensation, (2) develop a bacterial superinfection, (3) erode through the basement membrane and cause an inflammatory process, or (4) remain static.[2] Chin et al. suggest that concretions represent products of both epithelial and inflammatory cellular degeneration that occur with chronic conjunctivitis.[1]

Originally, concretions were termed lithiasis with the underlying assumption that they contained calcium; however, several studies showed an absence of calcium or oxalate salts, and the

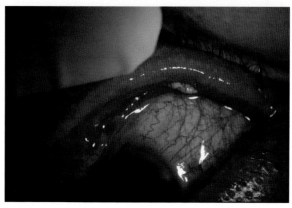

Fig. 11.1 A large exposed concretion can be seen on the left upper palpebral conjunctiva with eyelid eversion.

nomenclature was reversed.[1,2] On histological evaluation, conjunctival concretions are composed of degenerating epithelial cells and mucinous secretions from transformed conjunctival glands.[1] On electron microscopy, they consist of fine granular material and membranous debris in the subconjunctival epithelium.[1] Histochemical staining patterns showed strong positive staining for phospholipid and elastin and weak positive staining for neutral polysaccharides and lipid. There was negative staining for amyloid, collagen, glycogen, iron, mucopolysaccharides, RNA, and DNA.[1]

Case 1

A 70-year-old female presented with complaints of foreign body sensation in the left eye for several years. Her symptoms had been mild and intermittent for many years but worsened after cataract surgery. Her cataract surgery was reportedly uncomplicated in both eyes approximately 1 year prior to presentation, and her symptoms had been treated with a combination of ocular lubricants, including artificial tears, gels, and ointments. Her vision was 20/20 in each eye, and her examination was significant for scarring on both upper palpebral conjunctiva. She had more severe scarring on the left upper palpebral conjunctiva and had multiple conjunctival concretions, several of which were exposed (Fig. 11.1).

PROCEDURE: CONCRETION REMOVAL

Supplies

- Topical anesthetic
- Cotton-tip applicators
- Needlepoint forceps
- Optional: 30-gauge needle, curette

Procedure

Administer topical proparacaine and lidocaine gel 2% to achieve local anesthesia. Next, flip the eyelid to better visualize the concretions. Using a combination of a cotton tip for counterpressure and a needlepoint or jeweler forceps, the concretions are undermined and removed. The exposed concretions will easily express with minimal manipulation. The more embedded concretions will require "scooping" out with the tip of a needle. A sterile cotton-tip applicator can be utilized to achieve hemostasis. The patient is placed on topical antibiotics for 1 week (Video 11.1).

DISCUSSION

Treatment is commonly unnecessary for concretions since most patients are asymptomatic. If symptoms do arise, many different instruments can be used to remove the offending concretion such as a cotton tip, needlepoint forceps, curette, or 30-gauge needle. Hemostasis, if present, can be achieved with a cotton-tip applicator. A short course of postoperative antibiotics should be used to prevent secondary infection. Although treatment is rarely necessary, simple in-office excision is typically curative.

Conjunctival Cysts

Conjunctival cysts are benign, thin-walled sacs that contain clear serous fluid consisting of gelatinous mucus material or shed cells.[6] Cysts are common, and often, one or more cysts can be found in the inferior fornices of healthy patients. They are typically asymptomatic, but symptoms such as foreign body sensation, dry eye, and ocular discomfort can occur. The reduction of mobility has even been reported for very large cysts. For symptomatic cysts, surgical removal can be considered. Complete careful excision is necessary to prevent recurrence due to the secretory nature of the inner epithelial cyst lining and the fragility of the cyst capsule.[7]

EPIDEMIOLOGY, DEVELOPMENT, AND PATHOGENESIS

Conjunctival epithelial inclusion cysts account for 80% of all conjunctival cystic lesions and 6%–13% of all conjunctival lesions.[8] Cysts can be primary congenital or secondary acquired. Primary cysts typically start hidden in the fornices and then increase with age.[6] Congenital cysts are thought to develop when epithelial cells get sequestered in the subepithelial space.[9] Secondary cysts are much more common and can occur in both the bulbar and forniceal conjunctiva. They may develop naturally or with inflammatory conditions such as trachoma, vernal keratoconjunctivitis, trauma, and postsurgery. Common conjunctival surgeries associated with cysts include pterygium, strabismus, pars plana vitrectomy, and scleral buckling.[7] Acquired cysts typically form when a portion of the conjunctival epithelium is detached during surgery or trauma.[10]

Histologically, cysts are lined by nonkeratinizing conjunctival epithelium with goblet cells and are filled with fluid comprised of cellular debris.[11] On electron microscopy, the cyst epithelial cells have been shown to have fewer hemidesmosomes compared with normal epithelial cells, which may explain the mobility of the cysts.[12]

Case 2

A 74-year-old female presented with discomfort and irritation in the left eye for several months. Over the last 10 years, she experienced several brief episodes of irritation that were attributable to a conjunctival cyst, with all resolving spontaneously. This particular episode of irritation was similar in nature to her previous episodes except for its persistence. She had tried multiple topical lubricants with only temporary relief.

Her past ocular history was significant for primary open-angle glaucoma. She had undergone cataract and glaucoma surgery in the right eye. Both eyes had selective laser trabeculoplasty. Her visual acuity was 20/25 in the right eye and 20/40 in the left eye. Her slit-lamp examination revealed a large 5-mm by 4-mm conjunctival cyst in the nasal conjunctiva with mild surrounding hyperemia (Fig. 11.2).

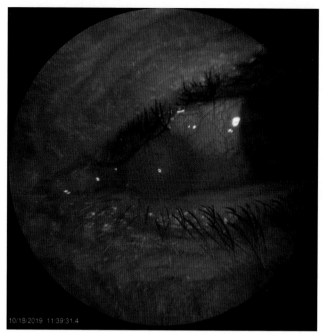

Fig. 11.2 A large conjunctival cyst is shown in the nasal conjunctiva of the left eye.

PROCEDURE: CONJUNCTIVAL CYST REMOVAL

Supplies

- Topical anesthetic
- Povidone-iodine
- Lid speculum
- Vannas scissors
- Nontoothed forceps
- 8-0 Vicryl suture
- Needle driver

Procedure

Administer topical proparacaine and lidocaine gel 2% to achieve local anesthesia. Clean the area with povidone-iodine. Next, create a small opening in the overlying conjunctiva with Vannas scissors. Perform careful dissection of the cyst with nontoothed forceps and Vannas scissors and remove the cyst in toto. A sterile cotton-tip applicator can be utilized to achieve hemostasis and the conjunctival defect left to close secondarily if the area is small. An 8-0 Vicryl suture can be used to close the conjunctival defect if necessary. The patient is placed on topical antibiotics for 1 week.

DISCUSSION

Many cysts are asymptomatic and can be managed solely through observation. If intervention is indicated, there are many ways to approach removal. For many surgeons, first-line treatment for conjunctival cysts is often simple aspiration using a 30-gauge needle. Although physicians tend to use this procedure as a primary step, it is not the preferred treatment, as recurrence is common due to the retention of the secretory epithelial cells that line the capsule. Preferred surgeries remove the cyst completely and may use the assistance of visualization dyes, lasers, or sclerosing agents.

Several novel techniques have been described. Ikeda et al. described a novel nonincisional extraction technique that can be performed at the slit lamp. After anesthetic was applied, a 26-gauge, 0.5-inch needle attached to a 1-mL syringe was inserted into the conjunctival cyst bevel up. The plunger was pulled up to extract the fluid by using negative pressure. After the fluid was drained, the negative pressure was still applied to suck up the inner walls of the cyst into the needle tip. While keeping the negative pressure applied, the needle was slowly removed. The collapsed cyst was grasped with forceps and excised. Occasionally, a small stump of the cyst remained behind. The benefits of this procedure are that it (1) uses topical anesthesia, (2) can be performed at a slit lamp, and (3) can be performed in under 3 minutes. This treatment is only indicated for freely mobile cysts. In this study of 11 eyes followed for 23.2 months, there was only one recurrence that responded to repeat extraction.[13]

Another group, Nishino et al., described a novel large cross-incision technique that can also be performed at a slit lamp. This technique can be successful with large, adherent cysts and cysts located deep in the fornices. In this technique, after anesthesia and a lid retractor were applied, a microknife was used to prick the cyst walls. The surrounding conjunctiva was held with non-toothed forceps, and Westcott scissors were inserted through the hole. The scissors were used to incise the cyst, creating a large cross incision, leaving the cyst completely open. The authors hypothesize that during the healing process, the inner lining of the cyst walls attach to the healthy conjunctival surface, preventing recurrence of the cyst wall. In this study, three patients were successfully treated with this technique, and no recurrence was seen in a follow-up of at least 12 months.[14]

Although conjunctival incisional surgery can be successful, if the cyst ruptures or collapses too early, the borders of the cyst and the surrounding tissue can become blurred, making total excision impossible. Many groups have described the use of visualization dyes to assist in the removal of these conjunctival cysts. Eom et al. described a sutureless small incision technique assisted by indocyanine green (ICG). In this procedure, after anesthesia was achieved, 0.05% ICG dye was injected into the cyst using a 30-gauge needle. Using a repeated aspiration and injection technique, approximately 0.05 mL of cystic fluid became mixed with 0.3 mL of ICG dye. After multiple rounds of aspiration and injection ending with cyst reduction, the needle was removed. The cyst was nicely defined. Next, 2% lidocaine was injected into the surrounding subconjunctival space to provide both releases of attachments and adequate anesthesia. Finally, a small 4.5-mm incision was made with Westcott scissors, and the cyst was removed with the assistance of a cotton-tip applicator.[11]

Another group explored cystectomy with the help of trypan blue dye and methylcellulose. After anesthesia was applied, 0.6 mg/mL of trypan blue was injected into the cyst using a 27-gauge needle. The least amount needed to achieve adequate staining was used. The needle was kept in place while the syringe was replaced with 2% methylcellulose. After the methylcellulose was injected, the anterior conjunctiva above the cyst was incised, and subconjunctival blunt dissection was performed. Finally, a clamp was placed at the cyst base, and the cyst was removed with scissors. The edge was cauterized, and the conjunctival defect was closed with 8-0 silk. This technique was used in three patients, two of which had no recurrence over a 2-year follow-up. One patient had a recurrence that necessitated a second surgery.[7]

Another strategy to perform a complete cystectomy is to use the assistance of heat or sclerosing agents. Although thermal cautery has been described and is fairly simple to perform, it is rarely used due to the considerable risk to the surrounding tissues. Similarly, injection of sclerosing agents, such as tetracycline or isopropyl alcohol, can also be simple to perform and curative, but damage to the surrounding tissues through drug leakage is a considerable risk. In one study by Bagheri et al., 10 patients followed for an average of 18.1 months had 100% successful cystectomy without complication. In this procedure, 10% trichloroacetic acid (TCA) was used to induce necrosis of the cells of the cyst walls. Because TCA is an analog of acetic acid, a careful application was paramount to prevent necrosis of surrounding tissues. After anesthetic application, a 27-gauge needle attached to a 2-mL syringe partially filled with TCA 10% was used to enter the cyst and aspirate the contents. The diluted TCA was then injected back into the cyst, and the process was repeated without moving the needle. The needle was then removed after the cyst was aspirated and collapsed, and the area was irrigated with copious amounts of normal saline.[15] Another group used foam sclerotherapy with 3% sodium tetradecyl sulfate (STS) to assist cystectomy in six patients. In this study, a 24-gauge needle attached to a 10-mL syringe was inserted into the cyst, and the contents were aspirated. Without changing the needle, a new syringe was attached containing 1 mL of 3% STS. The volume of the STS injected was approximately 20% of the aspirated fluid. All six patients had complete cyst resolution, and no cases of recurrence were reported over 15.6 months of follow-up.[16]

Laser assistance has also been described with conjunctival cystectomy. Argon laser photoablation was first described by Han et al.[17] Although argon laser achieves results through coagulation similar to thermal cautery or radio wave methods, the advantages of using argon laser are that the energy level can be controlled to achieve more selective ablations with delicate control. In the study by Han et al., 715 repetitions of an argon laser (power, 340–400 mW; duration, 0.1 s; spot size, 200 um) were needed for successful thermal photoablation of the cyst wall.[17] The use of argon laser can be curative, but often, extensive laser is needed to achieve success. In another paper, a modified method that used less argon laser was used to treat cysts. In this study by Han et al. of 17 cases with a mean follow-up of 13.3 months, 14 eyes achieved complete resolution. The other three cases achieved success with additional repeat treatment. No patients had any complications. After anesthesia was achieved, this technique used a purple marking pen to stain the surface of the cyst to increase the absorption of the argon beam and, in turn, decrease the required laser power. Next, the cyst was incised and drained using a 26-gauge needle. Finally, low-energy argon laser (532-nm argon green laser; spot size, 500 μm; power, 200–300 mW; duration, 0.3 s; ~100 shots) was applied to the cyst epithelial cells. Photoablation of the cyst epithelial cells was achieved as well as adhesions between the surrounding tissue and cyst capsule.[18]

Summary

Conjunctival cysts are benign and often asymptomatic. If symptoms do develop, there are multiple surgical techniques that can be used. Simple aspiration is often first-line treatment, although recurrence is common due to the retention of the secretory epithelial cells. Less recurrence is seen with complete cystectomy. Multiple variations of surgery have been described and may use the assistance of visualization dyes, sclerosing agents, or lasers.

References

1. Chin GN, Chi EY, Bunt AH. Ultrastructural and histochemical studies of conjunctival concretions. *Arch Ophthalmol*. 1980;98:720–724.
2. Chang SW, Hou PK, Chen MS. Conjunctival concretions. *Arch Ophthalmol*. 1990;108:405–408.
3. Haici P, Jankova H. Prevalence of conjunctival concretions. *Cesk Slov Oftalmol*. 2005;61(4):260–264.
4. Kulshrestha MK, Thaller VT. Prevalence of conjunctival concretions. Letters to the Journal. *Eye*. 1995;9:797–798.
5. Boettner EA, Fralick B, Wolter JR. Conjunctival concretions of sulfadiazine. *Arch Ophthalmol*. 1974;92:446–448.

6. Sherman SW, Cherny C, Suh L. Epithelial inclusion cyst of the bulbar conjunctiva secondary to scleral lens impingement managed with microvault. *Eye Contact Lens*. 2019;0:1–3.

7. El-Abedin Rajab GZ, Demer JL. Long-term results of surgical excision of conjunctival retention cyst using trypan blue with methylcellulose. *Am J Ophthalmol Case Rep*. 2019;14:28–31.

8. Kim DH, Khwarg SI, Oh JY. Atypical manifestation of conjunctival epithelial inclusion cyst: A case report. *Case Rep Ophthalmol*. 2014;5:239–242.

9. Gloor P, Horio B, Klassen M, Eagle RC Jr. Conjunctival cyst. *Arch Ophthal*. 1996;114:1020.

10. Thatte S, Jain J, Kinger M, Palod S, Wadhva J, Vishnoi A. Clinical study of histologically proven conjunctival cysts. *Saudi J Ophthal*. 2015;29:109–115.

11. Eom Y, Ahn SE, Kang SY, Kim HM, Song JS. Sutureless small-incision conjunctival cystectomy. *Can J Ophthal*. 2014;49(1):e17–e19.

12. Yang HK, Kim M, Lee SJ, Han SB, Hyon JY, Wee WR. Conjunctival cystectomy assisted by pattern scan laser photocoagulation. *Mil Med Res*. 2017;4:22.

13. Ikeda N, Ikeda T, Ishikawa H. In toto extraction of spontaneous conjunctival cysts without incision under slit-lamp microscopic view. *Can J Ophthalmol*. 2016;51(6):423–425.

14. Nishino T, Kobayashi A, Mori N, Masaki T, Yokogawa H, Sugiyama K. Clinical evaluation of a novel surgical technique (large cross incision) for conjunctival cysts. *Can J Ophthal*. 2018;53(1):e36–e39.

15. Bagheri A, Shahraki K, Yazdani S. Trichloroacetic acid 10% injection for treatment of conjunctival inclusion cysts. *Orbit*. 2020;39(2):107–111.

16. Dave T, Taneja S, Tiple S, Basu S, Naik MN. Conjunctival retention cysts: Outcomes of aspiration and sclerotherapy with sodium tetradecyl sulfate. *Ophthalmic Plast Reconstr Surg*. 2019;35(2):165–169.

17. Han SB, Yang HK, Hyon JY. Removal of conjunctival cyst using argon laser photoablation. *Can J Ophthalmol*. 2012;47:e6–e8.

18. Han J, Lee SH, Choi CY, Shin HJ. Treatment outcome of modified argon laser photoablation for conjunctival cysts. *Cornea*. 2019;0:1–5.

CHAPTER 12

Superior Limbic Keratoconjunctivitis

Lauren Chen ▦ Matthew Wade

Introduction

Superior limbic keratoconjunctivitis (SLK) is a relatively rare, chronic recurrent condition with remissions and exacerbations that can be associated with significant ocular surface symptoms and comorbidities. Episodes may last for a few days to more than a year, with remissions lasting a few weeks.[1] The average age of onset is at 50 years old, ranging from 20 to 67 years old. SLK is more common in females (3:1) and typically presents with bilateral symptoms, which may be asymmetrical.[1,2] Patients typically endorse having gradual onset of eye irritation, foreign body sensation, photophobia, burning, or pain. They may also have blepharospasm and mucoid discharge if filaments are present. However, visual acuity is not typically affected.

While the exact cause is unknown, the predominant theory is an inflammatory process from mechanical friction.[1,3] Continuous rubbing of the superior tarsal and bulbar conjunctiva induces chronic inflammatory changes such as keratinization and thickening of the conjunctiva, which are characteristic of SLK and perpetuate the inflammatory process. In addition, preexisting superior bulbar conjunctiva laxity may contribute to this process. Supporting a mechanical theory of pathogenesis, development of SLK has been seen after upper eyelid blepharoplasty, where there a is tighter approximation of the superior tarsal and bulbar conjunctiva.[4] Furthermore, treatments such as conjunctival resection and thermocauterization, which reduce bulbar conjunctiva laxity, have been shown to improve symptoms.[5]

A few clinical conditions are highly associated with SLK. History of thyroid dysfunction such as Graves disease has been reported to be present in 30%–64.9% of patients with SLK.[1,2,6–8] Conversely, the incidence of SLK in patients with Graves disease has been reported to be low at 3.3%.[9] SLK has also been suggested as a prognostic marker for decompression in Graves ophthalmopathy.[10] Globe protrusion may cause tighter approximation of the superior bulbar and tarsal conjunctiva, predisposing these patients to SLK. Dry eye disease (DED) has also been highly associated with SLK and reported to be present in 4.5%–54.5% of patients, with 24.2% having low Schirmer test results.[11–15] The increased friction between the tarsal and superior bulbar conjunctiva in DED contributes to the development of SLK. Additionally, secondary causes of dry eye conditions, such as ocular graft vs. host disease, have also reported SLK-like inflammation.[5]

Diagnosis

Diagnosis is dependent on classic symptoms with findings identified by slit lamp exam and corneal staining (fluorescein, lissamine green, or rose bengal) (Fig. 12.1). Theodore initially characterized SLK by having (1) marked inflammation of the tarsal conjunctiva of the upper lid, (2) inflammation of the upper bulbar conjunctiva, (3) fine punctate staining (fluorescein, rose bengal, or lissamine green) of the cornea at the upper limbus and the adjacent conjunctiva above the limbus between the 10 o'clock and 1 o'clock positions, (4) superior limbic proliferation, and (5) in some patients, filaments of the superior limbus or in the upper part of the cornea.[12] Of note, rose bengal staining of the superior conjunctiva by itself is not sufficient for diagnosis, as asymptomatic

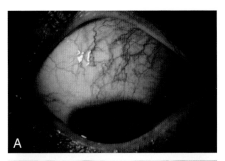

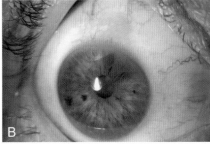

Fig. 12.1 (A) Inflammation of the superior bulbar conjunctiva in a patient with SLK. (B) Lissamine green staining of a patient with SLK.[17] (Photo credit with permission from Beeran Meghpara, MD).

patients can have similarly patterned staining.[16] Patients with SLK may also have low Schirmer tests, which can be confounded by preexisting DED.[13] Laboratory tests to rule out associated autoimmune disorders such as thyroid dysfunction, rheumatoid arthritis (anti cyclic citrullinated peptide), and Sjögren syndrome (SS) may also be warranted depending on clinical findings. Viral, bacterial, and fungal cultures are typically negative and are not helpful for diagnosis.

Treatment

While there is no gold-standard treatment of SLK, patients are typically started on topical medications such as preservative-free artificial tears and lubricating ointments to reduce friction, 0.5% cyclosporin A (Restasis),[18,19] or topical steroids (0.2% dexamethasone or 0.5% methylprednisolone four times a day).[11]

If refractory, a variety of other topical treatments have been reported to have variable efficacy: mast cell stabilizers (4% cromolyn sodium,[20] ketotifen fumarate,[21] lodoxamide tromethamine 0.1%[22,23]), autologous serum drops,[24,25] topical vitamin A (retinol palmitate),[26] 0.1% N-acetylcystine,[3] rebamipide,[27] and 0.03% tacrolimus.[28]

SLK was historically treated by applying 0.5% silver nitrate to the tarsal and superior bulbar conjunctiva[1,11] but would only have transient relief for 4–6 weeks and would require repeated treatments.[29] Additionally, one had to avoid high concentrations of silver nitrate to prevent caustic injury of the eye.

Currently, surgical conjunctival resection is a common procedure of choice to treat persistent or severe SLK.[14,30–33] A multitude of nontopical treatment procedure options have also been reported with different success rates and durations of response to treatment: lacrimal punctal occlusion with cautery and sutures[34,35] or punctal plugs,[36] pressure eye patching followed by soft contact lens wearing,[37] supratarsal triamcinolone injection,[38] botulinum toxin injection,[39,40] liquid nitrogen cryotherapy,[41] and thermocauterization.[15]

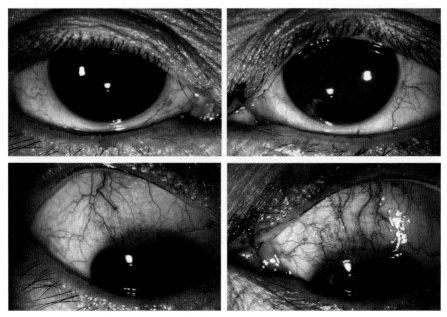

Fig. 12.2 Lissamine green staining of the superior bulbar conjunctiva left worse than right eye in a patient with asymmetric, bilateral superior limbic keratoconjunctivitis.

Case

A 62-year-old female presented with 2 weeks of left eye greater than right eye pain, 9 months post–bilateral blepharoplasty with bilateral upper lid levator resection for ptosis. Ocular history included bilateral blepharitis and keratoconjunctivitis sicca previously treated with bilateral lower lid punctal plugs.

Visual acuity, pupils, intraocular pressure (IOP), and external eye exam were normal. Notable findings included 2–3+ superior limbal staining with 1+ superficial punctate keratitis (SPK) of the right eye and superior limbal injection with 4+ punctate lissamine green staining (Fig. 12.2) without lid retraction, and 2–3+ inferior and superior superficial punctate keratitis of the left eye.

The patient continued to have persistent bilateral eye pain and left upper lid aching for 3 years despite trials of preservative-free artificial tears, lubricant ointment, autologous serum drops, and prescription antiinflammatory drops. As the patient was refractory to medical management, she underwent conjunctival resection with tenon capsule removal and AmnioGraft, with gradual improvement of symptoms.

Four months after conjunctival resection, she demonstrated recurrence of eye bilateral (left worse than right eye) irritation, superior limbal inflammation, and conjunctival staining despite aggressive lubrication and autologous serum drops. Given that she had failed medical and surgical management, the decision was made to proceed with in-office treatment with thermocauterization starting with the more affected eye. At her 1-week follow-up visit, the patient had marked symptomatic improvement, and therefore, thermocauterization was performed on the following eye. At follow-up 1 week and 3 months after thermocauterization, the patient remained clinically improved and stable.

PROCEDURE: THERMOCAUTERIZATION OF SUPERIOR BULBAR CONJUNCTIVA

Supplies (See Fig. 12.3)

- Low temperature, disposable microsurgery cautery
- Lissamine green stain
- 27- or 30-gauge needle
- 2% lidocaine with epinephrine or 2% xylocaine
- Eye speculum (optional)
- Topical erythromycin ointment

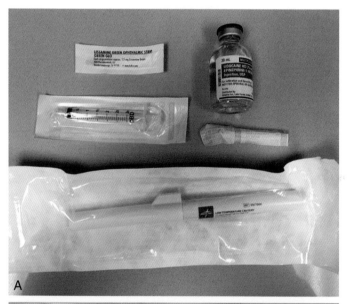

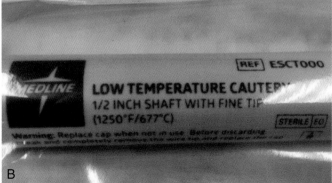

Fig. 12.3 (A–B) Instruments needed for thermocauterization of superior limbic keratoconjunctivitis procedure.

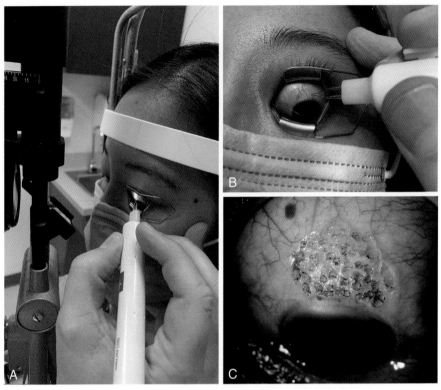

Fig. 12.4 (A) The positioning of the low-temperature microcautery at the slit lamp and (B) the proximity of the microcautery tip to bulbar conjunctiva. (C) Thermocauterization of superior bulbar conjunctiva treatment for superior limbic keratoconjunctivitis.[17] (Photo credit with permission from Christopher Rapuano, MD).

Procedure

The eye is prepped in the usual sterile fashion. Lissamine green is applied to stain the conjunctiva. Topical anesthetic proparacaine drops are instilled in the eye, and then with a 25-gauge or 30-gauge needle, 0.25 to 0.5 mL of 2% lidocaine with epinephrine 1:100,000 or 2% xylocaine is injected beneath the superior bulbar conjunctiva. A disposable microsurgery low-temperature cautery is applied to the superior bulbar conjunctiva briefly (approximately 1 second per spot) to create a light blanching of the tissue for 30–50 spots to cover the affected lissamine green–stained areas of the tissue (Fig. 12.4). Each application of the cautery should sufficiently burn the entire epithelial layer and produce stromal shrinkage without injuring the underlying sclera. Postprocedure, antibiotic drops or erythromycin ointment should be used for 1 week.

DISCUSSION

While the mechanism of thermocauterization in improving SLK is unknown, it is thought that cautery transiently increases vascularity, epithelial migration, and differentiation from the surrounding normal tissue and disrupts the inflammatory cycle, thereby restoring goblet cells.[15] The success rate of thermocauterization is reported to be at 73% (8 of 11 patients) with an average duration of response of 6.3 months, ranging from 2 months to 4 years per Udell.[15] In patients who develop recurrence despite initial treatment, improvement with a repeat thermocauterization was shown to be effective.[15] In cases that are partially responsive to treatment, adjunctive use of punctal occlusion or Bandage contact lenses (BCL) has shown to improve symptoms. Continued use of artificial tears may also be recommended for lubrication.

To ensure all affected areas are treated and to minimize chance of recurrence, we recommend using stains to identify and target the affected conjunctiva, as opposed to targeting the 10 o'clock and 2 o'clock positions from the limbus extending 8 mm posteriorly, as Udell originally described.[15] Thermocauterization is also a good alternative for patients who have failed silver nitrate therapy and are interested in a simple in-office approach prior to considering surgical conjunctival resection. Additionally, this case demonstrates its benefit in patients who have recurrence of symptoms after resection.

After thermocauterization treatment, patients typically experience mild ocular discomfort that resolves within 3 days, followed by symptomatic improvement of eye redness, irritation, and photophobia and clinical improvement of conjunctival inflammation and corneal filaments.

References

1. Wilson II FM, Ostler HB. Superior limbic keratoconjunctivitis. *Int Ophthalmol Clin.* 1986;26(4):99–112. https://doi.org/10.1097/00004397-198602640-00010.
2. Nelson JD. Superior limbic keratoconjunctivitis (SLK). *Eye (Lond).* 1989;3(Pt 2):180–189. https://doi.org/10.1038/eye.1989.26.
3. Wright P. Superior limbic keratoconjunctivitis. *Trans Ophthalmol Soc U K.* 1972;92:555–560.
4. Sheu MC, Schoenfield L, Jeng BH. Development of superior limbic keratoconjunctivitis after upper eyelid blepharoplasty surgery: support for the mechanical theory of its pathogenesis. *Cornea.* 2007; 26(4):490–492. https://doi.org/10.1097/ICO.0b013e3180303b02.
5. Sivaraman KR, Jivrajka RV, Soin K, et al. Superior limbic keratoconjunctivitis-like inflammation in patients with chronic graft-versus-host disease. *Ocul Surf.* 2016;14(3):393–400. https://doi.org/10.1016/j.jtos.2016.04.003.
6. Kadrmas EF, Bartley GB. Keratoconjunctivitis A prognostic sign for severe Graves ophthalmopathy. *Ophthalmology.* 1995;102(10):1472–1475. https://doi.org/10.1016/S0161-6420(95)30843-3.
7. Chelala E, El Rami H, Dirani A, Fakhoury H, Fadlallah A. Extensive superior limbic keratoconjunctivitis in Graves' disease: case report and mini-review of the literature. *Clin Ophthalmol.* 2015;9:467–468. https://doi.org/10.2147/OPTH.S79561.
8. Cher I. Clinical features of superior limbic keroconjunctivitis in Australia. A probable association with hyrotoxicosis. *Arch Ophthalmol.* 1969;82(5):580–586. https://doi.org/10.1001/archopht.1969.00990020582002.
9. Bartley GB. The epidemiologic characteristics and clinical course of ophthalmopathy associated with autoimmune thyroid disease in Olmstead County, Minnesota. *Transactions of the American Ophthalmological Society.* Vol 92. American Ophthalmological Society; 1994:477–588.
10. Kadrmas EF, Bartley GB. Superior limbic keratoconjunctivitis. A prognostic sign for severe Graves ophthalmopathy. *Ophthalmology.* 1995;102(10):1472–1475. https://doi.org/10.1016/s0161-6420(95)30843-3.
11. Corwin ME. Superior limbic keratoconjunctivitis. *Am J Ophthalmol.* 1968;66(2):338–340. https://doi.org/10.1016/0002-9394(68)92086-2.
12. Theodore FH. Superior limbic keratoconjunctivitis. *Eye Ear Nose Throat Mon.* 1963;42:25–28.
13. Nelson D. Superior Limbic Keratoconjunctivitis (SLK). Eye (Lond.). 1989;13:180–189.
14. Passons GA, Wood TO. Conjunctival resection for superior limbic keratoconjunctivitis. *Ophthalmology.* 1984;91(8):966–968. https://doi.org/10.1016/s0161-6420(84)34207-5.
15. Udell IJ, Kenyon KR, Sawa M, Dohlman CH. Treatment of superior limbic keratoconjunctivitis by thermocauterization of the superior bulbar conjunctiva. *Ophthalmology.* 1986;93(2):162–166. https://doi.org/10.1016/s0161-6420(86)33766-7.
16. Bainbridge JW, Mackie IA, Mackie I. Diagnosis of Theodore's superior limbic keratoconjunctivitis. *Eye (Lond).* 1998;12(Pt 4):748–749. https://doi.org/10.1038/eye.1998.185.
17. Meghpara B. Corneal Cases That No Clinician Should Miss. Collaborative Eye. July/August. 2018. https://collaborativeeye.com/articles/july-aug-18/corneal-cases-that-no-clinician-should-miss/.

18. Sahin A, Bozkurt B, Irkec M. Topical cyclosporine A in the treatment of superior limbic kerato-conjunctivitis: A long-term follow-up. *Cornea*. 2008;27(2):193–195. https://doi.org/10.1097/ICO.0b013e318033bd25.

19. Perry HD, Doshi-Carnevale S, Donnenfeld ED, Kornstein HS. Topical cyclosporine A 0.5% as a possible new treatment for superior limbic keratoconjunctivitis. *Ophthalmology*. 2003;110(8):1578–1581. https://doi.org/10.1016/S0161-6420(03)00538-4.

20. Confino J, Brown SI. Treatment of superior limbic keratoconjunctivitis with topical cromolyn sodium. *Ann Ophthalmol*. 1987;19(4):129–131.

21. Udell IJ, Guidera AC, Madani-Becker J. Ketotifen fumarate treatment of superior limbic keratoconjunctivitis. *Cornea*. 2002;21(8):778–780. https://doi.org/10.1097/00003226-200211000-00009.

22. Grutzmacher RD, Foster RS, Feiler LS. Lodoxamide tromethamine treatment for superior limbic keratoconjunctivitis. *Am J Ophthalmol*. 1995;120(3):400–402. https://doi.org/10.1016/S0002-9394(14)72177-4.

23. Rodriguez-Garcia A, Macias-Rodriguez Y, Gonzalez-Gonzalez JM. Efficacy and safety of 0.1% lodoxamide for the long-term treatment of superior limbic keratoconjunctivitis. *Int Ophthalmol*. 2018;38(3):1243–1249. https://doi.org/10.1007/s10792-017-0588-1.

24. Goto E, Shimmura S, Shimazaki J, Tsubota K. Treatment of superior limbic keratoconjunctivitis by application of autologous serum. *Cornea*. 2001;20(8):807–810. https://doi.org/10.1097/00003226-200111000-00006.

25. Azari AA, Rapuano CJ. Autologous serum eye drops for the treatment of ocular surface disease. *Eye Contact Lens*. 2015;41(3):133–140. https://doi.org/10.1097/ICL.0000000000000104.

26. Ohashi Y, Watanabe H, Kinoshita S, Hosotani H, Umemoto M, Manabe R. Vitamin A eyedrops for superior limbic keratoconjunctivitis. *Am J Ophthalmol*. 1988;105(5):523–527. https://doi.org/10.1016/0002-9394(88)90245-0.

27. Takahashi Y, Ichinose A, Kakizaki H. Topical rebamipide treatment for superior limbic keratoconjunctivitis in patients with thyroid eye disease. *Am J Ophthalmol*. 2014;157(4). https://doi.org/10.1016/j.ajo.2013.12.027.

28. Kymionis GD, Klados NE, Kontadakis GA, Mikropoulos DG. Treatment of superior limbic kerato-conjunctivitis with topical tacrolimus 0.03% ointment. *Cornea*. 2013;32(11):1499–1501. https://doi.org/10.1097/ICO.0b013e318295e6b9.

29. Theodore FH, Ferry AP. Superior limbic keratoconjunctivitis. Clinical and pathological correlations. *Arch Ophthalmol*. 1970;84(4):481–484. https://doi.org/10.1001/archopht.1970.00990040483016.

30. Donshik PC, Barry Collin H, Stephen Foster C, et al. Conjunctival resection treatment and ultra-structural histopathology of superior limbic keratoconjunctivitis. *Am J Ophthalmol*. 1978;85(1):101–110. https://doi.org/10.1016/S0002-9394(14)76673-5.

31. Yokoi N, Komuro A, Maruyama K, Tsuzuki M, Miyajima S, Kinoshita S. New surgical treatment for superior limbic keratoconjunctivitis and its association with conjunctivochalasis. *Am J Ophthalmol*. 2003;135(3):303–308. https://doi.org/10.1016/s0002-9394(02)01975-x.

32. Gris O, Plazas A, Lerma E, Guell JL, Pelegrin L, Elies D. Conjunctival resection with and without amniotic membrane graft for the treatment of superior limbic keratoconjunctivitis. *Cornea*. 2010;29(9): 1025–1030. https://doi.org/10.1097/ICO.0b013e3181d1d1cc.

33. Sun Y-C, Hsiao C-H, Chen W-L, Wang I-J, Hou Y-C, Hu F-R. Conjunctival resection combined with tenon layer excision and the involvement of mast cells in superior limbic keratoconjunctivitis. *Am J Ophthalmol*. 2008;145(3):445–452. https://doi.org/10.1016/j.ajo.2007.10.025.

34. Yang HY, Fujishima H, Toda I, Shimazaki J, Tsubota K. Lacrimal punctal occlusion for the treatment of superior limbic keratoconjunctivitis. *Am J Ophthalmol*. 1997;124(1):80–87. https://doi.org/10.1016/S0002-9394(14)71647-2.

35. Kabat AG. Lacrimal occlusion therapy for the treatment of superior limbic keratoconjunctivitis. *Optom Vis Sci*. 1998;75(10):714–718. https://doi.org/10.1097/00006324-199810000-00015.

36. Tai MC, Cosar CB, Cohen EJ, Rapuano CJ, Laibson PR. The clinical efficacy of silicone punctal plug therapy. *Cornea*. 2002;21(2):135–139. https://doi.org/10.1097/00003226-200203000-00001.

37. Mondino BJ, Zaidman GW, Salamon SW. Use of pressure patching and soft contact lenses in superior limbic keratoconjunctivitis. *Arch Ophthalmol*. 1982;100(12):1932–1934. https://doi.org/10.1001/archopht.1982.01030040912008.

38. Shen Y-C, Wang C-Y, Tsai H-Y, Lee Y-F. Supratarsal triamcinolone injection in the treatment of superior limbic keratoconjunctivitis. *Cornea.* 2007;26(4):423–426. https://doi.org/10.1097/ICO. 0b013e318030d230.

39. Kim JC, Chun YS. Treatment of superior limbic keratoconjunctivitis with a large-diameter contact lens and botulium toxin A. *Cornea.* 2009;28(7):752–758. https://doi.org/10.1097/ico.0b013e3181967006.

40. Mackie IA. Management of superior limbic keratoconjunctivitis with botulinum toxin. *Eye.* 1995; 9(1):143–144. https://doi.org/10.1038/eye.1995.25.

41. Fraunfelder FW. Liquid nitrogen cryotherapy of superior limbic keratoconjunctivitis. *Am J Ophthalmol.* 2009;147(2). https://doi.org/10.1016/j.ajo.2008.07.047.

CHAPTER 13

Conjunctivochalasis

Kate Xie ■ Kyoung Yul Seo ■ Stephen C. Pflugfelder

Introduction

Conjunctivochalasis (CCh) is redundant conjunctival folds characterized by loose, nonedematous bulbar conjunctiva that is typically found above the lower eyelid but can be observed in the superior and even the entire bulbar conjunctiva in some cases.[1,2] Pathogenesis of CCh involves degradation of elastic fibers in the substantia propria by matrix metalloproteinases whose expression is increased by inflammatory mediators and oxidative stress stimulated by dryness and mechanical trauma.[3–6] Bulbar lymphangiectasia has also been observed in histological sections of some cases.[7] Recently, CCh has been considered one of the friction-related diseases of the ocular surface, which also includes superior limbic keratoconjunctivitis and lid wiper epitheliopathy.[8]

Epidemiology

The prevalence of CCh increases after the third decade of life.[9] After the age of 60, the prevalence has been estimated to be between 44% and 90% based on large population studies of Chinese and Japanese patients.[9,10] The temporal conjunctiva is affected most frequently, followed by the nasal conjunctiva. The severity of CCh in these areas is strongly correlated with age.[11] It is more prevalent and tends to be more severe in females compared to males.[1,9] Associations have additionally been made between CCh and pinguecula, contact lens wear, Meibomian gland disease (MGD), and hyperopia.[1,12]

CCh has been associated with dermatochalasis and dry eye.[13] The exact relationship between these conditions remains to be determined. Because the prevalence and severity increase with age, it has been hypothesized that CCh results from the normal age-related loss of attachments of the bulbar conjunctiva to the sclera. The redundant conjunctiva is subject to chronic mechanical friction due to blinking, which, in turn, triggers an inflammatory response that includes increased production of matrix metalloproteinases, which exacerbate the degradation of elastin fibers. As CCh progresses, redundant conjunctival folds disrupt the inferior tear meniscus and may block the inferior punctum, resulting in delayed tear clearance and tear film instability.[1]

Typical Symptoms

CCh causes chronic eye irritation due to mechanical friction from blinking and from its negative impact on tear stability, distribution, and clearance.[1,11,13–15] Patients typically complain of foreign body sensation (particularly in the area of lid parallel folds [LPFs]), dryness, redness, blurred and fluctuating vision, and tearing.[16,17] Patients may also complain of frequent blinking.[18] Because these symptoms are similar to dry eye–associated symptoms, CCh is often misdiagnosed and treated as dry eye disease (DED). It often coexists with MGD, and symptoms may be more severe when both are present.[8,12,19] While treatments for DED/MGD may transiently improve symptoms, they generally do not provide adequate sustained relief. Surgical removal of CCh should be considered in patients who do not respond to medical therapy.[8,20,21]

Diagnosis of Conjunctivochalasis

CCh worsens with age and may be overlooked as a normal aging change. Patients with CCh have LPFs in the inferior bulbar conjunctiva above the lid margin that is typically most prominent in the nasal and temporal conjunctiva (Fig. 13.1A), conjunctival injection in this area, and increased tear meniscus height. Schemes for grading severity of LPFs from 1–3 have been reported and are described in Table 13.1. Severe cases have hooding of the inferior cornea and this area may stain with fluorescein or lissamine green dyes (Fig. 13.1B).[13,20] Patients may also experience recurrent subconjunctival hemorrhages.[22] Optical coherence tomography is a useful tool to measure tear meniscus height and the degree of conjunctiva prolapsing into inferior tear meniscus (Fig. 13.1C).[2,20,23] Signs of MGD, including lid margin injection/telangiectasia, orifice obstruction, and anterior displacement of the Marx line, may be observed.[12] Fluorescein tear breakup time is typically rapid.[12]

Medical Management

If asymptomatic, CCh does not need to be treated. For patients with dry eye symptoms, conservative management consisting of artificial tears and lubricating ointments may be sufficient to control their symptoms. If symptoms persist, then topical corticosteroids may be considered.[13] A study by Prabhasawat and Tseng showed that nonpreserved 1% methylprednisolone eye drops administered 3 times daily for 3 weeks resulted in both symptomatic improvement and objective improvement in delayed tear clearance.[24]

Other causes of tearing and irritation symptoms include Meibomian gland dysfunction, allergic conjunctivitis, trichiasis, nasolacrimal duct obstruction, and eyelid malposition, including entropion and ectropion.[17] These conditions may occur concomitantly and should be ruled out or treated before escalating to surgical management.

Case

The patient is a 75-year-old female with a 5-year history of worsening bilateral foreign body sensation that is worse in the right eye. She also complains of tearing and frequently wipes tears from her lateral canthus. She blinks frequently to clear her vision. She has experienced several subconjunctival hemorrhages in the right eye over the past year. Artificial tears provide temporary relief of irritation, but she has had no improvement from cyclosporine or lifitegrast. She had inferior punctal plugs placed in the past, but they worsened her tearing. Examination revealed bilateral CCh with grade 3 lid parallel (LIPCOF) folds. Fluorescein tear breakup was 4 seconds, and there was mild punctate fluorescein staining in the inferior cornea of both eyes. The conjunctiva occasionally hooded the inferior cornea after blinking. Optical coherence tomography showed an increased tear meniscus height in both eyes and prolapse of redundant conjunctiva into the inferior tear meniscus in the left eye.

The patient had in-office thermocautery of the inferior bulbar conjunctiva in both eyes and was treated with prednisolone acetate for 2 weeks postoperatively. She returned 1 month after the procedure and had almost complete relief of her foreign body sensation and resolution of her tearing. The inferior bulbar conjunctiva was smooth and tight, and no LPFs were noted.

PROCEDURES

Both thermocautery and radio wave electrosurgery are simple in-office procedures that have been reported to shrink the redundant conjunctiva.[2,25–27]

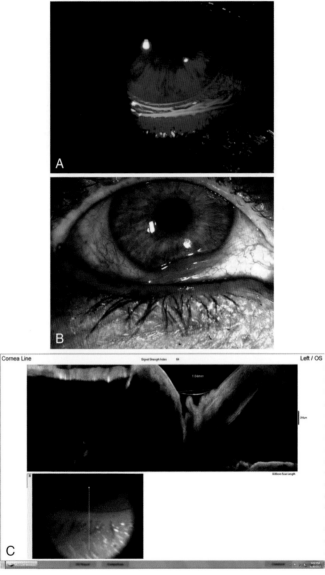

Fig. 13.1 (A) Severe conjunctivochalasis with Grade 3 lid parallel conjunctival folds (LIPCOF) noted with fluorescein dye. (B) Conjunctivochalasis riding up onto the inferior cornea and staining with lissamine green dye. (C) Anterior segment optical coherence tomography (OCT) showing redundant conjunctival folds with increased and anteriorly displaced tear meniscus.

Thermocautery

Medications and instruments used for thermocautery are described in Table 13.2. A video of the procedure is also provided (Video 13.1). After informed consent is obtained, the conjunctiva is anesthetized with two sequential instillations of lidocaine gel that provides excellent

TABLE 13.1 ■ LIPCOF Grading Scale for Conjunctivochalasis[20]

	LIPCOF Grade
No conjunctival folds	0
1 permanent and clear parallel fold	1
2 permanent and clear parallel folds (normally lower than 0.2 mm)	2
More than 2 permanent and clear parallel folds (normally higher than 0.2 mm)	3

TABLE 13.2 ■ Supplies for Conjunctival Thermocautery

Drug/Instrument	Vendor	Dose
Lidocaine gel	Akten lidocaine ophthalmic gel 3.5% (Akorn, Lake Forest, IL)	2 applications, 5 and 10 minutes prior to procedure
High-temperature battery cautery	Bovie high-temp cautery, fine tip (Bovie, Clearwater, FL)	
Tennant curved tying forceps	No. K5-5230 (Katena, Parsippany, NJ)	
Prednisolone or equivalent steroid eye drop	Brand or generic	QID for 1 week and BID for 1 week

BID, Twice daily; *QID*, four times daily.

anesthesia. Lids are either held open by an assistant or separated with a wire speculum. The redundant inferior bulbar conjunctiva is milked inferiorly away from the limbus with a closed curved tying forceps and then grasped such that the redundant tissue prolapses up between the blades (Fig. 13.2A). It is cauterized with the high-temperature battery cautery down to the blades, starting from the temporal bulbar conjunctiva near the lateral canthus and moving nasally. This usually requires cauterizing 3–4 segments to encompass the entire inferior bulbar conjunctiva (Figs. 13.2B and 13.2C). The CPT code for this procedure is 68115 (excision of conjunctival lesion > 1 cm).

Radio Wave Electrosurgery

Medications and instruments used for high-frequency radio wave electrosurgery are described in Table 13.3. A video of the procedure is also provided (Video 13.2). The same preparation for thermocautery as described above, topical 0.5% proparacaine is instilled in the conjunctiva for local anesthesia. The extent of the redundant inferior bulbar conjunctiva is determined (Fig. 13.3A). While the redundant conjunctiva is lifted with tying forceps, a fine-needle electrode is inserted into the target conjunctiva. One to two seconds of each ablation are used to produce shrinkage of the redundant tissue, starting from the temporal bulbar conjunctiva and moving nasally (Figs. 13.3B and 13.3C). Approximately 10 to 20 ablations are performed with the minimal power setting of 1 (of 100) in the coagulating mode. At the end of the procedure, the inferior bulbar conjunctiva shows a dusky white (blanching) color without prolapsed conjunctiva tissue (Fig. 13.3D).

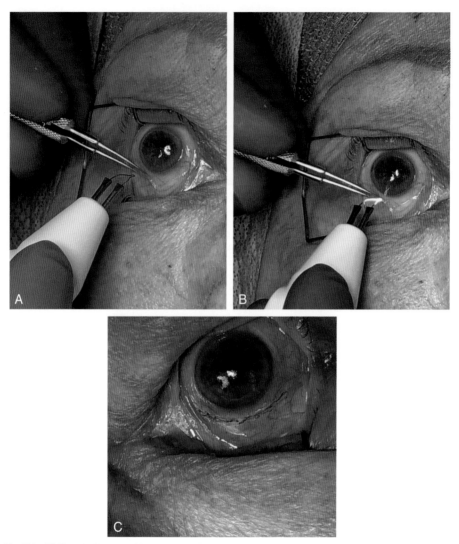

Fig. 13.2 (A) Eye is held open with a wire speculum. While the patient is looking up, the redundant conjunctiva in the inferior bulbar conjunctiva is grasped with the curved tying forceps, so the redundant conjunctiva prolapses up between the blades. (B) The prolapsed conjunctiva is cauterized with the high-temperature battery cautery down to the blades, starting from the temporal bulbar conjunctiva near the lateral canthus and moving nasally. This usually involved cauterizing 3–4 segments to encompass the entire inferior bulbar conjunctiva. (C) Thermocautery line in inferior bulbar conjunctiva at the completion of the procedure.

Conclusion

CCh is a very common and often overlooked underlying cause of irritation and unstable vision in patients. Careful evaluation for CCh should be undertaken in the workup for any patient with suspected ocular surface disturbance. When medical management is insufficient, office-based thermal cautery and radio wave electrosurgery are effective, simple to perform, and low-risk interventions that may be considered.

TABLE 13.3 ■ Supplies for Conjunctival Radio Wave Electrosurgery

Drug/Instrument	Vendor	Dose
0.5% Proparacaine eyedrops	Alcaine (Alcon Laboratories, Fort Worth, TX)	3–4 instillations just before the procedure
High-frequency radio wave electrosurgery system	Fine-needle electrode (fine insulated coated needle, 004 super fine) of the 4.0-MHz Ellman Surgitron Dual Frequency (Ellman International, Inc., Hewlett, NY)	
0.1% Fluorometholone and 0.5% moxifloxacin 0.5% (or equivalent steroid and antibiotic eye drop)	Brand or generic	QID for 2–4 weeks

QID, Four times daily.

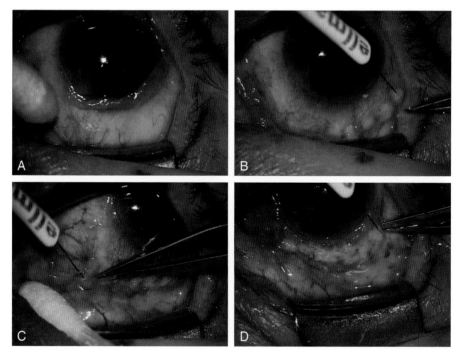

Fig. 13.3 (A) After instillation of 0.5% proparacaine, the extent of the redundant conjunctiva is determined using a cotton tip. (B) Using a fine insulated coated needle of the 4.0-MHz radio wave system, the target conjunctiva is ablated and shrunken without charring the tissue. (C) Approximately 10 to 20 ablations are usually performed, starting from temporal bulbar conjunctiva and moving nasally. (D) At the completion of the procedure, inferior bulbar conjunctiva shows a dusky white color (blanching) without prolapsed conjunctiva tissues.

Acknowledgment

Special thanks to Yong Woo, MD, for writing portions of and editing the video for the radio wave electrosurgery section.

References

1. Marmalidou A, Kheirkhah A, Dana R. Conjunctivochalasis: A systematic review. *Surv Ophthalmol.* 2018;63(4):554–564.
2. Gumus K, Crockett CH, Pflugfelder SC. Anterior segment optical coherence tomography: A diagnostic instrument for conjunctivochalasis. *Am J Ophthalmol.* 2010;150(6):798–806.
3. Ward SK, Wakamatsu TH, Dogru M, et al. The role of oxidative stress and inflammation in conjunctivochalasis. *Invest Ophthalmol Vis Sci.* 2010;51(4):1994–2002.
4. Harbiyeli II, Erdem E, Erdogan S, et al. Investigation of conjunctivochalasis histopathology with light and electron microscopy in patients with conjunctivochalasis in different locations. *Int Ophthalmol.* 2019;39(7):1491–1499.
5. Gan JY, Li QS, Zhang ZY, Zhang W, Zhang XR. The role of elastic fibers in pathogenesis of conjunctivochalasis. *Int J Ophthalmol.* 2017;10(9):1465–1473.
6. Acera A, Vecino E, Duran JA. Tear MMP-9 levels as a marker of ocular surface inflammation in conjunctivochalasis. *Invest Ophthalmol Vis Sci.* 2013;54(13):8285–8291.
7. Zhang XR, Liu YX, Sheng X, et al. [Clinical observation of lymphangiectasis in conjunctivochalasis cases]. *Zhonghua Yan Ke Za Zhi.* 2013;49(6):547–550.
8. Vu CHV, Kawashima M, Yamada M, et al. Influence of Meibomian gland dysfunction and friction-related disease on the severity of dry eye. *Ophthalmology.* 2018;125(8):1181–1188.
9. Mimura T, Yamagami S, Usui T, et al. Changes of conjunctivochalasis with age in a hospital-based study. *Am J Ophthalmol.* 2009;147(1):171–177.e171.
10. Zhang X, Li Q, Zou H, et al. Assessing the severity of conjunctivochalasis in a senile population: A community-based epidemiology study in Shanghai, China. *BMC public health.* 2011;11:198.
11. Gumus K, Pflugfelder SC. Increasing prevalence and severity of conjunctivochalasis with aging detected by anterior segment optical coherence tomography. *Am J Ophthalmol.* 2013;155(2):238–242.e232.
12. Pflugfelder SC, Gumus K, Feuerman J, Alex A. Tear volume-based diagnostic classification for tear dysfunction. *Int Ophthalmol Clin.* 2017;57(2):1–12.
13. Meller D, Tseng SC. Conjunctivochalasis: Literature review and possible pathophysiology. *Surv Ophthalmol.* 1998;43(3):225–232.
14. Chhadva P, Alexander A, McClellan AL, McManus KT, Seiden B, Galor A. The impact of conjunctivochalasis on dry eye symptoms and signs. *Invest Ophthalmol Vis Sci.* 2015;56(5):2867–2871.
15. Trivli A, Dalianis G, Terzidou C. A quick surgical treatment of conjunctivochalasis using radiofrequencies. *Healthcare (Basel).* 2018;6(1):14.
16. Balci O. Clinical characteristics of patients with conjunctivochalasis. *Clin Ophthalmol.* 2014;8:1655–1660.
17. Tse DT, Erickson BP, Tse BC. The BLICK mnemonic for clinical-anatomical assessment of patients with epiphora. *Ophthalmic Plast Reconstr Surg.* 2014;30(6):450–458.
18. Rahman EZ, Lam PK, Chu CK, Moore Q, Pflugfelder SC. Corneal sensitivity in tear dysfunction and its correlation with clinical parameters and blink rate. *Am J Ophthalmol.* 2015;160(5):858–866.e855.
19. Arita R, Mizoguchi T, Kawashima M, et al. Meibomian gland dysfunction and dry eye are similar but different based on a population-based study: The Hirado-Takushima study in Japan. *Am J Ophthalmol.* 2019;207:410–418.
20. Pult H, Riede-Pult BH. Impact of conjunctival folds on central tear meniscus height. *Invest Ophthalmol Vis Sci.* 2015;56(3):1459–1466.
21. Huang Y, Sheha H, Tseng SC. Conjunctivochalasis interferes with tear flow from fornix to tear meniscus. *Ophthalmology.* 2013;120(8):1681–1687.
22. Yamamoto Y, Yokoi N, Ogata M, et al. Correlation between recurrent subconjunctival hemorrhages and conjunctivochalasis by clinical profile and successful surgical outcome. *Eye Contact Lens.* 2015;41(6):367–372.
23. Bandlitz S, Purslow C, Murphy PJ, Pult H. Lid-parallel conjunctival fold (LIPCOF) morphology imaged by optical coherence tomography and its relationship to LIPCOF grade. *Cont Lens Anterior Eye.* 2019;42(3):299–303.
24. Prabhasawat P, Tseng SC. Frequent association of delayed tear clearance in ocular irritation. *Br J Ophthalmol.* 1998;82(6):666–675.
25. Marmalidou A, Palioura S, Dana R, Kheirkhah A. Medical and surgical management of conjunctivochalasis. *Ocul Surf.* 2019;17(3):393–399.
26. Ahn JM, Choi CY, Seo KY. Surgical approach with high-frequency radiowave electrosurgery for superior limbic keratoconjunctivitis. *Cornea.* 2014;33(2):210–214.
27. Youm DJ, Kim JM, Choi CY. Simple surgical approach with high-frequency radio-wave electrosurgery for conjunctivochalasis. *Ophthalmology.* 2010;117(11):2129–2133.

CHAPTER 14

Corneal Infectious Keratitis

Zaina Al-Mohtaseb ▨ Yvonne Wang

Introduction

Microbial keratitis is an ocular emergency that can cause significant visual impairment or blindness. The incidence has increased in developed countries in the past several decades due to the increase of contact lens usage. It is estimated that in the United States, microbial keratitis accounts for nearly 1 million clinical visits per year. The three main etiologies of microbial keratitis are bacterial, fungal, and amoebic. In developed countries, bacterial keratitis is the most common, accounting for up to 85%–98% of all microbial keratitis cases. This is related to risk in contact lens wearers. In developing countries, fungal keratitis may equal or even outpace bacterial keratitis. This may be related to the higher rates of agriculture-related ocular trauma in rural communities. Acanthamoeba keratitis accounts for 1%–3% of microbial keratitis. A risk factor for amoebic infections is exposure to contaminated water, commonly pools and hot tubs. Identifying the pathogen is crucial to the treatment of microbial keratitis.

Obtaining a pathogen is a pivotal step in the successful management of severe infectious corneal keratitis. While small corneal ulcers can be treated empirically, sight-threatening ulcers should be cultured as the first step in management. Ulcers can be categorized as low-risk or high-risk infections. Low-risk infections include small infiltrates that are located in the periphery and not sight threatening. High-risk infections include large infiltrates that are sight threatening. They also include infections associated with risk factors such as trauma, recurrent steroid use, ocular surface disease, and immunosuppression. Other high-risk features are limbal or scleral involvement, corneal thinning or melting, and atypical features such as satellite lesions or feathery borders. Additionally, ulcers that have not responded to empiric treatment should also be cultured. Early identification is important because a delay in treatment often leads to more scarring and poor visual outcomes.

CASE

PART 1

A 53-year-old male presented with a corneal ulcer in the right eye. He had a history of neurotrophic cornea secondary to herpes zoster keratitis and wore a scleral lens. His vision on presentation was hand motion. His exam showed a central 3.1-mm by 1.2-mm epithelial defect with a faint nonsuppurative infiltrate with surrounding white blood cell recruitment. There was 1+ corneal edema, 10% stromal thinning, and superior deep corneal neovascularization. The anterior chamber was deep with 3+ cell and a 2.5-mm layered hypopyon. The cornea was scraped and sent for culture. The patient was subsequently started on fortified antibiotics (Fig. 14.1).

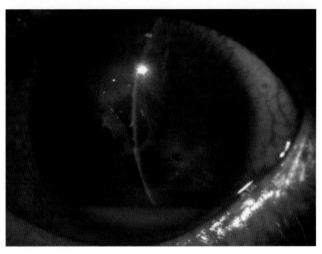

Fig. 14.1 Corneal ulcer with an epithelial defect, corneal infiltrate, and hypopyon.

CORNEAL CULTURE

If the patient has been started on antibiotics prior to culturing, or if a repeat culture needs to be done after the patient is started on empiric antibiotics yet has not improved, a 24-hour drug holiday could be done prior to culturing as long as the patient is not at risk for corneal perforation.

Having a corneal culture kit is a useful tool for any practice that sees corneal ulcers. Eye cultures are unique in that they allow identification of a pathogen from a very small sample. The kit should include tools needed to obtain a sufficient sample and culture media for aerobic and anaerobic bacterial, fungal, amoebic, viral, and atypical bacterial organisms.

PROCEDURE: OBTAINING A CORNEAL CULTURE (FIG. 14.2)

1. Lay out all material (Table 14.1), and label all plates.
2. Position patient at the slit lamp. The patient's lid should be held firmly open by the provider or an assistant to avoid contamination from the lashes or lid margin. A lid speculum can be used but is usually not necessary.
3. Using the Kimura spatula or the calcium alginate swab, scrape against the most active area of the ulcer, usually along the edge of the epithelial defect or where the infiltrate appears the densest. The scrape should be firm and indent the cornea slightly, aiming to obtain some of the stromal tissue. Avoid touching the lashes or surface of the conjunctiva to minimize contamination. A new swab should be used for each pass. The Kimura spatulas should be sterilized with a flame until red-hot and allowed to cool in between each pass for sterility.
4. Swipe on two glass slides first.
5. Repeat to inoculate the culture media. Make multiple rows of C-shaped streaks across the plates to help with differentiating a true-positive culture from a contaminant (Fig. 14.3). If there is limited infiltrate, inoculate for fungal or acanthamoeba first if suspected. Then the blood plate, then the chocolate.

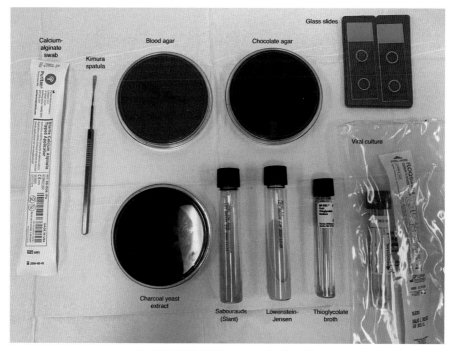

Fig. 14.2 Materials for a corneal culture kit.

6. Last, for the thioglycolate broth, pass the rim of the glass tube over a flame to sterilize the opening. Dip the calcium alginate swab into the tryptic soy broth, and then either wipe a cultured Kimura spatula on the tip or use the swab to directly culture the cornea. Break or cut off the swab tip into the thioglycolate broth. Keep this tube upright to maintain an oxygen gradient for aerobic growth at the top and anaerobic growth at the bottom.
7. After the culture is done, the patient is typically started on empiric antibiotics while waiting for the culture results. Use broad-spectrum fortified antibiotics in cases of severe ulcers or a fourth-generation fluroquinolone in cases of nonsevere ulcers.

CASE

PART 2

The patient's corneal cultures were negative. The patient's ulcer continued to worsen after 2 weeks of fortified antibiotic treatment (Fig. 14.4). A second culture was obtained after a drug holiday that was also negative. A decision was made to obtain a corneal biopsy. The biopsy results showed acanthamoeba cysts on pathology slides. The patient was started on antiamoebic treatment of brolene, polyhexamethylene biguanide, and chlorhexidine.

SUTURE PASS CULTURE AND CORNEAL BIOPSY

Superficial scrapings may be low yield if the corneal infiltrate is deep in the stroma and nonsuppurative or there is no overlying epithelial defect. Gram-positive bacterial, fungal, and atypical corneal infections, for example, may present with an intact epithelium. In addition, some organisms

TABLE 14.1 ■ Supplies for Corneal Culturing

Anesthetic Drop	Proparacaine or Tetracaine
Culturing instruments	• Platinum Kimura spatulas • Calcium alginate swabs • Curved blades (no. 15 or no. 69) • Cotton swabs wet with thioglycolate
Trypticase soy broth or brain heart infusion	• For dipping calcium alginate swab
Glass slides	• Gram stain for bacteria • Calcofluor stain for fungus and acanthamoeba • Acid-fast for mycobacteria and nocardia
Chocolate plate	• Aerobic and facultative anaerobic bacteria • Haemophilus influenza • Neisseria gonorrhea
Blood agar plate	• Most common pathogens • Aerobic and facultative anaerobic bacteria • Can also grow fungi and non-TB mycobacteria but takes a long time
Brucella agar plate	Anaerobic bacteria
Thioglycolate broth	• Aerobic and anaerobic bacteria • Fungi
Sabouraud (slant) tube	Fungal culture
Lowenstein-Jensen media	Tuberculosis or acid-fast bacterium
Escherichia coli over nonnutrient agar or buffered charcoal yeast extract	Acanthamoeba
Viral transport media	Herpes viral PCR

PCR, Polymerase chain reaction; *TB,* tuberculosis.

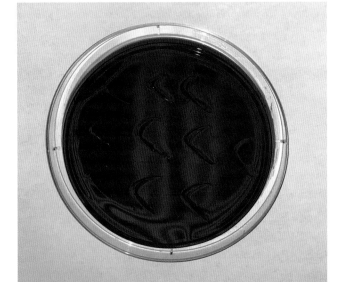

Fig. 14.3 C-streak pattern used to inoculate a blood agar culture plate.

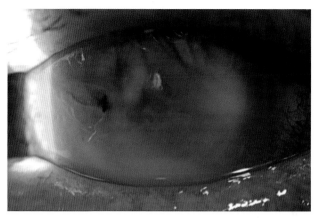

Fig. 14.4 Worsening corneal ulcer with diffuse opacification.

TABLE 14.2 ■ **Supplies for a Suture Pass Culture**

Sterile needle driver
Sterile scissors
Lid speculum
6-0, 7-0, or 8-0 vicryl suture cut to 1-inch long
Thioglycolate broth
Blood or chocolate plate (optional)

such as atypical bacteria and amoeba are very difficult to grow on culture. In cases when multiple cultures have been negative, a suture can be passed through the infiltrate to obtain a culture, or a corneal biopsy can be performed. If the infiltrate is in the center of the cornea, a suture culture can be attempted first. A biopsy obtains more stromal tissue to increase the likelihood of a positive culture and also allows for a pathologic evaluation of organisms. A biopsy should be done as far peripherally as possible while within the infiltrate because it may cause scarring and irregular astigmatism.

PROCEDURE: OBTAINING A SUTURE PASS CULTURE (VIDEO 14.1) ▶

1. Collect all materials (Table 14.2) and label culture media.
2. Position the patient at the slit lamp or lay them back in the exam chair under a microscope. The slit lamp is preferred to allow better judgment of depth.
3. Anesthetize the patient with topical proparacaine and place a lid speculum.
4. Cut the suture to about 1-inch long using sterile scissors. A long suture has a higher risk of getting contaminated across the skin.
5. Very slowly, pass the needle partial thickness through the cornea starting from outside the infiltrate and deep enough through the cornea to exit through the infiltrate. The suture should be pulled though very slowly to maximize yield. It is very important to avoid letting the suture touch the lashes or conjunctiva while passing the needle.

TABLE 14.3 ■ **Table of Supplies for Corneal Biopsy**

Lid speculum
Sterile 2-mm or 3-mm dermatologic punch
Sterile 0.12-mm forceps
Sterile crescent blade or Vannas scissors
Sterile paper (such as glove wrapper)
Formalin pathology specimen container
Sterile saline microbiology specimen container

6. Cut the suture and place in thioglycolate both.
7. (Optional) The needle can be cut off and used to inoculate a culture plate using C-streaks.

PROCEDURE: OBTAINING A CORNEAL BIOPSY (VIDEO 14.2)

1. Lay out all materials (Table 14.3), and label specimen containers.
2. Place a lid speculum after the eye is anesthetized with topical proparacaine. Position the patient at the slit lamp.
3. Use a 2.0-mm or 3.0-mm dermatological punch to slowly trephinate the cornea in the area of the infiltrate by gently twisting the punch with mild pressure against the cornea. The trephine should be done slowly, and the depth should be assessed at the slit lamp. Use the 0.12-mm forceps to lift or gape the edge to evaluate depth. Make sure to trephine deep enough to obtain adequate tissue containing the infiltrate, but not too deep as to cause excessive thinning.
4. Once you have trephinated deep enough, use the 0.12-mm forceps to hold the edge of the biopsy. Use the crescent blade or Vannas scissors to gently cut the biopsy.
5. Place the specimen on sterile paper and spread it out. Cut it in half using sterile scissors.
6. Place the specimen for pathology on the sterile paper, and place the paper in formalin. This allows easier identification of the small sample.
7. Place the specimen for microbiology in the sterile saline or directly into thioglycolate broth.
8. You can also use calcium alginate swabs to culture the floor of the biopsy site and send on additional culture media.
9. Remove the lid speculum.

Conclusion

While collecting the materials to prepare a kit, keep in mind that culturing materials may vary depending on the laboratory. It is important to establish good communication with your institution's pathologist and microbiologist to ensure prompt and accurate processing of your samples. This is especially critical for corneal biopsy specimens, as the media may differ depending on what testing you want to be done. Since eye cultures may only obtain small samples, it is helpful for the microbiologist to know what they should be looking for if you are suspicious of any particular microbe.

Positive culture results range from 32% to 62% in the reported literature.[1-3] This means that our current methods are not perfect and there is a high false-negative rate. If the corneal ulcer is worsening despite treatment, the provider should reevaluate the culture results and consider either a repeat culture or alternative therapy. If the initial culture is negative, the corneal culture should be repeated, and patient compliance with medication should be confirmed. Confocal microscopy can be used to evaluate for fungal hyphae or acanthamoeba cysts. If a repeat culture is still negative, a corneal biopsy can be considered. If a biopsy is also negative and the patient continues to worsen, a therapeutic keratoplasty is the last line of treatment.

If a culture is positive but the patient's infection shows no improvement or worsening despite treatment, the provider should consider resistant organisms, coinfections, or poor patient compliance. A repeat culture should be done after a 24-hour drug holiday. An alternate therapy should be tried, and a therapeutic keratoplasty is again the last line of treatment.

In summary, providers should strive to identify a causative organism as early as possible when presented with an infectious keratitis. If the culture is negative, a suture culture or corneal biopsy may be good options. A good set-up helps to maximize the efficiency of obtaining a culture and the chances of a positive result. Having a culturing kit is essential for any outpatient ophthalmology office that treats infectious corneal keratitis.

References

1. Green M, Apel A, Stapleton F. Risk factors and causative organisms in microbial keratitis. *Cornea*. 2008 Jan;27(1):22–27.
2. Tan SZ, Walkden A, Au L, et al. Twelve-year analysis of microbial keratitis trends at a UK tertiary hospital. *Eye (Lond)*. 2017 Aug;31(8):1229–1236.
3. Jin H, Parker WT, Law NW, et al. Evolving risk factors and antibiotic sensitivity patterns for microbial keratitis at a large county hospital. *Br J Ophthalmol*. 2017 Nov;101(11):1483–1487.

CHAPTER 15

Herpetic Corneal Disease

Neel Vaidya ▪ Shivani Majmudar ▪ Parag A. Majmudar

Introduction

Herpesviridae is a taxonomic family of DNA viruses that cause a variety of disease processes in human and animal hosts. This family of viruses includes herpes simplex virus (HSV, subtypes 1 and 2), varicella-zoster virus (VZV), Epstein-Barr virus, cytomegalovirus, and human herpes virus (subtypes 6, 7, and 8). HSV and VZV are most commonly implicated in ocular disease.[1]

Herpes Simplex Virus

HSV is a double-stranded DNA virus and is subcategorized into HSV-1 and HSV-2 viridae, which differ based on virus-specific antigens. Initial infection occurs with direct contact with infected skin or mucous membranes. The virus then spreads to neuronal cell bodies, where it can lay dormant for many years until reactivation. Ocular disease is most commonly caused by HSV-1. Herpetic keratitis can be subclassified based on the level of corneal tissue involved: epithelial keratitis, stromal keratitis, or disciform (endothelial) keratitis. Keratouveitis involves anterior chamber inflammation in addition to corneal involvement. Loss of corneal sensation and neurotrophic keratitis is a late sequela of prior herpetic infection.[1–3]

HSV epithelial keratitis usually presents with the classic epithelial dendrite, which can be seen with fluorescein staining under cobalt blue light (Fig. 15.1). Rose bengal staining of adjacent epithelium reveals a "terminal bulb" configuration. Dendritic lesions can coalesce to form geographic epithelial defects. Faint stromal opacities corresponding to epithelial dendrites can occur as well.

HSV stromal keratitis usually follows HSV epithelial keratitis, though it can also represent the primary manifestation of infection. HSV stromal keratitis occurs as a result of an intense immune response to herpetic infection. Examination of the affected cornea initially reveals mild stromal haze, which can progress to mid-to-deep stromal infiltrates and can be associated with stromal thinning and melt.

HSV disciform keratitis involves an endothelial immune reaction to HSV antigens and usually presents with diffuse corneal stromal edema. Rarely, corneal epithelial microcystic edema can be present. Up to 50% of cases of disciform keratitis present without prior history of epithelial keratitis.

Neurotrophic keratitis is a late manifestation of prior herpetic epithelial keratitis (among other mechanisms). Loss of corneal sensation leads to persistent epithelial defects, which classically appear with elevated, rounded, heaped-up borders. These persistent defects can lead to progressive scarring, as well as thinning and corneal melting. Neurotrophic defects are also prone to secondary infection and development of ulceration.[1,2,4]

DIAGNOSIS AND MEDICAL MANAGEMENT

The diagnosis of herpes simplex disease is often made clinically. Careful history taking is essential, as proper characterization of onset and quality of symptoms, as well as medical and ocular history,

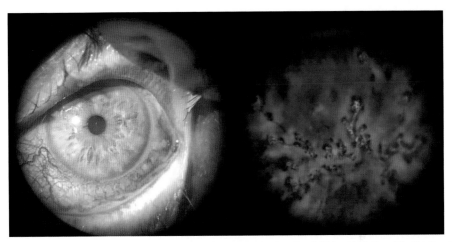

Fig. 15.1   External photograph of an eye affected with herpes simplex virus (HSV) epithelial keratitis (right) and blue light image of the same eye demonstrating classic dendritic-type staining pattern seen in HSV epithelial keratitis. (Images reproduced with the permission of Dean Ouano, MD.)

is crucial to appropriate diagnosis and timely treatment. Full ocular examination including slit lamp exam with corneal staining using lissamine green, rose bengal, and/or fluorescein stains. A dilated fundus examination is necessary as well to rule out posterior segment involvement. Additional diagnostic procedures such as anterior segment paracentesis with viral polymerase chain reaction (PCR) can help confirm a suspected diagnosis and is discussed later in this chapter.[5]

Management of herpes simplex keratitis depends on the type and location of disease. Both topical and systemic formulations of antiviral medications exist and have been used to treat epithelial keratitis. The mainstay of treatment for epithelial disease remains oral antiviral therapy (acyclovir 400 mg orally 5 times daily, valacyclovir 500 mg orally 3 times daily, or famciclovir 250 mg 3 times daily). Topical antiviral agents such as trifluridine drops or ganciclovir gel are also effective and can be used to treat epithelial disease; however, with prolonged use, these medications (specifically trifluridine) can be toxic to the corneal epithelium and limbal stem cells. Long-term (>1 year) prophylactic oral antiviral therapy has been shown to be effective at reducing disease burden in patients who exhibit recurrent epithelial disease.[6] Mechanical debridement of dendritic lesions can be of benefit and is described later in this chapter.

Treatment of stromal keratitis relies on topical steroid therapy with a slow taper to address the inflammatory reaction. Given the long-term toxicity of topical antiviral regimens, oral antiviral therapy is often preferred in conjunction with topical steroids for the treatment of stromal keratitis.[6] The treatment of endothelial (disciform) keratitis is similar to that of stromal keratitis.[6]

Varicella-Zoster Virus

VZV is a human herpes virus. Primary infection with VZV results in varicella ("chickenpox"), whereas herpes zoster (shingles) describes reactivation of VZV in the neurosensory ganglia. Following reactivation, VZV follows the ganglia it presided in and travels to the dermatome innervated by said ganglion. Herpes zoster ophthalmicus (HZO) is the term used when infection with herpes zoster affects the ophthalmic portion of the trigeminal nerve. HZO represents approximately 10%–25% of all cases of herpes zoster.[7]

Preliminary symptoms of herpes zoster include fever, malaise, and chills. A significant indicator of HZO is a vesicular rash that is distributed based on the affected dermatome. Another common manifestation is blepharitis, resulting in edema or inflammation of the eyelid, or conjunctivitis. Approximately 65% of patients develop corneal complications, which pose the greatest threat to vision loss. Patients generally will present with blurry vision, pain, and increased light sensitivity.[8]

DIAGNOSIS AND MEDICAL MANAGEMENT

Epithelial keratitis is one of the earliest ocular manifestations of HZO, presenting as early as 1 to 2 days after the onset of the rash. It appears as multiple swollen lesions upon slit lamp examination and can be stained with rose bengal or fluorescent dye. Dendrites can also appear, generally as elevated plaques of swollen epithelial cells, in contrast to the terminal bulb shape associated with HSV.

HZO stromal keratitis has two stages: anterior and deep. Early stromal involvement typically occurs in the second week after infection and appears as multiple granular infiltrates in the stroma layer of the cornea below the epithelial surface. Infiltrates are believed to arise as a result of the immune response to viral proliferation. Deep stromal keratitis is less common and tends to present approximately 4 months after infection. Most cases present with lesions that have localized areas of inflammation. Corneal edema in the anterior chamber can also be observed.

Neurotrophic keratopathy manifests as a result of virus-mediated nerve destruction, in which patients experience diminished corneal sensation, decreased lacrimation, and delayed epithelial healing. Corneal thinning can be a serious complication, of which the consequences include corneal perforation and increased risk of secondary bacterial infection.[9]

Long-term complications include recurrent neurotrophic ulcers, persistent keratitis that leads to progressive corneal scarring with decreased vision, and neuralgia. Pain that lasts over 1 month can be classified as postherpetic neuralgia and occurs in 10%–30% of patients with HZO. Postherpetic neuralgia is one of the most debilitating complications of HZO and significantly reduces patients' quality of life.

Oral antiviral treatment begun within 72 hours of onset of symptoms can effectively reduce the severity of the disease and minimize risks for long-term complications. Topical antivirals generally are not used. Oral acyclovir (800 mg 5 times daily), valacyclovir (1 g 3 times daily), or famciclovir (500 mg 3 times daily) can be administered at any stage of disease. Corticosteroids can be used to manage keratitis; however, tapering steroid treatment can be challenging. Use should be gradually discontinued, as rapid or abrupt discontinuation can increase the risk of rebound inflammation. Recombinant herpes zoster vaccine is recommended for all adults over the age of 50 years.[10]

Case 1

A healthy 34-year-old male presents with a 2-day history of worsening right eye photosensitivity, conjunctival injection, and blurred vision. The patient denies any history of trauma to the eye or contact lens wear. Visual acuity is 20/100 in the affected eye and 20/20 in the fellow eye. Corneal esthesiometry indicates decreased corneal sensation in the affected eye, and slit lamp examination with fluorescein staining reveals a typical dendrite. The remainder of the slit lamp examination, including fundus exam, is normal. The patient undergoes slit-lamp debridement of the corneal dendrite and is started on topical antibiotic therapy as well as systemic antiviral therapy. Repeat examination 2 weeks later reveals significant improvement in visual acuity (20/25), as well as resolution of the corneal dendrite.

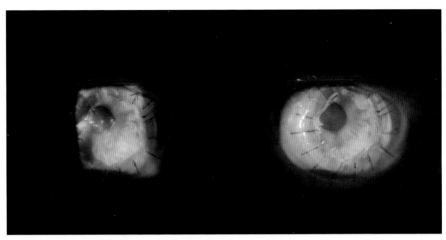

Fig. 15.2 Herpes simplex virus (HSV) epithelial keratitis with dendritic staining pattern prior to debridement (left) and postdebridement (right).

Prior to the advent of the topical antiviral therapies, mechanical debridement of the infected corneal epithelium was the mainstay of treatment for herpetic epithelial keratitis (see Fig. 15.2). With the development of numerous topical antiviral options over the last several decades, the role of epithelial debridement has significantly diminished. Numerous studies have compared mechanical epithelial debridement alone to topical antiviral therapy alone and a combination of debridement and topical antivirals.[11] Parlato et al. compared these procedures in a random-ized, nonplacebo, controlled trial in 1985 and found that debridement alone was statistically less effective than antiviral therapy (trifluridine) alone and combination antiviral therapy and debridement in the number of healed ulcers.[12] Several other studies (Jensen[13] and Herbort[14]), however, concluded that patients treated with a combination of topical antiviral therapy and debridement healed faster than patients treated with topical antiviral therapy alone. Given the paucity of well-powered randomized controlled studies and the variable results available in the published literature, the role of epithelial debridement in the treatment of herpetic epithelial keratitis remains unclear.

Numerous techniques utilizing a variety of commercially available instruments for epithelial debridement have been described. Each technique presents its own advantages and disadvantages; however, data comparing efficacy and complication rates of the various techniques are sparse.

PROCEDURE: VIRAL DEBULKING/DEBRIDEMENT (BOX 15.1A AND 15.1B)

See Video 15.1

POSTPROCEDURE CONSIDERATIONS AND COMPLICATIONS

Patients undergoing viral debulking should be initiated on topical antibiotic therapy in addition to antiviral therapy postprocedure to avoid secondary bacterial superinfection. Complications fol-lowing viral debulking are rare. Corneal haze/scar formation and recurrent epithelial erosions have been reported following epithelial debridement for other indications, including refractive ablations and basement membrane disease. Complications following epithelial debridement for herpetic keratitis have been poorly studied in the literature.[15,16]

BOX 15.1A ■ Supplies

5% povidone-iodine prep solution
Slit-lamp microscope
Lid speculum (optional)
Cotton tip applicator or sponge
Needle (21–25 gauge) (optional)
Blunt spatula (optional)
Kimura platinum spatula
Blade (optional)
    Beaver 57 or 64 blade (Beaver Visitec, Waltham, MA)
    Bard Parker 11 or 15 blade (BD Medical, Franklin Lakes, NJ)
Diamond burr (optional)

BOX 15.1B ■ Procedure

Anesthesia: topical
1. Prep the eye with 5% povidone-iodine solution.
2. Place lid speculum (optional).
3. Under visualization at slit lamp or under operating microscope, simple polishing of the surface of the dendrite with a cotton-tip applicator or blunt spatula is sufficient to debulk the diseased epithelium with active virus from the ocular surface.

Case 2

A 58-year-old female whose past ocular history is significant for corneal ulcer 30 years ago, with resultant scarring, underwent deep anterior lamellar keratoplasty in her left eye. Her best corrected visual acuity (BCVA) improved to 20/40 with a rigid contact lens. After 2 years, the deep anterior lamellar keratoplasty was repeated due to recurrent scarring. Four months following her second transplant, the patient presented with an epithelial dendritic keratitis. Her postoperative course was rocky with recurrent surface inflammation and opacity. Several years later, the patient presented with a central geographic ulceration, which initially responded to topical antivirals but later developed into a persistent epithelial defect. The most likely etiology of the keratopathy was attributed to neurotrophic disease due to a combination of prior HSV keratitis and prior corneal graft. Despite aggressive lubrication, followed by chronic bandage lens usage, there was no significant improvement in the size of the epithelial defect. The decision was made to place an amniotic membrane graft under a bandage contact lens. Two weeks following the procedure, the epithelial defect had resolved.

PROCEDURE: AMNIOTIC MEMBRANE PLACEMENT FOR HERPETIC CORNEAL DISEASE

Method to Affix Amniotic Membrane to Corneal Surface with Suture or Glue

POSTPROCEDURE CONSIDERATIONS AND COMPLICATIONS

For amniotic graft placement with glue or sutures, topical or subconjunctival steroid and antibiotic should be administered. The eye may be pressure patched to promote transplant adherence. Topical antibiotic and steroid drops should be administered for 4 to 6 weeks postprocedurally.

In the immediate postprocedural period, complications include transplant slippage/dehiscence and hematoma formation. Postamniotic membrane transplantation infections are rare but have been reported, with rates as low as 1.6% reported in the literature.[17] One case report of hypopyon development postamniotic membrane transplantation does exist in the literature.[18] Other

---

BOX 15.2A ■ Supplies

Operating microscope
5% povidone-iodine prep solution
Lid speculum
Needle driver
Needle holder
Caliper or ruler
Marking pen
Crescent blade
Vannas scissors
Bipolar cautery
Diamond burr or corneal knife (Tooke, Grieshaber, 64 blade)
Tying forceps
Amniotic membrane
    Fresh cryopreserved
    Dehydrated
8-0, 9-0, or 10-0 suture (absorbable or nonabsorbable)
Fibrin glue (Evicel, Tisseel)

BOX 15.2B ■ Procedure

Anesthesia: topical, subconjunctival, or retrobulbar block
1. Prep the eye with 5% povidone-iodine prep solution
2. Place lid speculum
3. Under visualization through operating microscope, remove affected corneal epithelium (scraping or burr)
4. Measure corneal diameter
5. Measure amniotic membrane: 2 to 3 mm larger than corneal diameter (if using dehydrated amniotic membrane, these will typically be precut to various diameters)
6. Place amniotic membrane graft over cornea stromal side down
7. Affix graft to limbus using interrupted or running suture or tissue glue
    ■ Avoid gaps between host conjunctiva and graft
    ■ Optional: 360-degree peritomy with suturing or gluing of graft to elevated conjunctiva
8. Trim excess graft tissue
9. If using dehydrated amniotic membrane, no glue or suture is required. A bandage contact lens is typically placed over the graft and left in place until the membrane is reabsorbed and epithelium has the corneal surface
    A self-retaining amniotic membrane consists of an amniotic membrane preanchored to a 360-degree polymethyl methacrylate ring that sits in the fornix and provides secure contact of the amniotic membrane with the cornea without the use of sutures, adhesive, or a contact lens.
    No need for microscope; patient can be sitting up in an exam chair.
1. Rinse the amniotic membrane with saline solution prior to insertion
2. Insert ProKera ring into upper and then and lower fornix
    ■ Orient convexity similar to contact lens placement

complications include pain, inflammatory episcleritis/scleritis, suture granuloma, symblepharon formation, premature degeneration of amniotic membrane, and recurrence of pathology. See Video 15.2.

Case 3 (Courtesy of Dean Ouano, MD)

A healthy 63-year-old male with no ocular history works in a cabinet factory and was struck in the left eye with projectile sawdust. He rinsed his eye immediately at a designated eyewash station. He was prescribed erythromycin ointment for a corneal abrasion by a local urgent care facility but developed pain and decreased vision over the next 3 days. The referring optometrist noted counting fingers visual acuity, an intraocular pressure of 42, and 3+ corneal edema. He was referred urgently for "keratitis OS of unknown etiology, r/o fungal."

Examination of the cornea revealed several round, overlapping stromal opacities in the superior cornea, an irregular epithelium inferiorly consistent with a recent corneal abrasion, diffuse stromal edema, and localized microcystic edema. Given the mechanism of injury, fungal keratitis was identified as the likely etiology of the exam findings. The elevated intraocular pressure, however, did not fit with this clinical picture. Given that a clear diagnosis was necessary to ensure appropriate treatment, anterior chamber tap with PCR evaluation for HSV was performed. The PCR returned positive for HSV-1. Following negative fungal culture results, the patient was started on topical steroids (in addition to systemic antiviral therapy and topical intraocular pressure–lowering therapy) with significant improvement in visual acuity and intraocular pressure after 2 weeks of therapy.

Herpes simplex keratouveitis represents a rare manifestation of herpetic ocular disease. HSV keratouveitis usually presents in conjunction with herpetic keratitis, though it can also occur in isolation. In addition to corneal involvement, herpetic keratouveitis can present with granulomatous or nongranulomatous inflammation, iris atrophy, and elevated intraocular pressure secondary to trabeculitis.[19]

While the diagnosis of herpetic keratouveitis is often made clinically, PCR testing for HSV DNA can be a valuable diagnostic tool in situations where a diagnosis is unclear or where diagnostic confirmation is required to drive treatment.[20,21] While studies have shown some utility of PCR of corneal epithelial scraping samples, PCR on aqueous humor has proven to be extremely sensitive and specific for the detection of herpes virus DNA given adequate sample volume and is therefore the preferred sample for this type of testing.[22]

PROCEDURE: ANTERIOR CHAMBER PARACENTESIS AND HERPES SIMPLEX VIRUS PCR TESTING

Method for Anterior Chamber Paracentesis for PCR (Box 15.3A and 15.3B).

Postprocedure Considerations and Complications

Currently, several commercial laboratories in the United States provide PCR testing options for HSV on ocular fluid samples, including Labcorp (Burlington, NC) and Viracor-Eurofins (Lee's Summit, MO). It is advisable to consult the individual laboratory for specific sample volume requirements and handling instructions to ensure the sample is appropriately handled.

Patients undergoing anterior chamber paracentesis should be started on topical antibiotic therapy in addition to antiviral therapy to prevent bacterial superinfection. Rare complications of this procedure include infection/endophthalmitis, hypotony, iris trauma/bleeding, and lens trauma/cataract formation.[20]

BOX 15.3A ■ Supplies

Slit-lamp or operating microscope
5% povidone-iodine prep solution
25-, 27-, or 30-gauge needle on 1cc tuberculin syringe
Paracentesis blade (optional)
27-gauge cannula (optional)
Balanced salt solution (BSS)
Sterile specimen container

BOX 15.3B ■ Procedure (with needle)

Anesthesia: topical
1. Prep the eye with 5% povidone-iodine solution
2. Place lid speculum (optional)
3. Remove plunger from syringe; keep sterile
4. Under visualization at slit lamp or under operating microscope, engage the peripheral cornea with 30-gauge needle with bevel facing posteriorly
5. Advance needle horizontally parallel to the iris plane, taking care to avoid engaging iris with needle tip
6. Monitor for flow of aqueous humor into the syringe. A minimum of 0.05 mL is necessary to ensure an adequate sample for PCR testing
7. Once adequate aqeuous fluid has been obtained, carefully remove needle from anterior chamber
8. Place needle and syringe into sterile specimen container
9. Reinsert plunger into syringe, thereby expelling syringe contents into sterile specimen container

Procedure (with Canula)

Repeat steps 1–2, as above
3. Under visualization at slit lamp or under operating microscope, make a peripheral paracentesis incision through clear cornea using a paracentesis blade
4. Gently enter the anterior chamber with a 27-gauge cannula on a 1-cc tuberculin syringe
5. Slowly withdraw aqueous fluid until a sufficient sample (0.1 mL) is obtained
6. Reform anterior chamber with balanced salt solution if needed
7. Stromal hydrate paracentesis wound if needed
8. Transfer aqueous sample from tuberculin syringe into sterile specimen container

---

References

1. AAO Basic and Clinical Science Course, External Disease and Cornea, 2016–2017, 205–239.
2. Saad S, Abdelmassih Y, Saad R, et al. Neurotrophic keratitis: Frequency, etiologies, clinical management and outcomes. *Ocul Surf.* 2019. *Ocul Surf.* 2019;18(2):231–236.
3. Valerio GS, Lin CC. Ocular manifestations of herpes simplex virus. *Curr Opin Ophthalmol.* 2019; 30(6):525–531.
4. Krachmer J, Mannis M, Holland E. *Cornea.* 2nd ed. Elsevier Mosby; 2005:1043–1074.
5. Azher TN, Yin XT, Tajfirouz D, Huang AJ, Stuart PM. Herpes simplex keratitis: Challenges in diagnosis and clinical management. *Clin Ophthalmol.* 2017;11:185–191.
6. Lee-White M, Chodosh J. Herpes simplex virus keratitis: A treatment guideline – 2014. AAO Clinical Statements. https://www.aao.org/clinical-statement/herpes-simplex-virus-keratitis-treatment-guideline. Accessed 29.06.20.
7. Saad Shaikh, Ta, Christopher N. Evaluation and management of herpes zoster ophthalmicus. *Am Fam Physician.* 2002;66(9):1723–1730.

8. Herpes Zoster Ophthalmicus. Herpetic corneal infections: Herpes zoster ophthalmicus, AAO Focal Points. Accessed 29.06.20.

9. Wakil SM, Ajlan R, Arthurs B. Herpes zoster ophthalmicus complicated by ipsilateral isolated Bell's palsy: A case report and review of the literature. *Can J Ophthalmol*. 2012;47(4):339–343.

10. Roat, Melvin I. Herpes Zoster Ophthalmicus - Eye Disorders. Merck Manuals Professional Edition. Rahway, NJ: Merck Manuals, Aug. 2018.

11. Wilhelmus KR, Coster DJ, Jones BR. Acyclovir and debridement in the treatment of ulcerative herpetic keratitis. *Am J Ophthalmol*. 1981;91:323–327.

12. Parlato CJ, Cohen EJ, Sakauye CM, Dreizen NG, Galentine PG, Laibson PR. Role of débridement and trifluridine (trifluorothymidine) in herpes simplex dendritic keratitis. *Arch Ophthalmol*. 1985;103(5):673–675.

13. Herbort CP, Buechi ER, Matter M. Blunt spatula debridement and trifluorothymidine in epithelial herpetic keratitis. *Curr Eye Res*. 1987;6:225–229.

14. Jensen KB, Nissen SH, Jessen F. Acyclovir in the treatment of herpetic keratitis. *Acta Ophthalmol (Copenh)*. 1982;60:557–563.

15. Mcgrath LA, Lee GA. Techniques, indications and complications of corneal debridement. *Surv Ophthalmol*. 2014;59(1):47–63.

16. Chaudhary O. How is corneal scraping surgery performed? AAO Ask an Ophthalmologist. https://www.aao.org/eye-health/ask-ophthalmologist-q/how-is-corneal-scraping-surgery-performed. 2016. Accessed 29.06.20.

17. Marangon FB, Alfonso EC, Miller D, Remonda NM, Marcus S, Tseng SC. Incidence of microbial infection after amniotic membrane transplantation. *Cornea*. 2004;23:264–269.

18. Gabler B, Lohmann CP. Hypopyon after repeated transplantation of human amniotic membrane onto the corneal surface. *Ophthalmology*. 2000;107:1344–1346.

19. Santos C. Herpes simplex uveitis. *Bol Asoc Med P R*. 2004;96(71–4):77–83.

20. Nakano S, Tomaru Y, Kubota T, et al. Evaluation of a multiplex strip PCR test for infectious uveitis: A prospective multi-center study. *Am J Ophthalmol*. 2019;213:252–259.

21. Fox GM, Crouse CA, Chuang EL, et al. Detection of herpesvirus DNA in vitreous and aqueous specimens by the polymerase chain reaction. *Arch Ophthalmol*. 1991;109(2):266–271. https://doi.org/10.1001/archopht.1991.01080020112054.

22. Chronopoulos A, Roquelaure D, Souteyrand G, Seebach JD, Schutz JS, Thumann G. Aqueous humor polymerase chain reaction in uveitis - utility and safety. *BMC Ophthalmol*. 2016;16(1):189.

CHAPTER 16

Neurotrophic Keratitis or the Nonhealing Epithelial Defect

Deepinder Kaur Dhaliwal ▓ Margaret C. Pollard ▓ Vishal Jhanji

Introduction

Neurotrophic keratitis (NK) is a degenerative corneal disease characterized by reduction or loss of corneal sensitivity due to trigeminal nerve impairment.[1] Etiologies include any ocular, neurological, or systemic process that affects the trigeminal nerve, from its origin in the pons, along its branches to the corneal nerve endings.[2] The most common entities causing NK are herpetic keratitis, which has been estimated to account for up to 1/3 of NK cases.[3] Other etiologies include chemical burns, corneal or limbal surgery, long-term topical medications, systemic diseases such as diabetes, and long-term contact lens wear. Often, the disease is multifactorial[3] (Table 16.1). NK is classified as an orphan disease with an estimated prevalence of less than 1.6 to 4.2 per 10,000 individuals.[1] NK is characterized by corneal epithelial changes ranging from punctate keratopathy to recurrent or persistent epithelial defects (PEDs), which can lead to corneal ulceration, melting, and perforation. Classification of NK based on severity was proposed by Mackie in 1995 and is still used today.[1] Table 16.2 lists the Mackie classification with corresponding clinical findings and treatment options.

Accurate diagnosis of NK is critical and is based on clinical exam. NK is often misdiagnosed as dry eye disease or herpetic keratitis. In a patient with severe epitheliopathy or with a PED, suspicion for NK should be high. Corneal sensitivity must be tested to confirm the diagnosis of NK. Quantitative assessment is performed with a Cochet-Bonnet esthesiometer. Qualitative assessment can be measured by touching the central and peripheral cornea with a cotton wisp or dental floss. Full eyelid evaluation should be performed, including lid position, blink rate, and presence of lagophthalmos. Tear film function and composition should be tested.

Vital dye staining with fluorescein or lissamine green can further evaluate the integrity of the conjunctiva and corneal surface and assist in detection of filaments.

Impression cytology of the cornea and conjunctiva has been used to characterize the epithelial changes associated with NK. In vivo confocal microscopy, though limited by reproducibility and user variability, can directly visualize decreased subbasal nerve plexus that may be present in some patients with NK.

Treatment of NK is notoriously difficult given the underlying loss of neuroprotective reflexes of the cornea and ocular surface. The pathogenesis and natural history are still not fully understood. Corneal nerves maintain ocular surface homeostasis and integrity by producing neurotrophins and facilitating tearing, blinking, and corneal reflexes. This homeostasis is disrupted with trigeminal nerve damage, leading to nerve and epithelial dysfunction. Patients often present in late stages since lack of corneal sensation typically makes this a painless process. Left untreated, NK progresses to severe stages, leading to perforation and vision loss.[4-6]

One breakthrough treatment is approval of recombinant human nerve growth factor. Cenegermin 0.002% (Oxervate) is the first US Food and Drug Administration–approved treatment specifically targeting NK. Its efficacy has been shown in NGF0212/REPARO and NGF0214 trials to improve lasting healing of corneal epithelial defects.[7] The drop is instilled six times daily

TABLE 16.1 ■ **Etiologies of Neurotrophic Keratitis.**

Infectious	Herpes simplex Herpes zoster Leprosy
Ocular pathologies	Chemical burns Chronic contact lens wear Chronic ocular surface injury and inflammation Prolonged use of topical medications and drug toxicity (topical anesthetics, timolol, topical NSAIDs, benzalkonium chloride) Corneal and anterior segment surgery (laser vision correction, corneal or limbal incisions, lamellar or penetrating keratoplasty) Corneal dystrophies, keratoconus
Central nervous system	Intracranial mass (neoplasm, aneurysm, neuroma) Stroke Postneurosurgical procedures (trigeminal neuralgia, acoustic neuroma, or other involving CNV1) Facial trauma
Systemic diseases	Diabetes Multiple sclerosis Vitamin A deficiency
Genetic	Riley-Day syndrome Goldenhar-Gorlin syndrome Mobius syndrome Familial corneal hypoesthesia

NSAID, Nonsteroidal antiinflammatory drug.

for 8 weeks and is approved for all stages of NK. This medical treatment is the only currently approved treatment to address the underlying cause of NK.

Case 1

A 66-year-old male presented for evaluation of a PED of 3 weeks duration. Seven weeks prior, he underwent phacoemulsification with intraocular lens implantation and developed a retinal detachment 3 weeks postoperatively. He underwent successful pars plana vitrectomy with cryotherapy. One week after retinal surgery, he developed an epithelial defect. He was being treated with topical antibiotics, steroids, and nonsteroidal antiinflammatory drugs (NSAIDs). His past ocular history was relevant for high myopia with long-term soft contact lens wear prior to cataract surgery. Initial exam showed a 3.5- by 2-mm central epithelial defect with stromal haze and edema without corneal infiltrate. There was moderate anterior chamber reaction without hypopyon. Peripheral corneal exam showed a mild superficial pannus bilaterally. Corneal sensation was diminished bilaterally both centrally and peripherally. At this time, the working diagnosis of his PED was NK due to multifactorial causes: chronic use of topical NSAIDs, multiple recent ocular surgeries, and long-term contact lens wear.

Initial management included herpes simplex virus 1 and 2 (HSV-1 and HSV-2, respectively) polymerase chain reaction (PCR) testing, which was negative. The edges of the epithelial defect were debrided, and a bandage contact lens was placed. Topical steroids and NSAIDs were stopped immediately, and frequent (every 2 hours) preservative-free artificial tears were initiated. One week later, his epithelial defect was marginally smaller in size. Autologous serum tears were started (50%), and a lower-lid silicone punctal plug was placed. One week later, the epithelial defect was significantly improved. Given PED after these interventions, a 9-mm dehydrated amniotic

TABLE 16.2 ■ Classification of Neurotrophic Keratitis by Stage with Associated Ocular Findings, Treatment Options, and Representative Clinical Photograph.

Stage	Ocular Findings	Treatment Modalities	Representative Image
Stage 1	Punctate keratopathy Superficial corneal haze Corneal edema Epithelial hyperplasia Superficial neovascularization Stromal scarring Decreased tear breakup time Increased viscosity of tear mucous	Discontinuation of topical drops Preservative-free artificial tears Punctal plug placement or punctal cautery Bandage contact lens placement Autologous serum tears Amniotic membrane Treatment of concurrent lid or ocular surface disorders Recombinant nerve growth factor drops (cenegermin)	
Stage 2	Recurrent or persistent epithelial defect Surrounding rim of loose epithelium	Treatment for stage 1 plus: Scleral therapeutic contact lenses Epithelial debridement of defect Tarsorrhaphy: temporary, permanent partial, or complete Sutured amniotic membrane transplantation	
Stage 3	Corneal ulcer Stromal melting Perforation	Treatment for stages 1 and 2 plus: Multilayer amniotic membrane transplantation Conjunctival flap Cyanoacrylate glue for small perforations Lamellar or penetrating keratoplasty	

membrane disc was placed on the cornea under a soft bandage contact lens. Two weeks later, his epithelial defect resolved. He was continued on topical antibiotic, autologous serum drops 50% concentration every 2 hours, and preservative-free artificial tears.

PROCEDURE: EPITHELIAL DEBRIDEMENT

Supplies

- Topical anesthetic drop
- Antibiotic drop
- Cotton-tip applicator
- Jeweler forceps
- Silicone hydrogel or other contact lens

The rolled edges of the epithelial defect act as a barrier to reepithelialization (Fig. 16.1A). Topical anesthetic drops and antibiotics are instilled. The rolled edges are debrided at the slit lamp with either a cotton-tip applicator (Fig. 16.1B) or jeweler forceps, extending to any epithelium that is poorly adherent and easily lifted. Care is taken to preserve as much adherent epithelium as possible given the compromised wound-healing capacity of the cornea. Bandage contact lens placement with concurrent use of fourth-generation fluoroquinolone for antibiotic coverage is recommended. Preservative-free antibiotic drops are preferred.

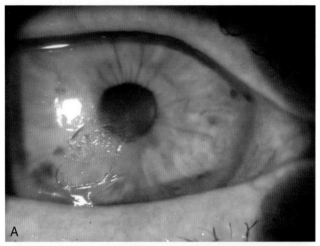

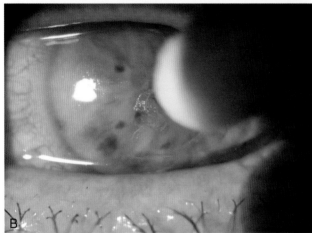

Fig. 16.1 (A–B) Clinical photograph of the rolled edges of an (A) NK epithelial defect and (B) debridement with a cotton-tip applicator.

PROCEDURE: DEHYDRATED AMNIOTIC MEMBRANE PLACEMENT

Supplies

- Topical anesthetic drop
- Antibiotic drop
- Lid speculum
- Jeweler forceps
- Dehydrated amniotic membrane
- Silicone hydrogel contact lens (larger than membrane diameter)

Dehydrated amniotic membrane transplantation (AMT) is a simple in-office procedure that can be implemented if serum drops and/or bandage contact lens alone are not sufficiently improving the size of a PED, or it can be used for severe epitheliopathy without an epithelial defect.[8] The amniotic membrane comes in various sizes, ranging from 8 to 15 mm. A speculum is placed, and a topical anesthetic is used if needed. The amniotic membrane can be placed directly on the PED after the cornea is sufficiently dried. It should be adherent after 2–5 minutes, and adherence can be tested with a dry spear sponge. A silicone hydrogel contact lens larger than the diameter of the AMT is then carefully placed. The patient is seen in approximately 1–2 weeks, and the AMT is generally disintegrated at this point. The bandage contact lens can be removed or kept in place, depending on the clinical picture. This procedure can be repeated as needed.

PROCEDURE: SELF-RETAINING CRYOPRESERVED AMNIOTIC MEMBRANE TRANSPLANTATION (PROKERA)

Supplies

- Topical anesthetic drop
- Blunt-tipped forceps (optional)
- Cotton-tipped applicator (optional)
- Cryopreserved-frozen amniotic membrane (Prokera, Prokera Slim, or other)
- Balanced salt solution (bottle or syringe, approximately 50–100 mL)

Prokera is comprised of a cryopreserved amniotic membrane graft fastened to an ophthalmic conformer; it is self-retaining. The membrane should be brought to room temperature in its packaging before opening, and an aseptic technique is used.

Peel back the inner pouch carefully. Pour out preservation media. Rinse thoroughly with sterile saline solution to remove the remaining preservation media (Video 16.1). A clear central retainer keeps the membrane in place while rinsing. Remove the membrane from its tray and further rinse on all sides. Thorough rinsing improves patient comfort and reduces stinging.

Topical anesthesia is applied. The patient is asked to look down (Fig. 16.2A). With a cotton-tipped applicator or finger, the upper lid is lifted. The Prokera is slid under the upper eyelid into the superior fornix (Fig. 16.2B). The lower eyelid is then pulled down, and the patient looks up. The lower rim is placed in the lower eyelid. Centration is checked at the slit lamp. A tape tarsorrhaphy over the lid can be placed. Antibiotic or other drops can be applied over the membrane. Fluorescein may be used with membrane in place to check healing. The membrane is generally kept in place for 1–2 weeks, and the retaining ring is removed.

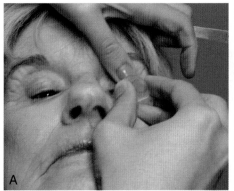
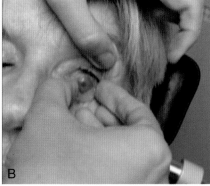

Fig. 16.2 Clinical photographs of (A) looking-down position for placement of a self-retaining cryopreserved amniotic membrane graft and (B) placement of the graft initially into the upper fornix.

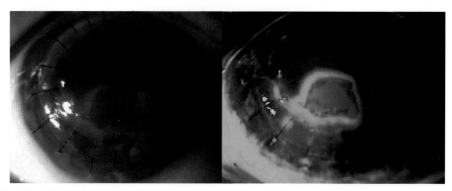

Fig. 16.3 Clinical photographs of neurotrophic epithelial defect with rolled epithelial edges.

DISCUSSION

This is an example of stage 2 NK. Stage 2 NK is characterized by recurrent and/or PED, typically with smooth and rolled edges caused by poor epithelial healing. The defect is classically in an oval or circular shape, most frequently localized centrally or in the superior half of the cornea (Fig. 16.3). The PED is typically surrounded by an area of poorly adherent, opaque, and edematous epithelium that can spontaneously detach and enlarge. Descemet membrane folds and stromal edema may be observed.

Initial conservative treatment includes discontinuation of all possible topical medications, use of frequent preservative-free artificial tears, and treatment of ocular surface diseases such as blepharitis and meibomian gland dysfunction.

Autologous Serum Tears

Autologous serum tears have been used for years for the treatment of severe ocular surface disorders, and multiple studies have shown a benefit in treating nonhealing epithelial defects.[9,10] The precise mechanism is not fully understood. Autologous serum tears have been shown to contain neural factors, including substance P and nerve growth factor, epidermal growth factor, and transforming growth factor β. There is no standardized protocol for the production of autologous serum-based eye drops in the United States. They are classified as blood products and therefore not regulated by the US Food and Drug Administration. In general, serum is obtained by peripheral blood draw with serum-separating tubes. The blood is allowed to clot, after which the serum and solid components of the blood are separated by centrifugation. The serum is then removed and may be diluted with sterile preservative-free normal saline or other eye-compatible solution. Concentration can range from 20% to 100% of serum concentration. Platelet-rich plasma preparations are also possible. Drops must remain frozen until ready for use and be refrigerated while in use. Patients generally instill drops 4–10 times daily.

HSV Testing

HSV should be ruled out in all cases of NK. If PCR is readily available, the conjunctiva can be swabbed with a cotton-tip applicator, or the epithelial defect can be sampled with an applicator or jewelers forceps and sent in viral media. Results typically are available in 24–48 hours. If easy access to PCR testing is not available, HSV-1 and -2 assays are also available. See Chapter 15 for more details.

Case 2

An 82-year-old female presented as a second opinion for a PED. She reported being treated for a corneal ulcer for 2 months. She had a history of V1 zoster with ocular involvement 13 years prior with significant scarring and poor vision in the affected eye for many years. She had no recent

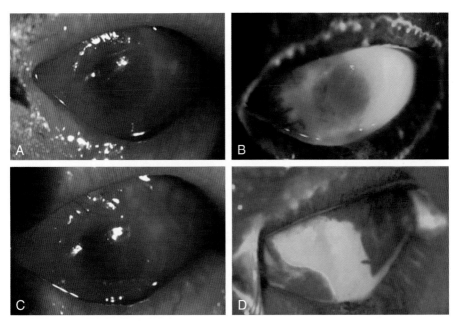

Fig. 16.4 (A–B) Stage 3 NK with significant stromal melting and large epithelial defect with temporary nasal tarsorrhaphy. (C–D) Clinical appearance 2 weeks after initiation of treatment with autologous serum tears. Note improvement in size of epithelial defect.

ocular flares. Her previous treatment included placement of a self-retained amniotic membrane followed by a temporary nasal tarsorrhaphy. On initial exam, her cornea revealed a large central epithelial defect with at least 50% melting with fibrinous material on the surface of epithelial defect. There was deep 360 degree stromal neovascularization with stromal haze and no active infiltrate. She had no corneal sensation in the affected eye (Fig. 16.4A and B).

She was started on 50% serum eye drops 6 times a day in the left eye (OS), moxifloxacin eye drops four times a day, and acyclovir 400 mg twice daily (BID). Viral PCR was negative. Two weeks later, her epithelial defect was improved in size (Fig. 16.4C and D). One month after onset, the initial epithelial defect healed; however, a new epithelial defect was noted. At this time, a complete tarsorrhaphy was performed, which was kept in place for 2 months. Following this time, the tarsorrhaphy was partially opened, and there was no frank epithelial defect. She was continued on serum drops, erythromycin ointment at bedtime, and moxifloxacin; prophylactic oral antiviral will be continued indefinitely.

PROCEDURE: BOTULINUM A TOXIN TARSORRHAPHY (BOTOX TARSORRHAPHY)

Supplies

- Alcohol prep pad or povidone-iodine
- Botulinum toxin A vial (50 units)
- Sterile saline vial
- 18-gauge needle
- 30-gauge needle or similar
- 1-mL syringe

Botulinum A toxin can be injected into the levator superioris palpebrae to induce temporary ptosis. The area is prepped and cleaned. The injection is performed at the level of the superior orbital rim in the mid-pupil plane. The botulinum toxin can be reconstituted with sterile saline. Typically, 50 units are in the vial. To achieve concentration of a 5 U/0.1 mL, 1 mL of sterile saline is drawn up with an 18-gauge needle and injected into the vial. The toxin should be gently reconstituted, not shaken vigorously. The reconstituted toxin is then drawn up in a 1-mL syringe with a 30-gauge needle or similar. The needle is introduced horizontally just below the superior orbital rim in the mid-pupillary plane. Then, 0.1–0.2 mL (5–10 U) of the reconstituted toxin is injected slowly into the levator palpebrae superioris muscle. During the injection, the eye can be kept open and in primary position. Five to 10 units can also be injected in a similar fashion to the lateral horn of the levator muscle. The amount needed for complete ptosis varies; 5–15 units are usually sufficient, but repeat injection may be necessary.

Complete ptosis takes, on average, 4 days to take effect and lasts for approximately 2–3 months. The benefits of this technique are the avoidance of incisions on the lid margin, which minimizes scarring and trichiasis. The eyelid can be easily lifted for examination of the cornea. Risks include temporary weakness of the superior rectus muscle. Patients may need to be followed initially to assess for complete ptosis. If incomplete ptosis, repeat injection may be necessary.

PROCEDURE: PERMANENT TARSORRHAPHY

Supplies (Fig. 16.5)

- Povidone-iodine
- Local anesthetic of choice (e.g., 2% lidocaine with epinephrine)
- 4- by 4-inch gauze pads and cotton-tipped applicators
- Needle driver
- 0.12-mm forceps
- Wescott scissors and/or no. 15 blade
- Suture: for posterior closure: 5-0 or 6-0 polyglactin. For anterior closure, 6-0 plain gut or polypropylene

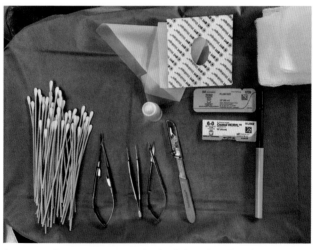

Fig. 16.5 Surgical tray setup for permanent tarsorrhaphy. Cotton-tipped applicators, needle driver, 0.12-mm forceps, Wescott scissors, no. 15 blade (optional), gauze pads, surgical drape, surgical marking pen, and choice of sutures.

Permanent tarsorrhaphy may be indicated for large epithelial defects or ulcers expected to persist long term. Permanent tarsorrhaphy may be placed at any point along the lid margin with varying degrees of lid closure. The desired length of the tarsorrhaphy should be marked first prior to injecting local anesthetic. The goal is to produce a permanent firm adhesion between the upper and lower eyelids. To do this, the epithelium of the eyelid margins must be removed either by splitting the anterior and posterior lamellae or removing the mucocutaneous junction along the posterior lamella without lid splitting. The authors prefer removing the posterior mucocutaneous junction without lid splitting (Fig. 16.6A and B). Generally, 5-0 or 6-0 polyglactin suture is used for the closure of the posterior lamellae in an interrupted fashion (Fig. 16.6C and D). The anterior lamella can be closed with a variety of suture materials; Nylon, polyglactin, polypropylene, plain gut, or silk suture can be used in an interrupted or running fashion, based on the surgeon's preference. If using nonabsorbable sutures, they may be removed in approximately 2 weeks. Permanent tarsorrhaphy can be surgically reversed, but the eyelid margin may sustain lid margin scarring, cicatricial entropion, trichiasis, and distichiasis.

PROCEDURE: TEMPORARY BOLSTER TARSORRHAPHY

Supplies

- Povidone-iodine
- Local anesthetic of choice (e.g., 2% lidocaine with epinephrine)
- 4- by 4-inch gauze pads and cotton-tipped applicators
- Needle driver
- 0.12-mm forceps
- Wescott scissors
- Suture: 4-0, 5-0, or 6-0 nonabsorbable suture (polypropylene, nylon, or silk)
- Bolster material: plastic, rubber, or foam material, cut into 2 by 2 cm lengthwise

Temporary bolster tarsorrhaphy is performed by placing horizontal mattress sutures with rubber or plastic bolsters through the upper and lower eyelids. The bolster simply prevents the suture from cutting into the skin when the knot is tied.

Anesthetize the upper and lower eyelids. Prep the area with povidone-iodine. Prepare two bolsters of equal size, approximately 2 cm lengthwise. The size can be larger or smaller depending on the size of the desired closure. Bolsters can be fashioned from a variety of materials: sterile plastic tubing, catheters, butterfly cannula, or foam inserts from suture material packaging.

Pass one needle of a double-armed nonabsorbable suture straight through one of the bolsters, approximately 2 mm from the end. Line up the bolster in the desired area of the eyelid and pass the same needle into the upper eyelid skin 3–4 mm above the lid margin, through the tarsal plate, and out of the gray line of the lid margin. Pass the same needle into the gray line of the lower lid, into the tarsal plate, and out of the skin 2–3 mm below the lower eyelid margin. Align the lower-lid bolster, and pass the needle through it 2 mm from the end. Pass the other needle of the double-armed suture in the same sequence: through the upper bolster, then the upper lid, then the lower lid, and, finally, through the lower bolster. If a single-armed suture is being used, the needle can be passed from the lower bolster back up to the upper bolster. The suture can either be knotted or tied in a slipknot so that the knot can be loosened for examination. The suture can be kept in place for 2–8 weeks. Depending on the degree and location of the epithelial defect, this can be performed nasally, laterally, or centrally. Generally, patients with NK will need long-term therapies, so temporary tarsorrhaphy may be of limited benefit.

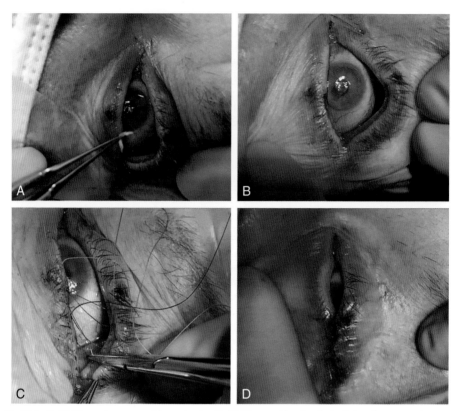

Fig. 16.6 (A–D) Steps of permanent tarsorrhaphy. (A–B) After marking the desired size, the mucocutaneous junction is removed with Wescott scissors (or no. 15 blade) on the upper and lower eyelids. (C) A polyglactin suture is passed through the tarsus in an interrupted fashion. For visualization, all sutures can be left long and tied at the end. (D) Final appearance of 50% tarsorrhaphy at completion of the procedure.

DISCUSSION

In this patient with a poor visual potential from a severe corneal scar and a history of herpetic keratitis, a tarsorrhaphy provides coverage of the ocular surface by immobilizing the lid and decreasing the width of the palpebral fissure.

Depending on the anticipated time needed for healing, a temporary or permanent tarsorrhaphy can be performed.

Case 3

A 58-year-old female presented to the emergency room with acute loss of vision and severe eye pain. Three days prior, she underwent superficial keratectomy with cryopreserved AMT and bandage contact lens placement for presumed corneal epithelial basement membrane dystrophy. She had been treated with chronic topical steroid drops in both eyes for 2 years for management of severe dry eye disease. Her past medical history was relevant for uncontrolled type 2 diabetes, (last HgBA1C, 12.8%), hypertension, morbid obesity, and current smoker of 1 pack per day for 40 years.

Initial exam of the affected eye showed light perception vision, 4+ conjunctival injection, and a total corneal epithelial defect total with corneal infiltrate. There was surrounding stromal haze and 1 mm hypopyon. B-scan ultrasonography showed no vitritis. She was started on moxifloxacin every 2 hours. Corneal cultures were obtained and returned growing *Pseudomonas aeruginosa* sensitive to ciprofloxacin and tobramycin; HSV PCR was negative. Due to her severe ulcer and inability to administer drops at home, she was admitted to the hospital for close observation and drop administration for 1 week. She was started on fortified tobramycin drops and ciprofloxacin drops every hour around the clock. For corneal wound healing, she was started on doxycycline 50 mg BID and vitamin C 1 g daily. Autologous serum tears were started 1 day later. Over the next 2 weeks, her large epithelial defect slowly improved but then acutely worsened (Fig. 16.7A and B). A dehydrated amniotic membrane was placed. She was continued on antibiotics and serum drops. Corneal sensation was tested in both eyes and found to be diminished bilaterally centrally and peripherally.

Six weeks after presentation, there was PED about 6 mm in diameter. The active corneal infiltrate was resolving, and there was early stromal thinning. Her inflammatory reaction was significant with circumferential stromal vascularization and fibrinous anterior chamber reaction. Given the improving infection but PED and inflammatory response, cryopreserved amniotic membrane was sutured over the cornea with a large-diameter contact lens (18 mm) placed. Ten days later, there was still a large epithelial defect and hypopyon/fibrinous clot in the anterior chamber, intrastromal hemorrhages from corneal vascularization, and progressive stromal melting. A multilayered amniotic membrane was glued and then sutured in a minor procedure room. Fourteen days later, the epithelial defect finally resolved. There were stable areas of stromal thinning (Fig. 16.7C). Once the epithelial defect was resolved, a topical steroid was started to control the intraocular and corneal inflammation. The patient was seen weekly for the next 2 weeks to monitor the cornea for recurrence of epithelial defect on topical steroids. Antibiotics were continued, and the bandage contact lens was removed. She was continued on serum drops. One month later, her epithelial defect remained resolved with almost total stromal opacification and improved corneal neovascularization (Fig. 16.7D). Steroids were tapered off and serum drops continued. Given her previous good vision in this eye, she is scheduled for full-thickness corneal transplantation with partial tarsorrhaphy and sutured amniotic membrane graft. Smoking cessation and glycemic control were stressed.

PROCEDURE: SUTURED SINGLE-LAYER AMNIOTIC MEMBRANE TRANSPLANTATION

Supplies

- Povidone-iodine
- Surgical drapes
- Anesthetic for subconjunctival injection (e.g., preservative-free lidocaine)
- Topical anesthetic drop
- Amniotic membrane of choice
- Tying or nontoothed forceps
- Colibri or 0.12-mm forceps
- Curved needle driver
- 8-0 polyglactin suture
- Spear sponges

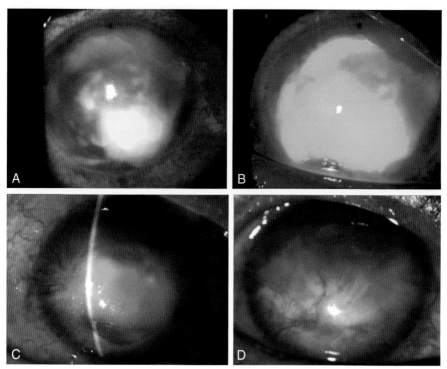

Fig. 16.7 (A–B) Severe *Pseudomonas* corneal infiltrate with large persistent epithelial defect 2 weeks after superficial keratectomy. (C) Two months later, stromal melting and neovascularization but healed epithelial defect. (D) Three months after presentation, epithelium remains healed; stromal neovascularization and inflammation is improved.

This procedure can be performed in an office minor procedure room with proper patient selection or in the operating room. The eye is prepped and draped in the usual sterile fashion. An eyelid speculum is placed. A perilimbal subconjunctival injection provides local anesthesia.

The amniotic membrane is the innermost, avascular layer of the placenta; it consists of a monolayer of cuboidal epithelium, basement membrane, and stromal layer. Cryopreserved amniotic membrane is thawed immediately before use. Generally, the epithelial layer is lost with cryopreservation. The tissue is stored on carrier paper within a peel pouch and can be cut to size for use. The stromal side of the tissue is attached to the carrier paper and should be oriented to face the cornea after peeling it from the carrier paper (Video 16.2). It is possible to determine the orientation of the graft after it has been removed; a dry surgical sponge will stick to the stromal side but not to the basement membrane side. Next, the membrane is gently smoothed using nontoothed instruments. Polyglactin or nylon sutures are placed at each corner and along each side of the membrane in an interrupted fashion or a running purse-string fashion. Typically, at least 8 sutures are necessary to keep the membrane taut. Episcleral or superficial scleral bites ensure adequate tension of the membrane. Tightness of sutures and membrane play an important role in fixation of the graft. A bandage contact lens should be placed over the membrane and sutures to protect it from mechanical trauma and improve patient comfort (Fig. 16.8).

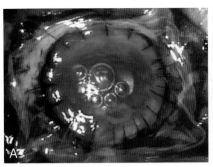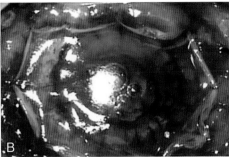

Fig. 16.8 (A–B) Sutured cryopreserved amniotic membrane transplantation. (A) Appearance of membrane after placement stromal-side down. Excess can then be trimmed before or after suture placement. (B) Appearance of membrane after suturing with polyglactin sutures with approximately 8 sutures, ensuring membrane is taut. Sutures are typically perilimbal; in this case with conjunctival scarring, a larger area was sutured. A bandage contact lens should be placed with a diameter large enough to cover all suture tails.

PROCEDURE: MULTILAYER SUTURED AMNIOTIC MEMBRANE TRANSPLANTATION

Supplies

- Povidone-iodine
- Surgical drapes
- Anesthetic for subconjunctival injection (e.g., preservative-free lidocaine)
- Topical anesthetic drop
- Amniotic membrane
- Tying forceps
- Colibri or 0.12-mm forceps
- Curved needle driver
- 8-0 polyglactin suture
- Fibrin glue
- Spear sponges

This procedure is similar to single-layer sutured amniotic membrane. The first layer of the amniotic membrane is cut to the size of the epithelial defect and peeled off the carrier paper. The amniotic membrane is then glued in place stromal-side down with fibrin glue; any loose edges should be trimmed. The fibrin glue is placed sparingly and sequentially via separate syringes of the thrombin and fibrinogen components. The authors prefer placing a small drop of the thicker component followed by a small drop of the thinner component, working quickly to smooth the membrane in place in the next 5 seconds after administration of glue. This step can be repeated multiple times to create a multilayered patch over an area of deep ulceration. Each layer much be fully dried and adherent before applying a new layer. The remaining larger amniotic membrane is smoothed over the cornea and sutured at the limbus with polyglactin or nylon sutures, and a bandage contact lens is placed. Since the uppermost layer is the only layer sutured in place, proper tension is key for maintaining the position of the glued layers underneath (Fig. 16.9A–E).

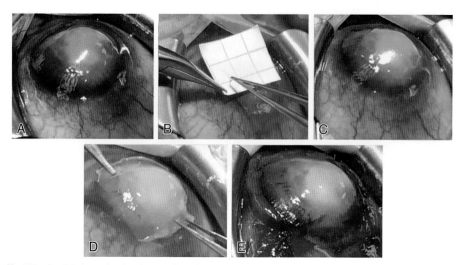

Fig. 16.9 Double-layer glued and sutured amniotic membrane. (A) Preoperative appearance with large central epithelial defect with stromal melting. (B) The amniotic membrane is cut to the size of the epithelial defect and peeled off the carrier paper. (C) The amniotic membrane is glued in place with fibrin glue. Any loose edges can be trimmed. (D–E) The remaining amniotic membrane is smoothed over the cornea (D) and is sutured securely at the limbus (E).

DISCUSSION

Stage 3 NK is characterized by a corneal ulcer with stromal involvement that may be complicated by stromal melting and progression to corneal perforation. In this case, an elective procedure created an epithelial defect that became severely infected and difficult to control. An inflammatory reaction in the anterior chamber may be present. Treatments are more invasive and are aimed at preventing progressive stromal melting and perforation.

In this severe case, it took almost 2 months for the epithelium to heal and to control the infectious keratitis. In prolonged epithelial healing, the immune response can be overwhelming. Topical steroids should be avoided until the epithelium is healed and atypical infection is ruled out (acanthamoeba, fungus).

In this case, corneal cultures were helpful in identifying the persistent bacterial isolate. Bacterial sensitivities helped tailor therapy and minimize unnecessary drop toxicity.

This case illustrates an important point: in severely dry ocular surfaces, corneal sensitivity must be tested prior to performing any elective surgery.

Partial or complete tarsorrhaphy may be necessary in some cases. Conjunctival flap should be considered in eyes with limited visual potential.

Microperforations and small perforations may be managed with cyanoacrylate glue. Deep ulcers with thinning and/or refractory to conventional treatments have been shown to stabilize with sutured single-layer or multilayer amniotic membrane placement. The exact mechanism of action of amniotic membrane is multifactorial and still being studied. The amniotic membrane contains trophic factors that regulate corneal wound healing. In addition, the membrane may integrate into the stroma and promote epithelialization and long-term stromal remodeling. This may delay or possibly avoid the need for incisional surgery. Ultimately, lamellar or penetrating keratoplasty may be necessary for large perforations. These are considered "last-resort" options given the higher failure rates of corneal transplantation in patients with NK.

Conclusion

NK is a degenerative corneal disease characterized by reduction or loss of corneal sensitivity due to trigeminal nerve impairment. Etiologies vary, including any ocular, neurological, or systemic process that affects the trigeminal nerve, with herpetic keratitis being the most common cause. Characteristic corneal epithelial changes range from punctate keratopathy to recurrent or PEDs to corneal ulceration, melting, and perforation. Accurate diagnosis of NK is critical and is based on clinical exam; corneal sensitivity must be tested to confirm the diagnosis. Treatment of NK is notoriously difficult given the underlying loss of neuroprotective reflexes of the cornea and ocular surface. Left untreated, NK progresses to severe stages, leading to perforation and vision loss.

References

1. Bonini S, Rama P, Olzi D, Lambiase A. Neurotrophic keratitis. *Eye (Lond)*. 2003;17(8):989–995.
2. Groos EB. Jr. Neurotrophic keratitis. In: Krachmer JH, Mannis MJ, Holland EJ, eds. *Cornea: Clinical Diagnosis and Management*. St Louis, MO, USA: Mosby; 1997.
3. Hsu HY, Modi D. Etiologies, quantitative hypoesthesia, and clinical outcomes of neurotrophic keratopathy. *Eye Contact Lens*. 2015;41(5):314–317.
4. Kaufman SC. Anterior segment complications of herpes zoster ophthalmicus. *Ophthalmology*. 2008;115 (2 Suppl):S24–S32.
5. Kowtharapu BS, Stachs O. Corneal cells: fine-tuning nerve regeneration. *Curr Eye Res*. 2019 Oct 18:1–12.
6. Mackie IA. Neuroparalytic keratitis. In: Fraunfelder F, Roy FH, Meyer SM, eds. *Current Ocular Therapy*. Philadelphia, PA, USA: WB Saunders; 1995.
7. Sheha H, Tighe S, Hashem O, Hayashida Y. Update on cenegermin eye drops in the treatment of neurotrophic keratitis. *Clin Ophthalmol*. 2019;13:1973–1980.
8. McDonald MB, Sheha H, Tighe S, et al. Treatment outcomes in the Dry Eye Amniotic Membrane (DREAM) study. *Clin Ophthalmol*. 2018 Apr 9;12:677–681.
9. Shtein RM, Shen JF, Kuo AN, Hammersmith KM, Li JY, Weikert MP. Autologous serum-based eye drops for treatment of ocular surface disease: A report by the American Academy of Ophthalmology. *Ophthalmology*. 2020 Jan;127(1):128–133.
10. Tsubota K, Goto E, Shimmura S, Shimazaki J. Treatment of persistent corneal epithelial defect by autologous serum application. *Ophthalmology*. 1999 Oct;106(10):1984–1989.

CHAPTER 17

Peripheral Ulcerative Keratitis

Julie Marie Schallhorn ■ Kareem Moussa ■ Miel Sundararajan

Introduction

The presentation of any patient with peripheral ulcerative keratitis (PUK) to the clinic may induce a sense of panic within the examining clinician, and not without good cause. Of all the conditions that may present to an ophthalmologist, PUK has the potential to be the most grave for both the patient and the eye. Appropriate management of the patient with PUK is essential to save vision and, in many cases, the patient's life.

Finding the Underlying Cause

The differential diagnosis for PUK is broad and encompasses many serious diseases (Table 17.1). Numerous systemic autoimmune disorders have PUK as a manifestation, as do many disorders that are localized to the eye. In addition to these systemic disorders, there are many infectious causes of PUK and scleritis that must be ruled out as well.

Approximately half the time, PUK is associated with a systemic vasculitic disease.[1] The most common systemic association is rheumatoid arthritis, but a number of other autoimmune etiologies have been implicated, including granulomatosis with polyangiitis (GPA, formerly known as Wegener vasculitis), polyarteritis nodosa, Coogan syndrome, systemic lupus erythematosus, relapsing polychondritis, eosinophilic GPA (Churg-Strauss syndrome), Behcet disease, inflammatory bowel disease, autoimmune hepatitis, and scleroderma.[2-5]

It is especially critical to properly diagnose patients with GPA, as patients with eye involvement in this condition have significantly elevated mortality—up to a 50% risk of mortality at 5 months.[6] A careful and systematic approach to evaluation and diagnosis is necessary to ensure that any potential serious diseases are properly diagnosed and infectious causes are properly treated.

Notably, infectious causes have also been implicated in PUK, including varicella-zoster virus (VZV) and herpes simplex viruses (HSV), acanthamoeba,[7] fungal infections, many bacterial species, syphilis, tuberculosis, as well as others.[3]

Mooren ulcer, which is thought to be an idiopathic cause of PUK, has been associated with hepatitis B and C as well as intestinal helminthiasis,[8-10] although the association with hepatitis C has been called into question.[11] Rosacea has also been associated with PUK and scleritis. In the postoperative setting, infectious and autoimmune causes should be ruled out; surgically induced necrotizing scleritis (SINS) is a diagnosis of exclusion.[12]

History and Exam

Once PUK is suspected, a careful history should be undertaken to elicit any other findings that could hold a clue to the underlying diagnosis. Symptoms of pain, redness, photophobia, and decreased vision should be assessed. Questions specific to the following should be included: a history of autoimmune or inflammatory disease, malignancy, infectious diseases (including

TABLE 17.1 ■ Differential Diagnosis of Peripheral Ulcerative Keratitis

Entity	Clinical Diagnoses
Vaculitic/autoimmune	Autoimmune hepatitis
	Behcet disease
	Coogan syndrome
	Eosinophilic granulomatosis with polyangiitis
	Granulomatosis with polyangiitis
	Inflammatory bowel disease
	Polyarteritis nodosa
	Relapsing polychondritis
	Rheumatoid arthritis
	Systemic lupus erythematosus
	Sarcoidosis
	Scleroderma
Infectious	Bacterial
	Fungal
	Herpes simplex
	Herpes zoster
	Acanthamoeba
	Syphilis
	Tuberculosis
Other	Rosacea
	Mooren ulcer
	Surgical-induced scleral necrosis
	Mechanical/dellen

sexually transmitted diseases, viral hepatitis, and intestinal parasites), recent illness, sinus disease or epistaxis, rashes or joint pains, travel, and consumption of raw or undercooked food. Specific questions pertaining to surgical history of intraocular surgery should be elicited given the potential for surgically induced necrotizing scleritis (SINS) or postoperative infectious keratitis and scleritis. The use of antimetabolites such as mitomycin C should be investigated. Any contact lens wear or trauma to the eye should be noted.

The patient's medications should be reviewed, as drugs such as bisphosphonates can be associated with scleritis.[13] A review of systems should also be undertaken to elicit signs of any new-onset autoimmune disorders. This should encompass all systems, as there is commonly multiorgan involvement. Specific questions pertaining to vasculitic processes, including arthralgia, new onset rashes, sinusitis or nosebleeds, tinnitus/hearing loss, cartilaginous tenderness over the nose and ears, and hemoptysis, should be included. Night sweats, fevers, weight loss, and general malaise should also be included, as these can be present in many autoimmune disorders as well as in tuberculosis.

A thorough ocular surface examination is appropriate in this setting. As rosacea can be associated with PUK, a careful exam of the lids, Meibomian glands, and lashes should be undertaken, with attention to lid position, lid margin telangectasias, blepharitis, or other lid irregularities. Lid eversion should be performed in all cases to evaluate for concurrent conjunctivitis or foreign bodies. The sclera and conjunctiva should be evaluated for concurrent scleritis or evidence of old scleritis, as PUK often travels hand in hand with this condition. The area of ulceration should be carefully examined with the slit lamp, and the epithelial defect should be measured. The degree of thinning should be noted, with Seidel testing if there is concern for perforation. Its location on the limbus should be examined with respect to the location of the lids. Infiltrate size and location, if present, should be noted and cultured (see Culture).

The remainder of the exam should be directed toward evaluating the rest of the eye for evidence of inflammatory disorders. A careful evaluation of the anterior chamber, iris, vitreous, and retina should be performed.

The location, nature, and associated findings of PUK can often give clues as to the underlying diagnosis. Inferior ulceration at the overlap of the lids on the limbus is more likely to represent an infectious cause or rosacea. Temporal or nasal ulceration in the setting of prior pterygium removal may represent infectious scleritis and keratitis but may also occur from heaping of the limbal tissue inducing a corneal dellen.

Imaging

Imaging of the cornea and sclera provides an objective measurement of tissue thinning, which is a hallmark feature of the disease, and can be used to assess disease severity and response to treatment. Anterior segment optical coherence tomography (AS-OCT), ultrasound pachymetry, and Pentacam Scheimpflug imaging are three distinct modalities that are commonly used to assess corneal thickness. In a recent study that compared corneal thickness estimation by fellowship-trained human graders to these three modalities, AS-OCT measurements were, on average, 10% thicker, ultrasound pachymetry measurements 20% thinner, and Scheimpflug measurements 10% thinner than human graders.[14] The reproducibility of these measurements was excellent, and AS-OCT, which is widely available in the United States, had the highest intraclass correlation coefficient. In a study of two patients with PUK followed longitudinally with AS-OCT, there was significant improvement in corneal thickness with control of the disease.[15]

Patients with PUK typically have concomitant involvement of the cornea and sclera. AS-OCT evaluation of the sclera in active anterior scleritis reveals scleral thickening and pockets of intrascleral edema.[16] In necrotizing scleritis, in which loss of tissue is a key feature, AS-OCT can be particularly helpful in evaluating the extent of tissue loss. Fig. 17.1A shows a case of active

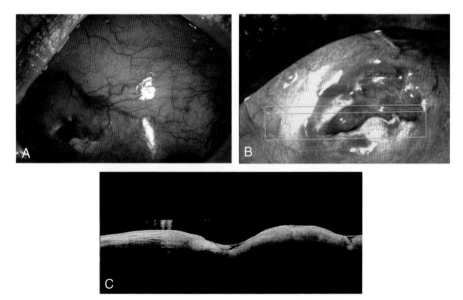

Fig. 17.1 Active scleritis in a patient with rheumatoid arthritis with scleral thinning without perforation demonstrated on color photograph (A) and anterior segment optical coherence tomography (AS-OCT) (B and C).

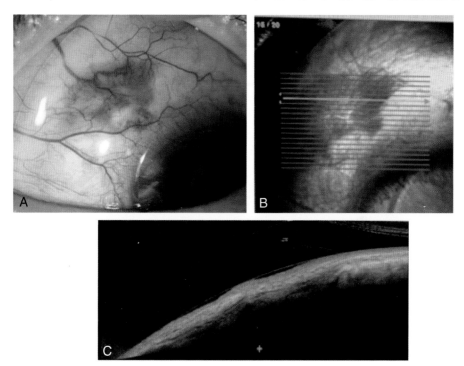

Fig. 17.2 Resolution of active scleritis of same patient as in Fig. 17.1. (A) The area of thinning is now epithelialized. (B–C) Note that the sclera looks much thicker on OCT. This is not due to regrowth of scleral fibers but, rather, to epithelialization and rehydration of the sclera.

necrotizing anterior scleritis in which it is difficult to determine if the sclera is thin and intact or perforated. Fig. 17.1B shows an AS-OCT image that confirms the sclera is quite thin but has not yet perforated. In the 3-month follow-up after treatment with oral corticosteroid and subcutaneous methotrexate injections, the scleritis has resolved on clinical exam (Fig. 17.2A), and AS-OCT shows significant improvement in scleral thickness in the area of previous necrosis (Fig. 17.2B). AS-OCT is a valuable tool for monitoring structural changes in the cornea and sclera in a wide variety of disorders, including PUK.

Culture

Microbial keratitis may also present with peripheral corneal melt or scleritis and should remain on the differential diagnosis, particularly in the postsurgical setting.[17–19] Thus, careful cultures of the affected area should be undertaken. Bacterial cultures should be performed on blood and chocolate agar. Fungal cultures may be taken on Sabouraud dextrose or potato flake agar. Acanthamoeba can be cultured using nonnutrient agar with *Escherichia coli* overlay. Viral agents such as herpes simplex and herpes zoster can be detected using polymerase chain reaction (PCR). Gram and fungal stain, i.e., via KOH (Potassium hydroxide) prep or Gomori methamine silver stain, should be sent as well for early identification of causative organisms. For refractory cases of scleritis, a scleral biopsy may be required to establish a diagnosis.[18]

TABLE 17.2 ■ Laboratory Studies for Peripheral Ulcerative Keratitis Workup

Laboratory studies
Complete blood count
Complete metabolic panel
Antinuclear antibody
Rheumatoid factor
Anticyclic citrullinated peptide antibodies
Antineutrophil cytoplasmic antibodies
Rapid plasma reagin
Fluorescent treponema antibody
Interferon-gamma release assay or purified protein derivative
Hepatitis B/C panel
Chest radiograph

Laboratory Workup

A thorough yet targeted laboratory investigation should be performed (Table 17.2). A baseline complete blood count and complete metabolic panel should be routinely performed to evaluate for renal and hepatic disease. Antinuclear antibody, rheumatoid factor, and anticyclic citrullinated peptide antibodies (anti-CCP) should be performed to assess for autoimmune conditions, particularly rheumatoid arthritis.[20–22] Antineutrophil cytoplasmic antibodies (ANCA) should be checked, as ANCA-associated vasculitides such as GPA may be associated.[21] A chest radiograph should be performed to evaluate for findings of granulomatous diseases, including sarcoidosis.[23] Infectious causes such as syphilis and tuberculosis should also be ruled out, specifically with both rapid plasma reagin and fluorescent treponema antibody for syphilis and interferon-gamma release assay or purified protein derivative for tuberculosis.[22,24–26] Viral hepatitis studies for hepatitis B and C should also be performed, given the possible association with Mooren ulcer.

Management

As with any ulcerative condition, the clinician's major directive for the cornea is to treat the underlying cause, assist epithelial healing, and prevent perforation.

MEDICAL THERAPY

Autoimmune Causes of PUK

Patients that are diagnosed with systemic autoimmune disease will require initiation or escalation of systemic immunosuppressive therapy to control their disease. This is of the utmost importance, as many conditions associated with PUK have a significantly elevated mortality risk. Prior to initiation, however, the clinician must rule out the coexistence of syphilis and tuberculosis, which can both masquerade as an autoimmune disease and are made significantly worse with immunosuppressive therapy. Likewise, hepatitis C should also be evaluated prior to starting systemic therapy and treated if present.

The initiation of oral prednisone, 1 mg/kg to start, will quickly bring most inflammatory conditions under control. However, for severe inflammation or pending perforation, pulse-dosed intravenous methylprednisolone (brand name Solumedrol), 1 gram per day for 3 days, can be given in-office or at an infusion center for more rapid effect. As the inflammation decreases, the prednisone can be tapered.

A frank discussion with patients regarding potential side effects of high-dose prednisone is necessary when initiating prednisone to prepare the patient for the common side effects of this drug. Symptoms such as insomnia, mood changes, and weight gain occur rapidly and are very noticeable to patients. Rare but serious risks include osteonecrosis of the femoral head and steroid-induced psychosis, which bear inclusion in patient counseling, as early diagnosis of these is important.

Most patients with autoimmune causes of PUK and scleritis will ultimately require long-term systemic immunomodulatory therapy. Consultation with a uveitis specialist or rheumatologist should be undertaken to select the appropriate agent and manage potential side effects.

INFECTIOUS CAUSES

If the diagnostic workup reveals syphilis or tuberculosis as the underlying cause, consultation with an infectious disease specialist should be undertaken to ensure proper treatment of the condition and compliance with reporting obligations. Other types of infectious agents should be treated with the appropriate therapy.

Case 1 Medical Therapy

A 44-year-old Indian female with perinuclear antineutrophil cytoplasmic antibody (p-ANCA)-associated cutaneous vasculitis presented with acute bilateral peripheral corneal thinning. The disease was incompletely controlled on oral steroids; thus, pulsed intravenous methylprednisolone followed by initiation of cyclophosphamide was required. Over the course of 6 months, her immunosuppressive regimen was transitioned to azathioprine, on which she was maintained thereafter (Fig. 17.3).

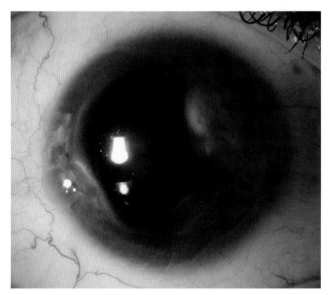

Fig. 17.3 Resolution of peripheral ulcerative keratitis in a patient treated with immunosuppression.

IN-OFFICE PROCEDURAL MANAGEMENT

During the initial management of PUK before control of the underlying disease process has been obtained, aggressive surgical interventions should be avoided unless absolutely necessary to save the globe. Performing surgery on an inflamed eye can result in further melting and destruction of tissue. Simple in-office management of any active ulcerations or small perforations while the underlying disease is being brought under control is the ideal initial step in treatment. Once the underlying process has been diagnosed and treated, definitive surgical treatment can be performed.

Case 2

A 64-year-old White female with a past medical history of Sjogren syndrome, non-Hodgkin lymphoma in remission, and bilateral herpes zoster ophthalmicus in the setting of immuno-compromise presented with new-onset redness and discomfort of the right eye for several days. Her past ocular history was also significant for neurotrophic keratopathy of the right eye in the setting of a past history of herpes zoster ophthalmicus, complicated by neurotrophic ulcer 1 year prior to this presentation.

On exam, the vision was noted to be counting fingers at 3 inches. The intraocular pressure was 5 mm Hg. A new 1.5-mm by 1.5-mm central epithelial defect with 90% thinning was noted. This area was Seidel negative. The remainder of the cornea demonstrated variable thinning, mid-stromal haze, peripheral neovascularization encroaching centrally in multiple clock hours, and rough keratopathy throughout. Corneal sensation was absent.

Bacterial and fungal cultures were performed, as were HSV and VZV PCR testing. Given the concern for impending perforation, corneal gluing of the focal area of thinning was undertaken.

PROCEDURE: CORNEAL GLUING

Supplies
■ Eyelid speculum
■ Topical anesthetic
■ Cyanoacrylate glue
■ Weck-Cel sponges
■ 1-cc tuberculin syringe
■ Short 30-gauge needle
■ Jeweler forceps
■ Bandage contact lens

Small corneal or limbal perforations (generally 3 mm or less) can be glued with cyanoacrylate glue.[27] Gluing is quite successful in small perforations, and in many cases, the cornea will reseal under the perforation, and no additional surgical intervention will be required. Multiple applications are sometimes required, and failure of the first application should not be taken as an indication that subsequent application will not work.[28]

Prior to gluing, cultures should be taken of the area to diagnose a potential infection and to debride any sloughing necrotic tissue. The epithelium surrounding the area of perforation should be removed, as cyanoacrylate does not adhere well to epithelium. This can be challenging near the limbus, but gentle abrasion of the adjacent conjunctiva will help glue adherence. The area of perforation should be dried carefully with a Weck-Cel, as cyanoacrylate glues

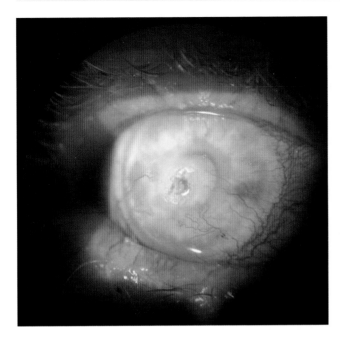

Fig. 17.4 Gluing of perforation in a patient with varicella zoster virus (VZV)–associated neurotrophic keratitis and corneal perforation. The patient ultimately went on to epithelialize and did not require surgical intervention for this perforation.

polymerize upon contact with aqueous and do not adhere to the cornea. Following this, glue should be applied.

There are multiple described methods for glue delivery.[29,30] The best method is the one in which the surgeon feels comfortable with delivering the glue in as accurate a fashion as possible. Especially with thinner cyanoacrylate glues such as Histoacryl, improper delivery can result in an excess of glue on the ocular surface and difficulty fitting a bandage contact lens. The authors of this chapter prefer to aspirate the glue into a 30-gauge needle on a tuberculin syringe for delivery. Fig. 17.4 demonstrates gluing in a patient with VZV-associated neurotrophic keratitis and corneal thinning with perforation.

After application, the glue should be allowed to dry until hard, generally 1 minute. Following this, a bandage contact lens should be placed. A large-diameter lens may be necessary to fully cover the glue. Uncovered glue is extremely abrasive and uncomfortable for the patient, and lid friction against uncovered glue may lead to dislodging and recurrence of a leak. Patients should be instructed to not rub their eyes and to wear a shield over the eye to prevent accidental trauma that might dislodge the glue.

The glue should be left in place until it becomes loose, which indicates that the corneal epithelium has healed underneath it and the perforation has sealed. This can be as short as 1 week to as long as several months but generally will become loose in 6–8 weeks.

CASE FOLLOW-UP

The patient was maintained on oral Valtrex and topical fluoroquinolone. The epithelium under the glue healed, and the glue fell off 3 weeks after gluing. The severe underlying corneal thinning had filled in, and the area was Seidel negative and stable.

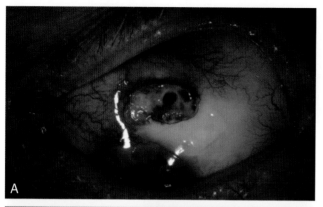

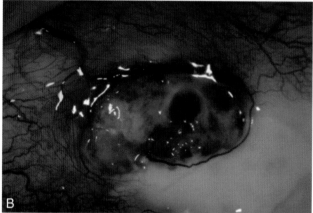

Fig. 17.5 (A–B) Necrotizing scleritis in a patient with anti–neutrophil cytoplasmic antibodies (ANCA)–associated vasculitis and prior mitomycin C application in setting of glaucoma drainage device. (B) Uveal tissue, visible at the base of the scleral defect.

Case 3

A 71-year-old White male presented with dull aching pain in the left eye for several weeks. His past medical history included ANCA-associated vasculitis characterized by lower-extremity myalgias and glomerulonephritis, controlled on rituximab and oral prednisone. Pertinent ocular history included primary open-angle glaucoma bilaterally, with a glaucoma drainage implant of the affected eye 2 years prior to presentation.

On exam, the vision was 20/25 in the affected eye, and the intraocular pressure was 7 mm Hg. A 6.4-mm by 3.3-mm scleral defect was noted adjacent to an area of blanched conjunctiva overlying Tutoplast coverage of a glaucoma drainage implant (Fig. 17.5A). At the base of the scleral defect, uveal tissue was visible (Fig. 17.5B). There was no epithelial defect. The remainder of the slit-lamp exam demonstrated several small granulomatous keratic precipitates of the inferior cornea and 0.5+ anterior chamber cells. The posterior segment was unremarkable except optic disc cupping.

The workup was notable for negative HSV and VZV PCR. Systemic workup was otherwise negative. Given the patient's underlying ANCA vasculitis, high-dose oral prednisone was initiated, and an additional rituximab dose was administered. Despite this intervention, the

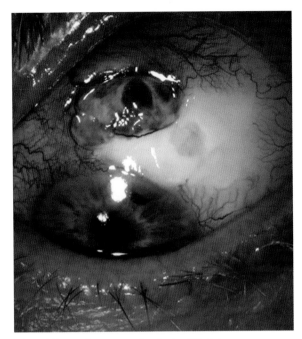

Fig. 17.6   Placement of amniotic membrane over site of scleral biopsy.

scleral thinning at the base of the defect began to progress. As a result, the patient underwent scleral biopsy with amniotic membrane overlay to attempt to identify an occult infectious cause (Fig. 17.6).

PROCEDURE: SCLERAL BIOPSY AND GLUED AMNIOTIC MEMBRANE

Supplies

- Topical anesthetic
- 3-mm skin biopsy punch trephine
- 0.12-mm forceps
- Crescent blade
- Amniotic membrane (cryopreserved)
- Tissue glue
- Vicryl suture (8-0 or 9-0)

The biopsy is performed in a lamellar fashion, sampling from the avascular sclera. A 3-mm skin punch is used to create a partial-thickness trephination through the avascular tissue, and this is carefully dissected using a crescent blade and 0.12-mm forceps. Cryopreserved fresh amniotic membrane is folded and placed into the defect and glued in place using fibrin glue. A second, larger piece of amniotic membrane can be placed over the site and glued into place. (For more detail, refer to Glued Amniotic Membrane in Chapter 16). Although not used in this case, it is possible to use Vicryl sutures to anchor the edges of the amniotic membrane if desired. In this case, using a fine suture such as 9-0 Vicryl is desirable so as to provoke minimal inflammation.

DISCUSSION

The amniotic membrane has a role as an adjuvant for epithelial healing in PUK when used in combination with therapies to treat the underlying cause.[31] Achieving epithelial healing is critical, as this signifies that the inflammatory process that caused epithelial sloughing has been resolved, and it prevents secondary infection and dessication of the exposed stroma. Denuded stroma also strongly expresses many inflammatory markers that may perpetuate the inflammation and stromal melting.[3]

Amniotic membrane placement in cases of Mooren ulcer has been shown to be useful to aid epithelialization; however, it is insufficient as primary therapy.[32,33] Literature regarding the use of amniotic membrane in other causes of PUK is sparse; however, it likely has a role in providing epithelial healing support.

Sutureless ring-supported cryopreserved amniotic membrane (Prokera; BioTissue) has been demonstrated to be useful in a number of ocular surface conditions, but its use has not been reported in PUK.[34] The ring-mounted structure of the membrane may preclude it from making good contact with the area of thinning in PUK; however, it may be useful in cases with more mild thinning. Dry amniotic membrane (Ambio Disk; IOP Ophthalmics) can be placed over the area of epithelial thinning in PUK and even folded to be placed into the PUK trough with a bandage contact lens placed over. Cryopreserved amniotic membrane can be placed in the areas of thinning and glued into place using fibrin glue.[31]

Bandage Contact Lens Placement

Bandage contact lenses can be useful to provide protection to areas of thinning and to prevent further dehydration of the corneal stroma from the dellen-like effect of significant thinning in severe PUK. Lenses can be placed with or without dried amniotic membrane as an adjuvant.

CASE FOLLOW-UP

Culture of the second biopsy specimen was again positive for *Cutibacterium acnes*. As a result, this was determined to be the true causative pathogen. Given low-grade intraocular inflammation on exam, the patient underwent explantation of the glaucoma drainage device and instillation of intravitreal clindamycin. A conjunctival flap was subsequently advanced over the defect site, and the patient healed well from the operation.

Case 4

A 32-year-old female presented with unilateral peripheral corneal thinning in a crescentic fashion (Fig. 17.7A). Serologies for syphilis, tuberculosis, and ANCA were negative, and the patient was diagnosed with Mooren ulcer. She was initiated on high-dose oral steroids at 1 mg/kg of prednisone, and conjunctival resection was performed in the area of crescentic thinning. Following the procedure, the patient experienced cessation of the melting and epithelialized the corneal and conjunctival defect. She remained healed 1 year after the resection (Fig. 17.7B).

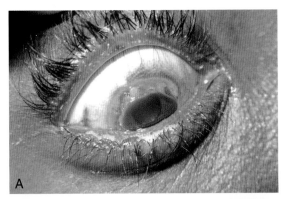

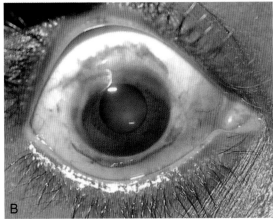

Fig. 17.7 Peripheral ulcerative keratitis (A) treated with conjunctival resection, leading to resolution (B). Case and photos courtesy of John Clements, MD.

PROCEDURE: CONJUNCTIVAL RESECTION

Supplies

- Eyelid speculum
- Topical anesthetic
- Subconjunctival anesthetic (lidocaine with epinephrine)
- Topical povidone-iodine 5%
- Westcott or Vannas scissors
- Castroviejo forceps, 0.12 mm
- Bipolar cautery

Conjunctival resection can be performed in-office under a procedural operating microscope. This procedure was previously considered to be the first-line treatment for Mooren ulcer.[35] However, it is now acknowledged that immunosuppressive therapy is more effective, but it can be considered in settings where immunosuppressive medications are unavailable or the patient is unable to take them.[36–38] The conjunctiva at the area of thinning and on two clock hours on either side should be resected 4 mm posterior to the limbus.[35] The conjunctiva surrounding the area of thinning is insufflated with lidocaine with epinephrine. A peritomy is then created using Westcott scissors, and the conjunctiva is resected to approximately 4 mm posterior to the limbus. Cautery is applied to blanch the episcleral vessels in this area. The residual epithelial defect was left open to heal. Cyanoacrylate glue and a bandage contact lens may be used in cases of significant thinning or perforation.[38]

Conclusion

PUK is a blinding condition that often is associated with severe systemic disease. Appropriate in-office management includes undertaking laboratory studies to determine the correct diagnosis as well as managing complications such as perforation that may occur. Several of these interventions, such as cyanoacrylate glue or amniotic membrane placement, can be performed in the office. Appropriate identification of the underlying etiology, whether infectious or autoimmune, is also critical to preventing progression of stromal necrolysis and resultant vision loss.

References

1. Knox Cartwright NE, Tole DM, Georgoudis P, Cook SD. Peripheral ulcerative keratitis and corneal melt: A 10-year single center review with historical comparison. *Cornea.* 2014;33(1):27–31.
2. Galor A, Thorne JE. Scleritis and peripheral ulcerative keratitis. *Rheum Dis Clin North Am.* 2007; 33(4):835–854. vii.
3. Dana MR, Qian Y, Hamrah P. Twenty-five-year panorama of corneal immunology: Emerging concepts in the immunopathogenesis of microbial keratitis, peripheral ulcerative keratitis, and corneal transplant rejection. *Cornea.* 2000;19(5):625–643.
4. Shiuey Y, Foster CS. Peripheral ulcerative keratitis and collagen vascular disease. *Int Ophthalmol Clin.* 1998; 38(1):21–32.
5. Eshraghi H, Mahtabfar A, Dastjerdi MH. A case of peripheral ulcerative keratitis associated with autoimmune hepatitis. *Case Rep Med.* 2017;2017:3939413.
6. Tarabishy AB, Schulte M, Papaliodis GN, Hoffman GS. Wegener's granulomatosis: Clinical manifestations, differential diagnosis, and management of ocular and systemic disease. *Surv Ophthalmol.* 2010; 55(5):429–444.
7. Moreira AT, Prajna NV. Acanthamoeba as a cause of peripheral ulcerative keratitis. *Cornea.* 2003; 22(6):576–577.
8. van der Gaag R, Abdillahi H, Stilma JS, Vetter JC. Circulating antibodies against corneal epithelium and hookworm in patients with Mooren's ulcer from Sierra Leone. *Br J Ophthalmol.* 1983;67(9):623–628.
9. Seino JY, Anderson SF. Mooren's ulcer. *Optom Vis Sci.* 1998;75(11):783–790.
10. Wei DW, Pagnoux C, Chan CC. Peripheral ulcerative keratitis secondary to chronic hepatitis B infection. *Cornea.* 2017;36(4):515–517.
11. Zegans ME, Srinivasan M, McHugh T, et al. Mooren ulcer in South India: Serology and clinical risk factors. *Am J Ophthalmol.* 1999;128(2):205–210.
12. Doshi RR, Harocopos GJ, Schwab IR, Cunningham Jr. ET. The spectrum of postoperative scleral necrosis. *Surv Ophthalmol.* 2013;58(6):620–633.
13. Clark EM, Durup D. Inflammatory eye reactions with bisphosphonates and other osteoporosis medications: What are the risks? *Ther Adv Musculoskelet Dis.* 2015;7(1):11–16.
14. Oatts JT, Keenan JD, Mannis T, et al. Multimodal assessment of corneal thinning using optical coherence tomography, Scheimpflug imaging, pachymetry, and slit-lamp examination. *Cornea.* 2017;36(4):425–430.
15. Garg A, De Rojas J, Mathews P, et al. Using anterior segment optical coherence tomography to monitor disease progression in peripheral ulcerative keratitis. *Case Rep Ophthalmol Med.* 2018;2018:3705753.
16. Shoughy SS, Jaroudi MO, Kozak I, Tabbara KF. Optical coherence tomography in the diagnosis of scleritis and episcleritis. *Am J Ophthalmol.* 2015;159(6):1045–1049.e1.
17. Yagci A. Update on peripheral ulcerative keratitis. *Clin Ophthalmol.* 2012;6:747–754.
18. Daniel Diaz J, Sobol EK, Gritz DC. Treatment and management of scleral disorders. *Surv Ophthalmol.* 2016;61(6):702–717.

19. Guerrero-Wooley RL, Peacock Jr. JE. Infectious scleritis: What the ID clinician should know. *Open Forum Infect Dis.* 2018;5(6):ofy140.
20. Akpek EK, Thorne JE, Qazi FA, et al. Evaluation of patients with scleritis for systemic disease. *Ophthalmology.* 2004;111(3):501–506.
21. Lin P, Bhullar SS, Tessler HH, Goldstein DA. Immunologic markers as potential predictors of systemic autoimmune disease in patients with idiopathic scleritis. *Am J Ophthalmol.* 2008;145(3):463–471.
22. Vignesh AP, Srinivasan R. Ocular manifestations of rheumatoid arthritis and their correlation with anti-cyclic citrullinated peptide antibodies. *Clin Ophthalmol.* 2015;9:393–397.
23. Harthan JS, Reeder RE. Peripheral ulcerative keratitis in association with sarcoidosis. *Cont Lens Anterior Eye.* 2013;36(6):313–317.
24. Yeh S, Sen HN, Colyer M, et al. Update on ocular tuberculosis. *Curr Opin Ophthalmol.* 2012;23(6): 551–556.
25. Ploysangam P, Mattern RM. Perforating peripheral ulcerative keratitis in syphilis. *Case Rep Ophthalmol.* 2019;10(2):267–273.
26. Sahin O, Ziaei A. Clinical and laboratory characteristics of ocular syphilis, co-infection, and therapy response. *Clin Ophthalmol.* 2016;10:13–28.
27. Jhanji V, Young AL, Mehta JS, et al. Management of corneal perforation. *Surv Ophthalmol.* 2011; 56(6):522–538.
28. Yin J, Singh RB, Al Karmi R, et al. Outcomes of cyanoacrylate tissue adhesive application in corneal thinning and perforation. *Cornea.* 2019;38(6):668–673.
29. Rana M, Savant V. A brief review of techniques used to seal corneal perforation using cyanoacrylate tissue adhesive. *Cont Lens Anterior Eye.* 2013;36(4):156–158.
30. Vote BJ, Elder MJ. Cyanoacrylate glue for corneal perforations: A description of a surgical technique and a review of the literature. *Clin Exp Ophthalmol.* 2000;28(6):437–442.
31. Hanada K, Shimazaki J, Shimmura S, Tsubota K. Multilayered amniotic membrane transplantation for severe ulceration of the cornea and sclera. *Am J Ophthalmol.* 2001;131(3):324–331.
32. Ngan ND, Chau HT. Amniotic membrane transplantation for Mooren's ulcer. *Clin Exp Ophthalmol.* 2011;39(5):386–392.
33. Schallenberg M, Westekemper H, Steuhl KP, Meller D. Amniotic membrane transplantation ineffective as additional therapy in patients with aggressive Mooren's ulcer. *BMC Ophthalmol.* 2013;13:81.
34. Suri K, Kosker M, Raber IM, et al. Sutureless amniotic membrane ProKera for ocular surface disorders: Short-term results. *Eye Contact Lens.* 2013;39(5):341–347.
35. Brown SI, Mondino BJ. Therapy of Mooren's ulcer. *Am J Ophthalmol.* 1984;98(1):1–6.
36. Feder RS, Krachmer JH. Conjunctival resection for the treatment of the rheumatoid corneal ulceration. *Ophthalmology.* 1984;91(2):111–115.
37. Agrawal V, Kumar A, Sangwan V, Rao GN. Cyanoacrylate adhesive with conjunctival resection and superficial keratectomy in Mooren's ulcer. *Indian J Ophthalmol.* 1996;44(1):23–27.
38. Lal I, Shivanagari SB, Ali MH, Vazirani J. Efficacy of conjunctival resection with cyanoacrylate glue application in preventing recurrences of Mooren's ulcer. *Br J Ophthalmol.* 2016;100(7):971–975.

CHAPTER 18

Corneal Perforation and Descemetocele

Elmer Y. Tu

Introduction

Both impending and frank corneal perforations represent an ocular emergency that can lead to permanent visual impairment or even loss of the eye. The loss of the barrier from extraocular elements exposes the intraocular contents to contamination, which can lead to infection or epithelial downgrowth. Further, ocular decompression of a corneal perforation can acutely result in loss of intraocular contents, including iris, lens, or intraocular lens implants, but even in their absence, the associated hypotony can lead to posterior segment complications, including expulsive choroidal hemorrhage, choroidal effusions, intraocular lens dislocations, and hypotony maculopathy. A more subacute complication is permanent secondary glaucoma, which occurs when the anterior chamber angle is occluded for more than a few days secondary to collapse of the normal anterior segment architecture and, consequently, the trabecular meshwork.

Presenting symptoms vary widely from being completely asymptomatic in the setting of a peripheral descemetocele to severe pain and acute visual loss. Prognosis depends largely on the size and location of the thinning/perforation as well as the condition of the surrounding tissue, other associated ocular abnormalities, and the underlying etiology of the perforation. Timely management of the perforation is critical to preserving the normal structure of the eye to prevent secondary complications.[1,2]

Pathogenesis and Epidemiology

The etiology of corneal perforations can be broadly characterized as traumatic or nontraumatic, although there can be some combination of the two, especially in areas of preexisting thinning.[2] Trauma does not generally lead to descemetocele formation but can include both surgical and nonsurgical penetration of the cornea. Nontraumatic causes originate with progressive loss of stromal tissue, including complications of microbial keratitis or noninfectious disorders, most commonly autoimmune, but also include forms of neurotrophic keratopathy. Descemetoceles are more common in these situations where there is a more subacute loss of corneal stroma while maintaining the integrity of the Descemet membrane. Although chemical burns, e.g., alkali or acid, could be considered traumatic, the pattern of stromal loss more closely follows the clinical course of nontraumatic injuries.

Studies of corneal perforations are less common, but recent publications addressing the value of corneal gluing reveal that the majority of perforations/descemetoceles have an association with microbial keratitis, 81% in Anchouche et al. and 55% in Yin et al.[3,4] It was noted that many of these patients also had concomitant noninfectious risk factors for corneal melting, so it is unclear whether the microbial keratitis was an inciting cause or secondary to preexisting corneal disease. Regardless, bacterial pathogens were the most common, followed by viral, primarily herpetic, disease. Despite their relative rarity in the geographic locations studied, fungal and amoebic infections were also reported in each study.[3,4]

In Yin et al., 35% of patients who received corneal gluing were considered sterile and non-traumatic, with the most common association being with rheumatoid arthritis, but also including graft vs. host disease (GVHD) and a myriad other autoimmune processes.[4] Anchouche et al. noted that 20% of their patients exhibited a neurotrophic keratopathy.[3] A significant number of corneal perforations and descemetoceles are multifactorial in nature. Traumatic injuries made up between 7% and 10% of patients receiving glue. These studies are significantly biased to perforations and descemetoceles that are amenable to in-office treatment, with the incidence of traumatic corneal perforation likely much higher.

Presentation and Diagnosis

Patients with acute perforations will often report a change in vision associated with a sudden "gush of tears," which corresponds to loss of aqueous humor from a corneal perforation. The "tearing" may either continue if the hole remains open or suddenly stop if plugged by the iris for other intraocular contents. The location and size of the defect will have an effect on change in vision where small and/or peripheral perforations that do not result in direct obstruction or anterior chamber shallowing will often demonstrate minimal visual disability and few other symptoms. Other associated symptoms include photophobia, pain, and redness, among others.

Presenting signs will include the finding of a corneal perforation or descemetocele. An area that is associated with thinning that does not bulge forward. In a patient without an active leak, the finding of pigment in the area of thinning strongly suggests that a perforation occurred at some point in the past. The presence of an epithelial defect in the bed of the stromal defect is often difficult to discern when fluorescein pools are in the base. Gentle irrigation or absorbing excess fluid with a cotton-tip applicator should determine whether a true epithelial defect remains. It is important to assess surrounding pathology, including size of the defect and surrounding abnormal tissue, size of the epithelial defect, quality of remaining corneal stroma, iris or other tissue incarceration in the perforation, depth of the anterior chamber, volume of flow through the perforation, and any abnormalities of the remainder of the eye. All of these will determine what options are available for stabilization and treatment.

Descemetoceles will appear to be very clear and thin upon slit-lamp examination, with a bulge forward from the normal posterior corneal curvature (Fig. 18.1). A very thin area that does not bulge forward indicates that there is still some stromal tissue or, perhaps, predescemetic layer remaining to provide structure (Fig. 18.2).[1] An intact predescemetic layer of 28–36 microns still provides significant resistance to perforation and can be observed over a true descemetocele, which is only 10 microns thick.[1] Corneal dellen due to stromal dehydration may mimic the appearance of a descemetocele but are distinguished by the lack of corneal ectasia and the lack of an epithelial defect. While extended dehydration may eventually lead to true corneal thinning, corneal dellen respond readily to topical lubricants. The Seidel test is the gold standard for determining whether a frank corneal perforation exists. This should be performed with 10% liquid fluorescein dropped carefully on the eye to avoid trauma. Observed under a cobalt blue filter, this concentration appears black. Dilution with leaking aqueous fluid will appear green as the concentration falls in the area of perforation. If the 10% solution is not available, a lower concentration, either liquid or strip, can be used, which will exhibit a similar phenomenon or exhibit a negative staining where the aqueous egress washes away all traces of the fluorescein from the area of the leak. Generally, checking intraocular pressure is not advisable in an open globe, but some patients with a corneal perforation will have extremely high pressure secondary to pupillary/anterior chamber angle block.

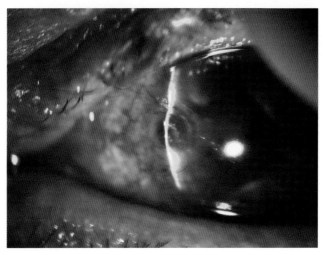

Fig. 18.1 Patient with a peripheral autoimmune melt and descemetocele due to rheumatoid arthritis. Note the bulging forward of the central portion of the thinned cornea.

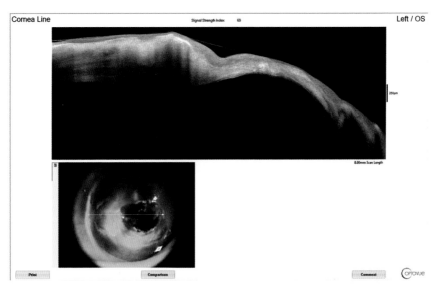

Fig. 18.2 An optical coherence tomograph (OCT) of an 89-year-old male with a bulging descemetocele with some residual thickness to the stroma underneath a contact lens. (Courtesy of Rachel Epstein, MD.)

Management

The primary goal in managing a critical loss of corneal integrity is to restore or prevent the loss of a watertight barrier and thereby prevent secondary complications of infection and hypotony. In severe corneal thinning without perforation, all attention should be directed toward controlling underlying disease and optimizing the ocular surface to heal the epithelium, as progression of corneal thinning is highly unusual in the presence of an intact epithelium. Concurrently, investigation and treatment of the systemic or local disease contributing to the corneal melting need to be addressed to improve the outcome of any intervention. Culturing and empiric therapy should be instituted if infection is suspected either as a primary or secondary process. Herpetic keratitis commonly presents with a triad of nonhealing epithelial defects, neurotrophic keratopathy, and stromal inflammation, which can cause a wide range of presentations, both peripheral and central. Noninfiltrative ulcers should prompt a detailed history and systemic workup for autoimmune diseases such as rheumatoid arthritis, systemic lupus erythematosus, and more aggressive disorders such as GVHD or Stevens-Johnson syndrome. Local factors that inhibit healing, including lid disorders, ocular surface disease, dry eye syndrome as well as inflammatory and allergic disorders, need to be investigated and addressed. Hypovitaminosis A can rapidly lead to descemetocele and corneal perforation and should be suspected in patients with nutritional deficiencies or absorption defects such as is seen with bariatric surgery. Isolated ocular disorders such as Terriens marginal degeneration, corneal dellen, and Fuchs keratitis should also be in the differential.[1,2]

If the anterior chamber and the rest of the eye remain formed with a reasonable intraocular pressure, smaller perforations can be closely observed possibly with the addition of patching, a Bandage contact lens, and/or application of ocular hypotensive medications to reduce flow. Many surgery-related perforations are suture track leaks or small wound leaks in an otherwise normal stromal bed that can be managed successfully with conservative management or polyethylene glycol hydrogel–based sealants. Similarly, repair of perforations with iris incarceration and a formed eye, if chronic, can be scheduled in the operating room, especially if the iris has been epithelialized. If the iris incarceration is more acute, even with a formed eye, the perforation should be resolved before epithelialization and ischemia of the involved iris occur, usually within days.

Corneal gluing is an in-office procedure that can be used to either temporarily or permanently treat corneal perforations and act to stabilize corneas with severe thinning and impending perforation, including descemetoceles. Tissue adhesives can act as a bridge to stabilize an eye until definitive treatment, usually a corneal transplant and/or sterilization, can be achieved. These glues may also result in long-term stability of the cornea, as the underlying cornea scars and the epithelium heals under its protective cover.

A number of corneal adhesives have been described in the management of corneal thinning and perforation. Most share the property of polymerizing once they come in contact with moisture. The only product that is approved specifically for ophthalmic use in the United States is ReSure sealant, which is a polyethylene glycol hydrogel indicated for sealing clear corneal cataract wounds, while OcuSeal has a similar approval in Europe.[5,6] Categorized as a sealant, it will penetrate any gaps to create a watertight seal. The substance dissolves within 1–3 days, limiting its utility in settings where there is significant tissue loss, tension on the wound edges, or the need for longer-term closure of a defect. Fibrin tissue glue has been shown to create a reasonable seal, especially when used in conjunction with a tissue patch of amniotic membrane, but like ReSure sealant, the product lasts a short time and can be unpredictable in its dissolution.

Cyanoacrylate adhesives are the most common form of tissue adhesive utilized for closing corneal wounds.[7,8] While they are not specifically indicated for ophthalmic use, a number of compounds are approved and commercially available for closing skin defects that have been applied to the eye (Table 18.1).[1–5,9] They vary in properties of polymerization time and flexibility. Cyanoacrylates are categorized as glues, so they act to bind tissues together. After contact with water, these glues release formaldehyde as part of the curing process, which causes significant local toxicity both to microbial pathogens and local tissue. Cyanoacrylate glues have been shown to be effective at closing wounds 3 mm or less in diameter. Larger wounds can also be amenable to cyanoacrylate application but are less stable and harder to seal completely. Other poor predictive factors include a high-flow aqueous egress, which can make control of the polymerization and precise application of volume and location difficult, and extensive necrosis of the host cornea. The latter results in a mobile glue patch and unstable adhesion that can shorten the life of the adhesive. Cyanoacrylate glues provide good closure once in place with a high burst pressure. Studies vary

TABLE 18.1 ■ Compounds described for sealing corneal perforations

Compound Class	Compound	Commercial Name
PEG-based sealants	PEG plus trilysine acetate	ReSure
	Poly(glycerol succinic acid) and PEG-aldehyde	Ocuseal
Cyanoacrylates	2-Octyl-cyanoacrylate	Dermabond SurgiSeal Octylseal
	N-2-butyl-cyanoacrylate	Histoacryl/Histoacryl Blue Indermil Liquiband
Fibrin tissue glue		Tisseel Evicel Hemaseel

PEG, Polyethylene glycol hydrogel.

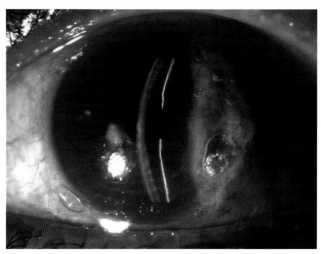

Fig. 18.3 A female with a history of peripheral ulcerative keratitis and perforation consistent with Mooren ulcer with a customized cyanoacrylate glue application to avoid the conjunctiva. Note the peaked pupil, which indicates probable iris incarceration, either past or current.

on the success rate of corneal gluing, largely because of disparate definitions of success, but range from 22% to 94%.[3,4,10] Multiple applications are often needed as the glue patch loosens and, for most cases, acts as a bridge to eventual corneal grafting. Cyanoacrylate glues do not, however, adhere well to conjunctiva and should be applied only to the cornea in cases of peripheral ulcerative keratitis (Fig. 18.3). Because the surface of the adhesive is often rough, a Bandage contact lens is placed at the end of the procedure.

Large perforations with extensive loss of corneal tissue and/or extrusion of intraocular contents, including iris, are best managed with tectonic keratoplasty. If transplant-grade corneal tissue is not available, other sterile human tissues, e.g., cryopreserved corneal tissue, pericardium, etc., can be used to seal the perforation until transplant tissue is available. Multilayer amniotic membrane can also be customized to fill the corneal defect and fixated with fibrin tissue glue,

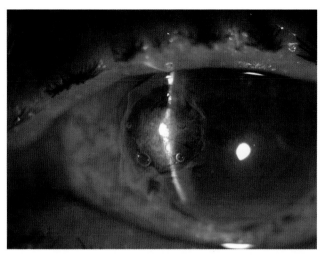

Fig. 18.4 A patient with paracentral Sjogren syndrome–associated melt who has undergone multilayer amniotic membrane transplantation (AMT) grafting with an overlying contact lens.

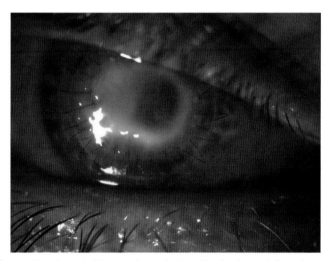

Fig. 18.5 A 40-year-old male treated for acanthamoeba keratitis showing an infiltrate in a previous corneal transplant.

with a larger section of amniotic membrane covering and protecting it while it epithelializes and integrates into the stroma (Fig. 18.4).[11,12]

Case 1

A 40-year-old male with keratoconus with a history of corneal transplantation in the right eye and subsequent contact lens wear presented with an acanthamoeba keratitis involving his right eye. He was treated for 4 weeks with improvement in the appearance of the infiltrate but with continued thinning of the central cornea (Fig. 18.5). Optical coherence tomography revealed a progressive predescemetocele centrally (Fig. 18.6).

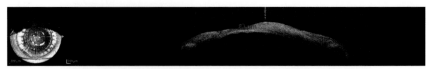

Fig. 18.6 An optical coherence tomograph (OCT) from Case 1 demonstrating critical thinning in the central cornea. (Courtesy of Rachel Epstein, MD.)

PROCEDURE: CORNEAL GLUING

Supplies

- 2-Octyl-cyanoacrylate (Dermabond)
- Topical anesthetic
- Eye spear sponges
- Tuberculin syringe with small-gauge needle, 27 or 30 gauge
- Bandage contact lens
- Eyelid speculum

PROCEDURE

Corneal gluing can be performed at the slit-lamp microscope or under a minor procedure room microscope. The glue ampoule is broken and squeezed out to form a droplet, which is suctioned into the needle and syringe. The glue syringe with a small-gauge needle is brought to the field and the plunger advanced minimally until a small droplet of glue is clinging to the needle tip. The cornea is dried meticulously with the spear sponges. The droplet of glue is then placed on the descemetocele and surrounding cornea, allowing it to polymerize in 1–2 minutes. A Bandage contact lens is placed over the cornea, and the speculum is removed.

DISCUSSION

Patients with either frank descemetoceles or progressive near descemetoceles are at risk for acute perforation, either spontaneously or with minor trauma. Risks of irreversible visual loss rise significantly with an acute perforation and should be avoided. Corneal gluing can stabilize the eye in the short term and encourage scarring and neovascularization enough to be a long-term solution. In an eye with modest corneal clouding, optical coherence tomography (OCT) can be helpful to define the amount of corneal stroma that remains present. Applying a corneal adhesive in a nonperforated eye is also simpler in that there is no active flow to disturb the even polymerization of the glue. When applied in this fashion, it may be done at either the slit lamp or supine at an operating microscope, but it is easier in a minor procedure room, as the application of the glue can be more precise and not as dependent on gravity. Limiting the amount of glue will improve its contour and longevity on the surface. A contact lens is required because most glues will have a rough surface after hardening.

Case 2

A 65-year-old male with GVHD status post penetrating keratoplasty for a previous perforation and subsequent complex retinal detachment repair with a pars plana vitrectomy and scleral buckle with silicone oil 4 months prior presents with a complaint of increased tearing and discomfort of the left eye. He is 20/1000 in the right eye and Hand Motions in the left. An

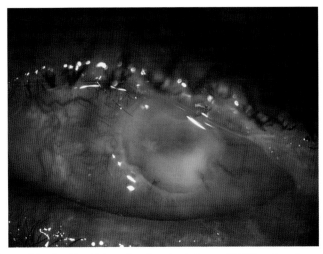

Fig. 18.7 A 65-year-old male with a history of graft vs. host disease (GVHD) and previous penetrating keratoplasty for corneal perforation who presents with a severe suppurative keratitis and extrusion of silicone oil.

acute suppurative, necrotic corneal ulcer involving the entire corneal transplant with an acute perforation nasally of approximately 1.5 mm is found to be leaking silicone oil (Fig. 18.7). The anterior chamber appears flat, but the view is poor. The patient had been seen 2 weeks earlier with an intact transplant.

PROCEDURE: CORNEAL GLUING WITH A PATCH

Supplies

- 2-Octyl-cyanoacrylate (Dermabond)
- Topical anesthetic
- Cotton-tip applicators
- Ophthalmic ointment
- Clear plastic surgical drape
- Dermatologic skin biopsy punch, 3-mm size
- Forceps
- Eye spear sponges
- Tuberculin syringe with small-gauge needle, 27 or 30 gauge
- Sterile gloves
- Fluorescein strip or 10% liquid fluorescein
- Bandage contact lens

PROCEDURE

(Video 18.1) A small sterile field is set up to prepare the glue applicator. A small amount of sterile ophthalmic ointment is squeezed onto a corner of the field. The rest of the materials are opened onto the sterile field, and sterile gloves are donned. The glue ampoule is broken and squeezed out to form a droplet, which is suctioned into the needle and syringe and set aside. The drape is punched through the folded drape using the dermatologic punch so that multiple 4-mm discs are created. A cotton-tip applicator is held by the cotton tip, lightly touching the flat end of the handle to the ophthalmic ointment and any excess ointment removed. The same flat end, now with a minimal amount of ointment as a releasable adhesive, is used to pick up a single plastic disc created from the drape. A thin layer of glue is placed on the exposed side of the plastic drape disc and set aside.

The patient is then placed into the slit lamp, the eye opened (optionally with a speculum), and the area around the perforation dried meticulously with an eye surgical spear after anesthetizing the eye topically. The preassembled cotton-tip applicator is then used to quickly apply the glue and disc precisely over the perforation, holding it for several seconds to allow the moisture to polymerize the glue while holding the eyelids away until the process is complete, usually 30–60 seconds.

A Seidel test is performed to confirm sealing of the perforation and a Bandage contact lens placed. The patient is examined later to confirm repressurization of the eye, deepening of the anterior chamber, and seal of the leak. If the leak is not sealed, the glue can be removed with a forceps and the process repeated. A Bandage contact lens can then be placed over the glued patch.

DISCUSSION

Microbial keratitis is the most common cause of corneal melting, and when presenting acutely with a corneal perforation, especially with an undiagnosed and untreated infection, stabilization of the eye to allow medical treatment prior to corneal transplantation is desirable. Tectonic, therapeutic grafts in this situation can be challenging and have devastating consequences if the infection recurs. Corneal gluing can stabilize the globe and avoid intraocular complications of hypotony while control or sterilization of the cornea is achieved. Polymerization of the glue and its consequential release of toxic compounds like formaldehyde onto the ocular surface has also been shown to have significant antimicrobial effects.[13,14]

These perforations present several challenges to corneal gluing, including an unstable surrounding necrotic ocular surface and often persistent flow of aqueous from the perforation. For adherence of the glue, it is vitally important that it is anchored well to tissue and that the glue polymerizes as simultaneously as possible all around the perforation. Asymmetric application will only force the flow of aqueous to one side, which will cause the glue to harden and form a channel for egress around the glue, creating a persistent leak. The method forementioned allows the glue to be applied to the entire area at once, preventing flow. The drape material is left behind as additional tectonic support and presents a smooth surface that will minimize irritation and loosening.

Conclusion

Impending and frank corneal perforation represent an urgent or emergent situation. A broad range of small to medium corneal defects can be successfully managed with corneal gluing, utilizing commonly available medical-grade adhesives in a simple in-office setting. Gluing can both represent a valuable bridge to treat underlying disease until more definitive surgical treatment can be applied and, in some cases, a long-term solution in high-risk patients if the glue can remain in place until scarring and fibrosis occur.

References

1. Agarwal R, Nagpal R, Todi V, Sharma N. Descemetocele. *Surv Ophthalmol*. 2021;66(1):2–19.
2. Jhanji V, Young AL, Mehta JS, Sharma N, Agarwal T, Vajpayee RB. Management of corneal perforation. *Surv Ophthalmol*. 2011;56(6):522–538.

3. Anchouche S, Harissi-Dagher M, Segal L, Racine L, Darvish-Zargar M, Robert MC. Cyanoacrylate tissue adhesive for the treatment of corneal thinning and perforations: A multicenter study. *Cornea.* 2020;39(11):1371–1376.

4. Yin J, Singh RB, Al Karmi R, Yung A, Yu M, Dana R. Outcomes of cyanoacrylate tissue adhesive application in corneal thinning and perforation. *Cornea.* 2019;38(6):668–673.

5. Guhan S, Peng SL, Janbatian H, et al. Surgical adhesives in ophthalmology: history and current trends. *Br J Ophthalmol.* 2018;102(10):1328–1335.

6. Tong AY, Gupta PK, Kim T. Wound closure and tissue adhesives in clear corneal incision cataract surgery. *Curr Opin Ophthalmol.* 2018;29(1):14–18.

7. Webster Jr. RG, Dohlman CH, Refojo MF. The use of adhesives in anterior segment surgery. *Trans Pac Coast Otoophthalmol Soc Annu Meet.* 1969;50:121–135.

8. Webster Jr. RG, Slansky HH, Refojo MF, Boruchoff SA, Dohlman CH. The use of adhesive for the closure of corneal perforations. Report of two cases. *Arch Ophthalmol.* 1968;80(6):705–709.

9. Tan J, Foster LJR, Watson SL. Corneal sealants in clinical use: A systematic review. *Curr Eye Res.* 2020;45(9):1025–1030.

10. Loya-Garcia D, Serna-Ojeda JC, Pedro-Aguilar L, Jimenez-Corona A, Olivo-Payne A, Graue-Hernandez EO. Non-traumatic corneal perforations: Aetiology, treatment and outcomes. *Br J Ophthalmol.* 2017;101(5):634–639.

11. Kruse FE, Rohrschneider K, Volcker HE. Multilayer amniotic membrane transplantation for reconstruction of deep corneal ulcers. *Ophthalmology.* 1999;106(8):1504–1510, discussion 1511.

12. Nubile M, Carpineto P, Lanzini M, Ciancaglini M, Zuppardi E, Mastropasqua L. Multilayer amniotic membrane transplantation for bacterial keratitis with corneal perforation after hyperopic photorefractive keratectomy: Case report and literature review. *J Cataract Refract Surg.* 2007;33(9):1636–1640.

13. Dogan C, Aygun G, Bahar-Tokman H, et al. In vitro antifungal effect of acrylic corneal glue (N-butyl-2-cyanoacrylate). *Cornea.* 2019;38(12):1563–1567.

14. Eiferman RA, Snyder JW. Antibacterial effect of cyanoacrylate glue. *Arch Ophthalmol.* 1983;101(6):958–960.

CHAPTER 19

Acute Chemical Burn

Alex P. Beazer ▪ Natalie A. Afshari

Introduction

Acute chemical burn to the eye represents one of the few true ophthalmic emergencies. It can result in a spectrum of damage ranging from mild irritation to severe anterior segment devastation with permanent vision loss or loss of the eye. Young adult males represent the majority of victims, while children under 2 years old are also at particular risk. Fortunately, most cases are mild exposures with an excellent prognosis. Prototypical offending agents include cleaning solutions such as bleach and ammonia, battery fluid, fertilizers, and fireworks.

Presentation is often confounded by thermal injury to the ocular surface and skin; orbital trauma, such as retained intraocular foreign body; and lid and adnexal injury. Prognosis depends largely on the nature of the injury and causative agent as well as timely treatment response by the patient and care team. This begins with immediate copious irrigation. Prognosis after severe injury is poor due to both direct damage and serious vision-threatening sequelae. Prudent measures toward early reepithelization of the ocular surface are crucial.

EPIDEMIOLOGY

Of all ocular trauma, 7.7%–18% is attributed to chemical injury.[1] Men constitute 56% of total events, with a median age of 32 years.[2] The vast majority of ocular chemical injuries are accidental, with approximately two-thirds occurring in the workplace and one-third at home, oftentimes from domestic cleaning agents.[3] A small subset is due to assault. Most workplace accidents occur on construction sites, in factories, or chemical plants. Eye protection has been shown to be more effective at home than the workplace in these cases, where industrial chemicals often overwhelm even robust personal protective equipment.

Children under 2 are also at particular risk of accidental chemical injury.[2] This grim reality of preventable events highlights the importance of proper storage and education regarding common household cleaning supplies, including the emergence of laundry detergent pods.

INCITING AGENTS

Alkali agents are typically more destructive to the eye and are more ubiquitous in everyday life. With the ability to saponify cell membranes, certain alkali agents such as ammonia can reach the anterior chamber within 15 seconds.[4] A pH level of >11.5 has been shown to produce irreversible damage to the anterior segment.[5] Lime plaster found in cement and mortar is the most common alkaline offender. Other agents include ammonia, potassium hydroxide, sodium hydroxide (lye), and magnesium hydroxide (see Table 19.1). Each entity presents unique obstacles to the respondent clinician: combining water with lye can release toxic fumes, magnesium hydroxide in fireworks is often accompanied by thermal injury, and lime is comparatively less toxic but is associated with particulates, which continue to release noxious chemicals until meticulously removed.

Acids classically cause more limited damage than alkalis, due partly to the immediate barrier created by precipitation of epithelial proteins. These act as a buffer against further penetration through tissue and can neutralize the low pH. The most common acidic agent in ocular injury is sulfuric acid, frequently from an automobile battery explosion. Others include sulfurous acid found in bleach, acetic acid found in vinegar, and hydrochloric acid (see Table 19.1). Hydrofluoric acid is exceptional in its ability to act like an alkali and rapidly penetrate the cornea. It offers particular challenges in exposure management and can result in severe stromal scarring, vascularization, and anterior segment damage.

Diagnosis and Grading

A thorough history is the first step in adequately diagnosing and managing acute chemical injury. Identifying the causative agent can be valuable in gauging severity. Included in the history is the nature of the exposure, duration, and the velocity and temperature of the agent when available.

Several classification systems of ocular chemical injuries exist for the purposes of treatment and prognosis. The Roper-Hall system (see Table 19.2) is a widely used and simple I–IV grading system that offers relatively accurate prognostic value. It is based on the extent of corneal involvement and observed limbal ischemia, which is a marker of limbal stem cell damage. The extent of limbal stem cell damage is an indicator of long-term prognosis. The Dua et al. system (see Table 19.3) has been developed to take into account conjunctival involvement and may offer a more accurate prognosis in severe chemical burns.[6] It expands the Roper-Hall grade IV injury into

TABLE 19.1 ■ **Chart of Acids and Alkalis**

Common Acids	Chemical Composition	pH (0.1 M Solution)	Example
Sulfuric acid	H_2SO_4	1.2	Car battery fluid
Sulfurous acid	H_2SO_3	1.5	Bleach
Acetic acid	CH_3COOH	2.9	Vinegar
Hydrochloric acid	HCl	1.1	Swimming pool cleaner
Hydrofluoric acid	HF	2.1	Glass polisher, silicone production

Common Alkalis	Chemical Composition	pH (0.1 M Solution)	Example
Ammonia	NH_3	11.1	Household cleaning agents, fertilizer
Lye	NaOH	13	Drain cleaner
Potassium hydroxide	KOH	12	Caustic potash
Magnesium hydroxide	$Mg(OH)_2$	10.5	Fireworks, incendiaries
Lime	$Ca(OH)_2$	12.4	Plaster, mortar, cement

TABLE 19.2 ■ **Roper-Hall Classification System**

Grade	Corneal Findings	Limbal Findings	Prognosis
I	Epithelial damage	No limbal ischemia	Good
II	Haze, iris details visible	<1/3 limbal ischemia	Good
III	Total epithelial defect, stromal haze, iris details obscured	1/3–1/2 limbal ischemia	Guarded
IV	Opaque, iris, and pupil details obscured	>1/2 limbal ischemia	Poor

TABLE 19.3 ■ Dua et al. Classification System

Grade	Limbal Involvement	Conjunctival Involvement (%)[a]	Analogue Scale (%)[b]	Prognosis
I	0 clock hours	0	0	Very good
II	<3 clock hours	<30	0.1–3/1–29.9	Good
III	3–6 clock hours	30–50	3.1–6/31–50	Good
IV	6–9 clock hours	50–75	6.1–9/51–75	Good to guarded
V	9–12 clock hours	75–100	9.1–11.9/75.1–99.9	Guarded to poor
VI	Total limbus	Total conjunctiva	12/100	Very poor

[a]Conjunctival involvement calculated for bulbar conjunctiva only, including the fornices.
[b]Analogue scale records the amount of limbal involvement in clock hours of affected limbus/percentage of conjunctival involvement.

grades IV to VI and assesses fluorescein staining of the limbus rather than perilimbal ischemia. Interestingly, the Dua et al. system does not account for corneal involvement.

Accurate clinical grading is confounded by poor consistency, even among cornea specialists. Hence, anterior segment photography and, in some cases, angiography remain important tools to track progression or improvement.

Management

The management of chemical injury changes as the phases of healing progress. Immediate management hinges on timely and copious irrigation. Focus in the acute phase (days 1–7) is on epithelial healing, inflammation control, and infection prevention. The early reparative phase (days 7–21) varies greatly from full resolution in grade I injuries to persistent epithelial defects or sterile ulceration in severe injury. Treatment focuses on preventing melt by encouraging collagen synthesis while minimizing inflammation-mediated collagenase activity. The late reparative phase (day >21) result is often based on limbal stem cell involvement. Grade I injuries will have fully recovered with a normal corneal epithelium. Grade II injuries can demonstrate focal conjunctivalization in areas of limbal stem cell loss, while grades III and beyond likely require surgical management to even reach the somber goal of a completely conjunctivalized yet structurally stable cornea (Fig. 19.1).

The phase-dependent management described previously can include topical corticosteroids to control inflammation, aggressive lubrication, cycloplegia for patient comfort, and topical antibiotics. Depending on severity, adjunctive topical and oral vitamin C supplementation can promote collagen synthesis, and oral tetracyclines help to prevent ulceration and stromal melt. Topical intraocular pressure-lowering agents may be needed. Debridement and amniotic membrane transplantation are beneficial in promoting epithelization, as will be discussed. Grades III and higher injuries often require surgery for acute and long-term management.

Case 1

A 34-year-old male presents urgently to the clinic for eye pain. He was applying lime plaster on an internal wall at a construction site across the street, and it splashed into his right eye about 20 minutes prior. He was not wearing safety glasses. He states that he splashed some water on it without improvement. There is visible plaster debris on his right brow and upper eyelid. He is immediately seated in a minor procedure room for irrigation.

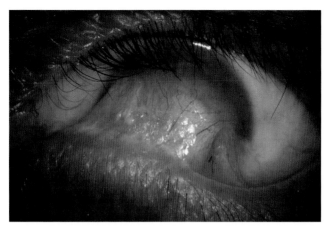

Fig. 19.1   Alkali burn that has resulted in severe ocular surface disease with symblepharon formation, dense conjunctivalization of the cornea, and limbal stem cell loss.

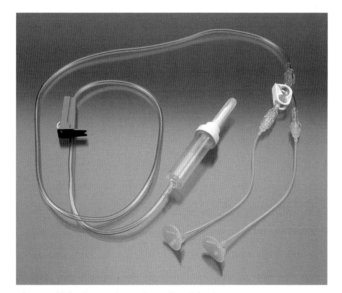

Fig. 19.2   Morgan lens and irrigation set for ocular surface irrigation.

PROCEDURE: OCULAR IRRIGATION

Supplies

- Isotonic saline or Ringer lactate (clean tap water is an acceptable alternative in the acute setting)
- Topical anesthetic
- Cotton-tip applicators
- pH paper, expanded range
- Eyelid speculum
- Morgan lens and standard intravenous (IV) set if available (Fig. 19.2).
- 500-mL kidney basin
- Jeweler forceps

Procedure

Seat the patient with head back and tilted to the affected side. Apply topical anesthetic. Place an eyelid speculum, and begin irrigation with the fluid flowing nasal to temporal, avoiding runoff onto the unaffected eye. Alternatively, use a Morgan lens and standard IV set to assist with irrigation, if available (Fig. 19.2). A kidney basin can be positioned against the patient to limit irrigation of the chemical agent further onto the skin or clothes. Ask the patient to look in all directions to ensure penetration of the fluid to the conjunctival cul-de-sac. Rapid irrigation with any clean fluid takes precedence over all the listed supplies.

After a minimum of 30 minutes (1–3 L of fluid), stop the fluid and allow the tear film to normalize for 5 minutes. Check the pH by applying pH paper to the inferior tear lake. If abnormal, resume irrigation for another 1–3 L of fluid. Compare to the fellow eye.

After pH normalization (7.0–7.2), perform a complete eye exam. Evert the eyelids and sweep the fornices with a cotton-tip applicator to remove any solid chemical debris. Recheck the pH every 15–30 minutes to ensure that it stays within normal limits. If pH fails to normalize, examine the patient under the slit lamp and use jeweler forceps to remove any further chemical particulates hidden in the fornix or embedded in the conjunctiva.

DISCUSSION

In this procedure, time is truly of the essence. By the time the ophthalmologist is examining the patient, the patient has likely already undergone irrigation in the field or with assistance of others in the care team, such as emergency room providers. This should not lull the astute clinician into a state of complacency. Rapid and copious irrigation takes precedence over history taking, visual acuity measurement, slit-lamp biomicroscopy, or any other routine exam maneuver. Handheld irrigation with IV tubing is a common practice in the emergency room and can be enhanced with a contact lens attachment (Morgan lens). The Morgan lens can increase patient comfort and can overcome blepharospasm. A minimum of 30 minutes and several liters of fluid are often required while erring on the side of excessive. Allowing the tear film to normalize ensures the most accurate physiologic pH measurement undiluted by rinsing or anesthetic agents. Comparison to the fellow eye is beneficial, as slight alterations in pH paper color can be subtle.

Do not delay at the expense of irrigation type. It can be argued that water may enable deeper penetration of the chemical agent due to its osmolarity.[7] In an ideal scenario, the use of specialized buffered irrigating agents can most rapidly normalize the intracameral pH and may decrease reepithelization time, yet their long-term clinical benefit is unproven.[8] Topical anesthesia can arguably augment penetration of the offending agent by increasing epithelial fragility. However, in most situations, the benefit of efficient irrigation facilitated by topical anesthesia far outweighs the risks associated with its short-term use.

Removing chemical particulates is crucial, especially with lime plaster, as they may be eluting further chemical onto the ocular surface. Measure the intraocular pressure, as chemical burn is associated with acute pressure spikes. Carefully assess the ocular surface, paying special attention to the limbus and conjunctiva. In a completely deepithelized cornea, delayed or poor fluorescein uptake into the Bowman membrane can fool the rushed observer.

Case 2

A 21-year-old male was seen in the emergency department for an acidic chemical burn of the left eye 3 days prior. His eye was irrigated, pH normalized, and his injury was managed with topical corticosteroids, antibiotics, and a cycloplegic. He missed his same-day follow-up appointment and presents today with continued irritation, photophobia, redness, and decreased vision. Slit-lamp examination reveals a large inferior corneal epithelial defect involving the limbus with rolled-up borders and irregular necrotic material partially obscuring the view to the anterior chamber.

PROCEDURE: EPITHELIAL DEBRIDEMENT

Supplies
■ Eyelid speculum ■ Topical anesthetic ■ Cotton-tip applicators ■ Cellulose eye sponges (Weck-Cel) ■ Jeweler forceps ■ Optional: Kimura spatula, no. 15 or 67 blade

Procedure

Administer topical anesthesia and insert the eyelid speculum. Position the patient at the slit lamp. Use a cotton-tip applicator or dry eye sponge to gently identify and remove loose or necrotic epithelium. Consider tissue forceps, a Kimura spatula, or blade to assist with necrotic material excision. Irrigate generously to ensure removal of any chemical debris embedded in damaged tissue.

DISCUSSION

Epithelial debridement can be beneficial in grade II or higher chemical burns. Early debridement is thought to shorten the time to reepithelization. Necrotic ocular tissue can seed the area with inflammatory mediators, which inhibit normal healing.[9] Severe injuries may require serial debridement. Extreme care must be taken not to perforate the cornea during this procedure, given the propensity for corneoscleral melt in high-grade chemical burns. Underlying scleral ischemia in severe injuries will contribute to nonhealing epithelial defects. If epithelial growth does not begin despite repeated debridement, placement of an amniotic membrane is likely indicated.

Case 3

A 30-year-old male with a grade III alkali injury to the right eye 10 days prior presents for evaluation. He demonstrated a complete corneal epithelium defect during initial evaluation, including 3 clock hours of conjunctival involvement. He has been managed on frequent topical corticosteroids and a topical antibiotic. Today, the epithelial defect shows no improvement. Topical steroids will be tapered. After undergoing epithelial debridement at the slit lamp, the decision is made to place amniotic membrane on a conformer ring.

PROCEDURE: PLACEMENT OF SUTURELESS AMNIOTIC MEMBRANE

Supplies

- Eyelid speculum
- Topical anesthetic
- Amniotic membrane on a conformer ring (cryopreserved) or dehydrated amniotic membrane
- Blunt forceps
- Saline solution
- Clear Transpore surgical tape
- Bandage contact lens

Procedure

Administer topical anesthesia. Remove properly sized amniotic graft on a conformer ring (Prokera) from packaging and rinse with sterile saline solution per manufacturer recommendations. Retract the upper eyelid and ask the patient to look down. An eyelid speculum may be used but is not necessary. Using blunt forceps, insert the conformer ring into the superior fornix. Release the upper eyelid and retract the lower eyelid, inserting the inferior portion of the ring into the inferior fornix. Check centration under the slit lamp. Apply a tape tarsorrhaphy horizontally over the upper eyelid crease to narrow the palpebral fissure and improve patient comfort.

Alternatively, dehydrated amniotic membrane (such as AmbioDisk) can be applied directly to the ocular surface and covered with an overlying Bandage contact lens. Ensure the graft is oriented stromal side down so the watermark is properly oriented per manufacturer recommendations.

DISCUSSION

Amniotic membranes act as antiinflammatory scaffolds for the regrowth of corneal and conjunctival epithelium, as well as barriers to inflammatory mediators. The rate of epithelial healing has been shown to be significantly higher in eyes with amniotic membrane placement, especially in moderate chemical burns.[10] A conformer system is low risk and also functions as a symblepharon ring. Longevity will vary depending on the extent of injury. The membrane will typically dissolve within 3–5 days after insertion, after which it can be beneficial to insert a new membrane. However, it is argued that the amniotic membrane longevity in inflamed eyes can be low and the significant cost of placement does not justify its use. Furthermore, amniotic membrane transplantation cannot overcome complete limbal stem cell loss. In high-grade chemical exposures, more definitive treatments in the operating room may be warranted, such as sutured amniotic membrane transplantation, tenonplasty, or limbal stem cell transplantation. The long-term result of successful amniotic membrane placement after moderate-severe injury can still be a completely vascularized conjunctivalization of the cornea. This represents a trade-off for avoiding corneoscleral melt in these severe cases and may require late-penetrating keratoplasty after structural stabilization.

Conclusion

Ocular chemical burns offer unique challenges and can result in significant ocular morbidity. Proper medical and surgical management can optimize visual outcomes in this potentially blinding event. Early in-office procedures play a considerable role in promoting repair and preventing corneal melt.

References

1. Pfister RR. Chemical injuries of the eye. *Ophthalmology*. 1983;90(10):1246–1253.
2. Haring RS, Sheffield ID, Channa R, Canner JK, Schneider EB. Epidemiologic trends of chemical ocular burns in the United States [published correction appears in *JAMA Ophthalmol*. 2017 Apr 1;135(4):404]. *JAMA Ophthalmol*. 2016;134(10):1119–1124. https://doi.org/10.1001/jamaophthalmol.2016.2645.
3. Blackburn J, Levitan EB, MacLennan PA, Owsley C, McGwin Jr. G. The epidemiology of chemical eye injuries. *Curr Eye Res*. 2012;37(9):787–793. https://doi.org/10.3109/02713683.2012.681747.
4. Gérard M, Louis V, Merle H, Josset P, Menerath JM, Blomet J. Experimental study about intra-ocular penetration of ammonia. *J Fr Ophtalmol*. 1999;22(10):1047–1053. https://PubMed.gov/10617842.
5. Pfister RR, Friend J, Dohlman CH. The anterior segments of rabbits after alkali burns. Metabolic and histologic alterations. *Arch Ophthalmol*. 1971;86(2):189–193. https://doi.org/10.1001/archopht. 1971.01000010191013.
6. Dua HS, King AJ, Joseph A. A new classification of ocular surface burns. *Br J Ophthalmol*. 2001; 85(11):1379–1383. https://doi.org/10.1136/bjo.85.11.1379.
7. Kuckelkorn R, Schrage N, Keller G, Redbrake C. Emergency treatment of chemical and thermal eye burns. *Acta Ophthalmol Scand*. 2002;80(1):4–10. https://doi.org/10.1034/j.1600-0420.2002.800102.x.
8. Rihawi S, Frentz M, Schrage NF. Emergency treatment of eye burns: Which rinsing solution should we choose? *Graefes Arch Clin Exp Ophthalmol*. 2006;244(7):845–854. https://doi.org/10.1007/s00417-005-0034-3.
9. Reim M. The results of ischaemia in chemical injuries. *Eye (Lond)*. 1992;6(Pt 4):376–380. https://doi.org/10.1038/eye.1992.77.
10. Tandon R, Gupta N, Kalaivani M, Sharma N, Titiyal JS, Vajpayee RB. Amniotic membrane transplantation as an adjunct to medical therapy in acute ocular burns. *Br J Ophthalmol*. 2011;95(2):199–204. https://doi.org/10.1136/bjo.2009.173716.

CHAPTER 20

Acute Stevens-Johnson Syndrome

Austin S. Nakatsuka ■ Amy Lin

Introduction

Stevens-Johnson syndrome (SJS) and its severe counterpart, toxic epidermal necrolysis (TEN), is a dermatologic emergency characterized by bullous lesions of the mucosal tissues and epidermis with potential for severe ophthalmic sequelae. SJS involves less than 10% of the total body surface area, while TEN involves greater than 30%.[1] The pathophysiology of the disease involves widespread apoptosis of epidermal keratinocytes mediated by cytotoxic T cells and natural killer cells. These immune mediators release granulysin, a protein that disrupts the cellular membrane of target cells, leading to mitochondrial damage and eventual apoptosis.[2–4] In 75% of cases, the inciting agent is a drug or drug metabolite that is processed by the epidermal keratinocytes, leading to this cascade of cell-mediated events. Medications from multiple drug classes have been implicated in this disease, although the association with sulfa-based antibiotics is one of the most well-known.[5,6] The remaining 25% of cases are thought to be directly related to infectious etiologies, with *Mycobacterium pneumoniae* being the most commonly implicated organism.[7]

The goals of systemic treatment for SJS include immediate identification and removal of the offending agent, if possible, and initiation of essential life support. Due to the significant loss of epidermal tissues, patients are frequently admitted to a burn unit where protocols for sepsis prevention and treatment for hypovolemia are implemented to counteract loss of the natural skin barrier. Systemic use of high-dose steroids is controversial due to high risks of life-threatening infections, masking of septicemia, and delayed reepithelialization of tissues.[1,8] The use of intravenous immunoglobulin has also produced equivocal results. A few case reports and one case series have shown some benefit with the use of systemic cyclosporine, but overall, no prospective randomized controlled studies have been done to show superiority of systemic treatments over supportive care.[9] Despite treatment options, mortality rates for this disease are significantly high, approaching 40%.[10–16]

The acute phase of SJS lasts about 8 to 12 days and initially manifests in ocular tissues as bilateral conjunctivitis with purulent discharge, often occurring independently of dermatological findings.[6,17] This can progress to the formation of conjunctival pseudomembranes, ulceration, and hemorrhages. Eventually, these changes lead to cicatricial changes in the conjunctiva and lid margin. Corneal changes in the acute phase of SJS range from superficial punctate epithelial erosions to large epithelial defects that can lead to ulceration and even perforation. Uveitis is a less common but potentially devastating complication.[18]

Chronic, long-term complications of SJS include debilitating symblepharon, limbal stem cell failure, and lid keratinization leading to perpetual irritation. Even recurrent trichiasis caused by forniceal destruction can be difficult to treat, leading to corneal thinning and ulceration. Permanent dry eye can result due to destruction of goblet cells, Meibomian gland orifices, and lacrimal gland ductules.[19] Medical management largely involves lubrication and local control of inflammation, while surgical intervention with amniotic membrane to cover the eyelids is key to prevent the aforementioned complications. One study showed that early surgical intervention with the amniotic membrane in patients with at least moderate SJS ocular disease was effective in preventing severe vision loss.[20] Thus, recognition and prevention of the early findings in acute SJS are key to avoiding the potentially irreversible late manifestations of this disease.[1]

Management

The management of SJS involves daily bedside exams, with special attention to the cornea and conjunctiva. Because of the logistical difficulty of performing a traditional slit-lamp examination in an inpatient setting (and if a portable slit lamp is not available), the exam is often accomplished with an indirect ophthalmoscope with or without a magnifying lens. A 20- or 28-diopter lens can be used in conjunction with the indirect unit to magnify the image and thus improve the diagnostic utility of the examination. If an indirect ophthalmoscope or other similar device (such as a direct ophthalmoscope) is not available, a penlight or even a smartphone light can suffice as a backup option. Downloadable smartphone apps have been designed with cobalt blue light, which can be used to identify fluorescent staining. Fluorescein dye with strips or fluorescein solution should be used daily to stain the cornea and conjunctiva in order to assess disease severity and follow progression. Forniceal sweeps with a glass rod, lidocaine-soaked cotton tip, or scleral depressor can be done every 1 to 2 days to remove pseudomembranes (Fig. 20.1), although this has not been unequivocally proven to prevent formation of symblepharon.[9]

A grading system for disease severity was created by Gregory and published in *Ophthalmology* in 2016.[21] The system involves assessment and staining of the cornea, conjunctiva, and lid margin to classify the ocular involvement of the disease process. With this system, additional medical and/or surgical options are advised (Table 20.1).

Ophthalmic medical management of acute SJS involves infection prophylaxis, aggressive lubrication, and prevention of inflammation. Patients are typically started on a triad of topical steroids (e.g., loteprednol 0.5% or dexamethasone 0.1%), fluoroquinolones (e.g., moxifloxacin 0.5%), and lubricating drops or ointment. Medications without preservatives are preferred to limit ocular

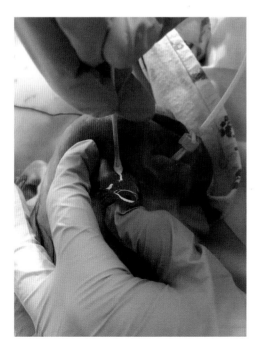

Fig. 20.1 Forniceal sweeps to remove pseudomembranes can be done with a lidocaine-soaked cotton-tip swab, glass rod, or scleral depressor.

TABLE 20.1 ■ Ophthalmologic Grading Criteria and Treatment Recommendations for Acute Steven-Johnson Syndrome

Staining Location and Treatment Recommendations	Severity of Eye Involvement			
	Mild	Moderate	Severe[a]	Extremely Severe[b]
Lid margin	No stain	Stain <1/3 of lid margin length	Stain <1/3 of lid margin length on at least 1 lid	Stain <1/3 of lid margin length on more than 1 lid
Cornea	No stain	No stain	Any epithelial detect more than punctate staining	Any epithelial defect more than punctate staining
Conjunctiva (bulbar and palpebral)	Hyperemia, without stain	(+)Stain, <1 cm in greatest diameter	(+)Stain >1 cm	Multiple areas of stain >1 cm
Treatment recommendations	Medical	Medical and close observation	Medical and urgent AMT	Medical and urgent AMT (may require repeat AMT)

[a]A case was considered severe if there was severe involvement of the lid margin, cornea, or conjunctiva. It was not required that all 3 areas have severe involvement simultaneously.
[b]Extremely severe cases had multiple areas of extensive fluorescein staining simultaneously.
AMT, Amniotic membrane transplantation.
Taken from Gregory DG. New grading system and treatment guidelines for the acute ocular manifestations of Stevens-Johnson syndrome. *Ophthalmology*. 2016;123(8):1653–1658.

surface irritation. Topical cyclosporine 0.05% can be utilized for its lacrimal-stimulating and mild immunomodulating effects. To prevent symblepharon and promote corneal healing, a symblepharon ring fused to the amniotic membrane, such as Prokera (BioTissue), is often placed over the cornea and within the fornices.[9]

Case

A 64-year-old male presented to the emergency department for diffuse rash, mucous membrane lesions, and sloughing bullae of his extremities after taking a 7-day course of sulfamethoxazole-trimethoprim (Bactrim) for cellulitis. He was admitted for care after dermatology confirmed the diagnosis of acute SJS, and he was immediately treated with high-dose intravenous steroids (1 gram methylprednisolone daily initially).

Upon initial ophthalmologic assessment, the patient was noted to be 20/20 best corrected visual acuity (BCVA) in both eyes, with mild punctate epithelial corneal staining and patchy bulbar conjunctival staining bilaterally. He was noted to have discontinuous staining of the upper and lower eyelid margins of the right eye, involving approximately 1/3 of the lid margin.

Treatment was initiated with a course of topical preservative-free loteprednol 0.5% (Lotemax) ointment four times a day, topical cyclosporine 0.05% (Restasis) two times a day, tobramycin 0.3%-dexamethasone 0.1% (Tobradex) drops two times a day, and frequent lubrication with preservative-free artificial tears every 1 to 2 hours. Over the next few days, the eyelid margin staining of the right eye began to slowly progress to greater than 1/3 of the margin, and pseudomembranes began to form. Daily sweeps of the fornices were initiated, and the patient was transitioned to preservative-free dexamethasone 0.1% eye drops. After progression of eyelid margin staining and pseudomembrane formation despite the treatment alterations, the decision was made to perform amniotic membrane transplantation to the right upper and lower eyelids.

Following amniotic membrane placement to the right upper and lower fornices and Prokera placement, the patient was monitored daily until discharge. The membranes had completely dissolved by postoperative day 14, and the sutures were removed in the office. At this point, the patient appeared to be improving, with resolution of pseudomembranes and improvement in eyelid staining, as well as systemically. The steroid eye drops were tapered, and the patient ultimately did fairly well, with very mild symblepharon formation that did not significantly affect function or quality of life.

PROCEDURE: SYMBLEPHARON LYSING AT THE BEDSIDE

Supplies

- Scissors: Westcott, sharp or blunt
- Toothed forceps (e.g., 0.12- or 0.3-mm Castroviejo forceps with teeth)
- Lidocaine 4% gel
- Handheld high-temperature cautery
- Symblepharon ring or amniotic membrane with symblepharon ring (e.g., Prokera)

Procedure Details

1. Place copious amounts of lidocaine 4% gel over the eye and in the fornices for at least 5 to 10 minutes.
2. Identify areas of symblepharon.
3. Using toothed forceps and Westcott scissors, incise and release conjunctival attachments from the globe.
4. Use handheld cautery as needed to achieve hemostasis, taking care not to cause too much conjunctival burning, as this can create more scar tissue.
5. Place a symblepharon ring or amniotic membrane with a symblepharon ring to prevent further adhesions.

PROCEDURE: PLACEMENT OF SYMBLEPHARON RING OR SELF-RETAINING AMNIOTIC MEMBRANE GRAFT

Supplies

- Symblepharon ring or amniotic membrane with symblepharon ring, (e.g., Prokera)
- Proparacaine or tetracaine topical drops
- Long cotton-tip applicator

Procedure Details

1. Instill at least 2–3 drops of topical anesthetic (e.g., proparacaine or tetracaine) into the eye, including into the deep fornices.
2. Remove the symblepharon ring or amniotic membrane with symblepharon ring from the packaging.

3. If using the amniotic membrane with symblepharon ring, rinse with balanced salt solution or saline, as the packaging fluid can be irritating to the ocular surface.
4. While the patient is looking inferiorly, insert the ring in the deep superior fornix, using the cotton-tip applicator to evert the upper eyelid as needed.
5. Have the patient then look superiorly, and then insert the ring into the inferior fornix, using a fingertip or cotton-tip applicator to evert the lower eyelid as needed.
6. Center the ring and ensure that it is resting deep within both fornices. If an amniotic membrane is present on the ring, make sure that the entire cornea is covered.

In moderate to severe cases, surgical intervention is often indicated to prevent significant conjunctival scarring. This involves the placement of amniotic membrane grafts over the eyelids, conjunctival fornices, and sometimes the cornea. Although techniques have been described using cyanoacrylate glue,[22] small-caliber sutures to secure the grafts to the underlying tissues may provide greater security of the graft. Because of the fine suturing required for the procedure and the length of surgical time needed to apply membrane to all of the eyelids, we recommend that this procedure be done under general anesthesia in the operating room, if possible. Others have advocated for bedside surgical intervention,[23] but we have found that the requirements of at least moderate sedation, a cooperative patient, and a semisterile environment free from accessories and equipment around the head of the bed are rarely possible with these severely ill patients. Regardless of where the procedure takes place, discussion should be done first with the primary burn service and the anesthesiologists involved.

PROCEDURE: OCULAR SURFACE RECONSTRUCTION WITH SUTURED AMNIOTIC MEMBRANE GRAFTING

Supplies (Fig. 20.2)

- Forceps, Castroviejo, 0.12 mm with teeth
- Forceps, Castroviejo, 0.3 mm with teeth
- Forceps, Castroviejo, 0.5 mm with teeth
- Caliper, Castroviejo, 20 mm
- Needle holder, curved, with or without lock
- Surgical marker
- Cyclodialysis spatula
- Muscle hook, Jameson or Graefe
- Scissors, Westcott, sharp
- Scissors, Westcott, blunt
- Retractor, Desmarres (optional)
- Forceps, Kelman McPherson, tying (optional)

Sutures
- Two double-armed Prolene sutures (5-0 or 6-0) per eyelid
- 8-0 nylon suture

Additional
- One 5-cm × 5-cm sheet of cryopreserved amniotic membrane per eye (half sheet per eyelid) or two 3.5-cm × 3.5-cm sheets per eye (1 sheet per eyelid)
- Bolsters: intravenous (IV) tubing cut into 1-cm sections or cut pieces of Styrofoam from suture packet
- Amniotic membrane with symblepharon ring (e.g., Prokera) or IV tubing (21 or 18 gauge) with additional suture to create a symblepharon ring

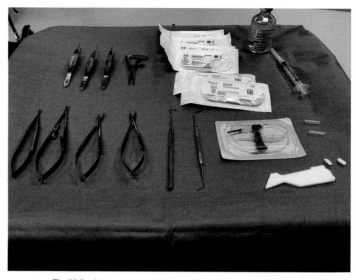

Fig. 20.2   Instrument tray for amniotic membrane placement.

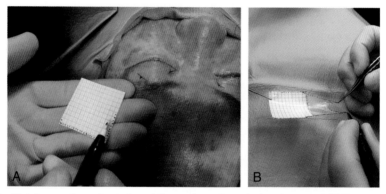

Fig. 20.3   (A) A 5-cm × 5-cm sheet of amniotic membrane is marked and prepared. (B) Two tying forceps without teeth are used to gently remove the membrane from the underlying card, and the stromal side is placed downward, overlying the palpebral conjunctiva.

- 2% lidocaine with epinephrine
- 3- or 5-cc syringe with 27-gauge needle

Ocular Surface Reconstruction With Amniotic Membrane Grafting

Technique

1. Employ standard preoperative protocol, including instillation of antiinfective and anesthetic drops or ointment.
2. Use alcohol to clean the eyelid(s) and inject 2% lidocaine with epinephrine 1:100,000 to achieve local anesthesia, approximately 3 cc per eyelid.
3. Apply 5% povidone-iodine solution and apply sterile drapes to the operative eye(s).
4. Cut the lashes of the eyelid(s) to the base with Wescott scissors.
5. Cut the 5-cm × 5-cm amniotic membrane in half. All edges of each half should be completely marked to facilitate visualization of the membrane once it has been removed from the paper backing. Each 5-cm × 2.5-cm half can be used for an eyelid (Fig. 20.3).

6. Lay the amniotic membrane segment over the eyelid. Secure the amniotic membrane edge to the eyelid skin approximately 2 mm anterior to the lash line with 8-0 running nylon suture.

7. Use a muscle hook or other blunt instrument to bury the free edge of the amniotic membrane as deep as possible into the fornix. A Desmarres retractor or muscle hook can be used to evert the eyelid if this helps.

8. At the medial aspect of the eyelid, use a double-armed 5-0 or 6-0 Prolene suture to secure the free edge of the amniotic membrane into the deep fornix, passing the needle through the membrane and then through the fornix and out through the skin. Bolsters are used to secure the knot to the eyelid skin to avoid late cheese wiring through the tissue.

9. Repeat this suture at the lateral aspect of the eyelid so that the amniotic membrane is covering as much of the eyelid margin, the palpebral conjunctiva, and the fornix as possible (Fig. 20.4).

10. Repeat the procedure for all eyelids involved.

11. Antibiotic/steroid ointment can be placed in the fornices and overlying the sutures on the skin.

12. Place the amniotic membrane with symblepharon ring (i.e., Prokera) over the cornea and ensure that it is centered and secured by the eyelids (Fig. 20.5).

Creation of Amniotic Membrane Symblepharon Ring Intraoperatively (if Prokera is not available or sizing is not appropriate) (Fig. 20.6):

Measure the approximate size of IV tubing needed to create the ring. The tubing can be placed within the fornices and adjusted as needed. The fit should be large enough to fit deep within the fornices but not too large that it would cause unbearable discomfort or incomplete lid closure.

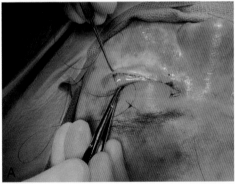

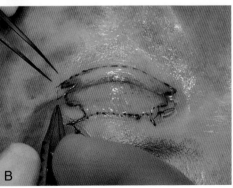

Fig. 20.4 (A) After eyelashes are removed, the membrane is secured to the eyelid skin anterior to the lash line. (B) The membrane is buried deep within the fornix, and a Prolene suture is used to secure the edge to the deep fornix.

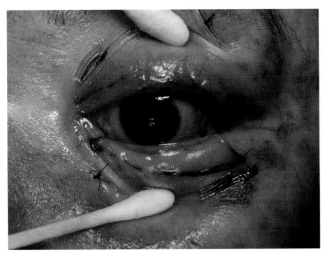

Fig. 20.5 An amniotic membrane with symblepharon ring (e.g., Prokera) is placed over the cornea after the membranes overlying the eyelids have been completed.

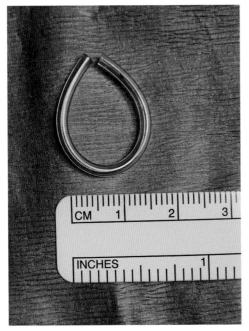

Fig. 20.6 Symblepharon ring made from intravenous (IV) tubing and Prolene suture.

1. Cut the tubing with heavy, straight scissors.
2. Run a suture through the tubing. Prolene is likely the easiest to do this; however, silk or nylon will also work.
3. Tie the suture at the ends of the tubing. The knot needs to be as tight as possible.
4. Rotate the suture so that the knot is within the tubing. The ring will be slightly elliptical in shape.

5. Place the symblepharon ring within the fornices and position with the tied ends sitting posterior to the lateral canthus. The elliptical shape of the ring should allow it to fit appropriately within the space of the globe, palpebral conjunctiva, and canthi, which is larger horizontally than vertically.

(Cyanoacrylate glue or a connector made from a piece of larger-gauge IV tubing can also be used to secure the ends together instead of suture.[22])

Conclusion

SJS and TEN have severe ocular implications ranging from mild keratoconjunctivitis to severe corneal vascularization and symblepharon formation. In the acute phase of SJS-TEN, it is estimated that 80% of patients will have some ocular involvement, and up to 60% of adult survivors will develop chronic ocular changes secondary to the disease.[1,6] Medical management of the ocular findings in acute SJS includes aggressive lubrication, suppression of inflammation, infection prophylaxis, and pseudomembrane removal. Surgical management in the acute phase involves amniotic membrane placement to prevent cicatricial changes of the eyelids and fornices. This also provides growth factors to heal and prevent further corneal changes caused by inflammation and scarring. Early recognition and intervention are key to preventing devastating sequelae that can often be irreversible in this rare but debilitating disease.

Acknowledgments

Special thanks to Christina Mamalis, MD, and Severin Pouly, MD, for their assistance with images.

This was supported in part by an unrestricted grant from Research to Prevent Blindness, New York, New York, to the Department of Ophthalmology & Visual Sciences, city of University of Utah, Salt Lake City, Utah.

References

1. Nirken MH, High WA, Roujeau J-C. Stevens Johnson syndrome and toxic epidermal necrolysis: Pathogenesis, clinical manifestations, and diagnosis. UpToDate website. August 2015. Accessed 11/14/2023. https://www.uptodate.com/contents/stevens-johnson-syndrome-and-toxic-epidermal-necrolysis-pathogenesis-clinical-manifestations-and-diagnosis.
2. Chung WH, Hung SI, Yang JY, et al. Granulysin is a key mediator for disseminated keratinocyte death in Stevens-Johnson syndrome and toxic epidermal necrolysis. Nat Med. 2008;14(12):1343–1350.
3. Wei HM, Lin LC, Wang CF, Lee YJ, Chen YT, Liao YD. Antimicrobial properties of an immuno-modulator-15 kDa human granulysin. PLoS One. 2016;11(6):e0156321.
4. Saeed HN, Chodosh J. Immunologic mediators in Stevens-Johnson syndrome and toxic epidermal necrolysis. Semin Ophthalmol. 2016;31(1-2):85–90.
5. Wander AH, Kroger J. Stevens-Johnson Syndrome. American Academy of Ophthalmology, EyeWiki. Last updated 9/11/2023. Accessed 11/14/2023. https://eyewiki.org/Stevens-Johnson_Syndrome#cite_note-wetter_3-3.
6. Chantachaeng W, Chularojanamontri L, Kulthanan K, Jongjarearnprasert K, Dhana N. Cutaneous adverse reactions to sulfonamide antibiotics. Asian Pac J Allergy Immunol. 2011;29(3):284–289.
7. Wetter DA, Camilleri MJ. Clinical, etiologic, and histopathologic features of Stevens-Johnson syndrome during an 8-year period at Mayo Clinic. Mayo Clin Proc. 2010;85(2):131–138.
8. Sriram A, Sreya K, Lakshmi PN. Steven Johnson syndrome and toxic epidermal necrolysis: A review. Int J Pharmacol Res. 2014;4(4):158–165.
9. Gregory DG. The ophthalmologic management of acute Stevens-Johnson syndrome. Ocul Surf. 2008;6(2):87–95.

10. Haber J, Hopman W, Gomez M, Cartotto R. Late outcomes in adult survivors of toxic epidermal necrolysis after treatment in a burn center. *J Burn Care Rehabil.* 2005;26:33–41.
11. French LE. Toxic epidermal necrolysis and Stevens Johnson syndrome: our current understanding. *Allergol Int.* 2006;55:9–16.
12. Power WJ, Ghoraishi M, Merayo-Lloves J, et al. Analysis of the acute ophthalmic manifestations of the erythema multiforme/Stevens-Johnson syndrome/toxic epidermal necrolysis disease spectrum. *Ophthalmology.* 1995;102:1669–1676.
13. De Rojas MV, Dart JK, Saw VP. The natural history of Stevens-Johnson syndrome: Patterns of chronic ocular disease and the role of systemic immunosuppressive therapy. *Br J Ophthalmol.* 2007;91:1048–1053.
14. Mittman N, Chan B, Knowles S, et al. Intravenous immunoglobulin use in patients with toxic epidermal necrolysis and Stevens-Johnson syndrome. *Am J Clin Dermatol.* 2006;7:359–368.
15. Ahmed AR, Dahl MV. Consensus statement on the use of intravenous immunoglobulin therapy in the treatment of autoimmune mucocutaneous blistering diseases. *Arch Dermatol.* 2003;139:1051–1059.
16. Schneck J, Fagot J, Sekula P, et al. Effects of treatments on the mortality of Stevens-Johnson syndrome and toxic epidermal necrolysis: A retrospective study on patients included in the prospective EuroSCAR study. *J Am Acad Dermatol.* 2008;58:33–40.
17. Catt CJ, Hamilton GM, Fish J, Mireskandari K, Ali A. Ocular manifestations of Stevens-Johnson syndrome and toxic epidermal necrolysis in children. *Am J Ophthalmol.* 2016;166:68–75.
18. Jain R, Sharma N, Basu S, et al. Stevens-Johnson syndrome: The role of an ophthalmologist. *Surv Ophthalmol.* 2016;61(4):369–399.
19. Lin A, Patel N, Yoo D, DeMartelaere S, Bouchard C. Management of ocular conditions in the burn unit: Thermal and chemical burns and Stevens-Johnson syndrome/toxic epidermal necrolysis. *J Burn Care Res.* 2011 Sep-Oct;32(5):547–560.
20. Hsu M, Jayaram A, Verner R, Lin A, Bouchard C. Indications and outcomes of amniotic membrane transplantation in the management of acute Stevens-Johnson syndrome and toxic epidermal necrolysis: A case-control study. *Cornea.* 2012 Dec;31(12):1394–1402.
21. Gregory DG. New grading system and treatment guidelines for the acute ocular manifestations of Stevens-Johnson syndrome. *Ophthalmology.* 2016;123(8):1653–1658.
22. Shanbhag SS, Chodosh J, Saeed HN. Sutureless amniotic membrane transplantation with cyanoacrylate glue for acute Stevens-Johnson syndrome/toxic epidermal necrolysis. *Ocul Surf.* 2019 Jul;17(3):560–564.
23. Saeed HN, Chodosh J. Ocular manifestations of Stevens-Johnson syndrome and their management. *Curr Opin Ophthalmol.* 2016 Nov;27(6):522–529.

CHAPTER 21

Limbal Stem Cell Deficiency

Taylor W. Starnes ■ Ali R. Djalilian

Introduction

Limbal stem cell deficiency (LSCD) is the result of damage or dysfunction of the limbal stem cell niche, which is the microenvironment that functions to maintain the health of the limbal stem cells. The limbal stem cells reside in the Palisades of Vogt, where they are supported by capillary networks, nerves, mesenchymal cells, melanocytes, and a variety of signaling molecules and growth factors. These various components create the niche, and disrupting them through trauma or inflammation can compromise the function of the limbal stem cells.[1,2] When the limbal niche and limbal stem cells are not functioning properly, they no longer inhibit conjunctival and vascular growth onto the cornea, leading to the typical finding of corneal conjunctivalization.[3] This abnormal corneal epithelium impairs visual acuity due to its decreased clarity and irregular refracting surface.

In early disease, there may be a mixture of normal corneal epithelium, metaplastic corneal epithelium, and conjunctival epithelium. In this stage, the predominant clinical sign is punctate staining with fluorescein. This staining differs from that seen in dry eye due to its location (can be present in any part of the cornea rather than just interpalpebral) and size (larger puncta than in dry eye).[1,3] As LSCD progresses, the proportion of conjunctival epithelium increases. The conjunctival epithelium is thinner and more opaque than the corneal epithelium, which gives the affected areas a hazy, irregular appearance. Neovascularization also develops as LSCD progresses. Additionally, because of the greater permeability of conjunctival epithelium to fluorescein, there is late staining of this epithelium that follows a characteristic whorl pattern. In later stages of LSCD, subepithelial scarring and recurrent or persistent epithelial defects may occur.[4-6]

While LSCD is predominately a clinical diagnosis, adjunctive techniques may be used for confirmation. Impression cytology can be performed to assess for conjunctival epithelial cells or goblet cells, which should not be present in normal corneal epithelium.[7] Confocal microscopy and anterior segment optical coherence tomography can also differentiate normal and conjunctival epithelium based on morphology.[8,9]

A consensus group recently developed a staging system for LSCD based on the degree of conjunctivalization and pannus covering the cornea. In stage I, the central 5 mm of the cornea is clear. When the central 5 mm is affected, the patient is stage II, and when the entire cornea is affected, the patient is stage III.[3]

In early disease, when there are viable limbal stem cells remaining, improving their function requires optimizing the health of the limbal niche. This may be done by removing toxic substances, suppressing inflammation, and replacing growth factors. In advanced disease, limbal transplantation procedures may be needed to restore the limbal niche and healthy corneal epithelium.[1,10] Here, we describe procedures that may be performed in the clinic to optimize the health of the limbal niche and restore corneal clarity in patients with partial LSCD.

Case 1

A 39-year-old male was referred for cornea consultation for LSCD in the left eye. He sustained a chemical injury with battery acid in the left eye 5 months prior to our evaluation. The right eye was unaffected. Treatment of the acute injury was performed at an outside institution. At the time of our evaluation, he noted blurry vision and redness in the left eye. He denied any pain or irritation. He was being treated with prednisolone acetate 1% four times per day and ofloxacin 0.3% two times per day.

Best corrected visual acuities were 20/20 and 20/100 in the right and left eyes, respectively. The right eye had a clear cornea with healthy epithelium. The conjunctiva of the left eye was mildly injected, and there was a pseudopterygium extending onto the nasal aspect of the cornea. Centrally and inferiorly, there was raised and irregular epithelium that stained in a pattern consistent with LSCD. Approximately 30% of the limbus was affected. There was mild stromal haze temporally (Fig. 21.1). The remainder of the exam was unremarkable.

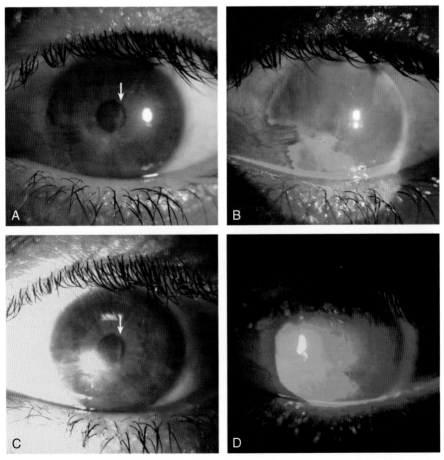

Fig. 21.1 Slit-lamp photos of the left eye from the patient described in Case 1. (A–B) Appearance prior to initiating treatment with serum tears without (A) and with (B) fluorescein. Note the ridge of abnormal epithelium extending into the central cornea (A, *white arrow*). (C–D) Slit-lamp photos after 2 months of treatment with serum tears. Note the improved corneal clarity in the central and paracentral cornea and the decreased prominence of the epithelial ridge.

Our patient met the criteria for stage II LSCD because of central corneal involvement with 8 clock hours of healthy limbus. Because of the moderate degree of LSCD, we felt that the patient was a good candidate for medical treatment with autologous serum tear drops.

PROCEDURE: OBTAINING AUTOLOGOUS SERUM TEARS

The procedure for obtaining serum tears varies by institution. Patients will need to have blood collected in red-top Vacutainer or equivalent tubes with silica coating designed for serum collection. This may be performed by a nurse in clinic or at a participating phlebotomy lab. The blood is then transferred to a local compounding pharmacy that makes the serum tears product. Some pharmacies require testing for bloodborne pathogens prior to compounding serum tears.

To produce serum tears, blood is collected and left at room temperature for approximately 2 hours to achieve complete clotting. The tubes are then centrifuged at $3000 \times g$ for 15 minutes to separate the serum from the clotted blood. The serum is then collected and diluted with saline to achieve the desired concentration.[11] Serum tears are most commonly produced in strengths ranging from 20% to 50%, but they can be made at various concentrations up to 100% serum.[4,5,12,13] An important consideration for LSCD patients is minimizing the preservative burden on the ocular surface due to the epithelial toxicity of common ophthalmic preservatives, such as benzalkonium chloride.[14–16] Therefore, we recommend preservative-free formulations of serum tears for LSCD patients whenever possible. We typically recommend instillation of serum tears 4–6 times per day, but a wide range of dosing regimens from 4 times per day to every 1 hour have been studied.[13]

CASE FOLLOW-UP

We continued to treat our patient with prednisolone acetate 1% four times per day and added preservative-free 50% autologous serum tears four times per day. After 2 months of treatment, the patient's best corrected vision improved to 20/40 in the left eye. The pseudopterygium remained stable in appearance. There was significant improvement in the central epithelial irregularity, with only a small paracentral epithelial ridge remaining.

We plan to maintain the patient on serum tears until his vision and epithelial clarity plateau. Based on his early response, he may continue to improve with continued serum tear therapy. If the epithelial ridge does not resolve, we may treat him with a superficial keratectomy or scleral contact lens. We hope to avoid surgical intervention in this patient. However, he would be a good candidate for a right eye-to-left eye conjunctival limbal autograft or simple limbal epithelial transfer should we experience difficulty in maintaining epithelial clarity in the future. Fortunately, he did not have any chemical injury to the right eye. If a limbal autograft is being considered, it is important to assess the health of the corneal epithelium and Palisades of Vogt in the noninjured eye preoperatively. In some cases, the fellow eye may have a subclinical LSCD with clear epithelium, and harvesting a limbal autograft could precipitate symptomatic LSCD.

DISCUSSION

Serum tears have been used as an off-label treatment for many ocular surface diseases, including LSCD, dry eye syndrome, Sjogren syndrome, and neurotrophic keratitis.[13,17] The benefits of serum tears result from the presence of soluble growth factors, cytokines, and vitamins that are not available in standard artificial tears. Factors present in serum tears with proven benefits in epithelial healing and homeostasis include epidermal growth factor, nerve growth factor, transforming growth factor-β1, and vitamin A.[13,16–19] Epidermal growth factor is normally produced by both the lacrimal gland and corneal epithelial cells and induces proliferation and migration of epithelial cells. In addition to promoting corneal nerve growth and regeneration, nerve growth factor also acts directly on limbal stem cells to promote survival and expansion.[20,21] While many isolated components of serum have demonstrated efficacy in promoting epithelial healing, the powerful benefits of serum tears are likely a result of multiple factors that closely mimic the composition of natural tears to promote the health of the limbal niche.

There are no large, controlled studies evaluating the efficacy of serum tears in patients with LSCD. Visual acuity and corneal clarity improved in patients with partial LSCD due to aniridia who were treated with serum tears for 2 months. Patients with more advanced disease had improved epithelial stability, and there was improvement in squamous metaplasia across all degrees of LSCD.[22] Additionally, serum tears have demonstrated efficacy in a variety of other ocular surface conditions. Serum tears appeared to be beneficial in healing persistent epithelial defects in studies with mixed populations of ocular surface disease.[4,5,12] Serum tears have also been used to improve epithelial healing after refractive surgery and corneal transplantation and in patients with neurotrophic keratopathy.[19,23,24] Controlled trials of serum tears in dry eye found improvement in both symptoms and clinical signs.[25,26] Overall, there is substantial evidence across the spectrum of ocular surface disease that serum tears promote a stable corneal epithelium. Plasma tears (i.e., platelet-rich plasma) have likewise been studied extensively in patients with ocular surface disease. While we use serum and plasma tears interchangeably, there may be additional factors in plasma tears that may be advantageous in certain clinical scenarios.

Both serum and plasma tears have a very favorable safety and tolerability profile. Because they are a compounded medication, there is a risk of contamination leading to infection, although this appears to be fairly rare. Some patients have reported discomfort, redness, and swelling when using serum tears.[4,5,13,23,24]

Case 2

A 56-year-old male was referred for management of LSCD in the right eye due to soft contact lens wear. He had a 36-year history of soft contact lens wear and reported using monthly disposable lenses. Prior to our initial evaluation, he had been instructed to cease using soft contact lenses. He was treated with cyclosporine 0.05% two times per day and artificial tears in both eyes. The right eye also received fluorometholone 0.1% drops daily. He had also been treated with a superficial keratectomy in the right eye to remove the abnormal epithelium, but this was unsuccessful in improving his vision, as there was a recurrence of irregular epithelium in his visual axis.

At the time of his initial presentation in our clinic, the best corrected visual acuities were 20/70 and 20/20 in the right and left eyes, respectively. In the right eye, the Palisades of Vogt were poorly defined superiorly and inferiorly affecting 70% of the limbus, and conjunctivalized epithelium grew onto the cornea from these areas. There was abnormal corneal epithelium centrally, which was consistent with stage II disease (Fig. 21.2). The left eye demonstrated poorly defined Palisades of Vogt and mild superficial pannus formation affecting 25% of the limbus superiorly, but the cornea remained clear centrally (stage I). The remainder of the anterior segment exam was unremarkable.

After starting doxycycline and serum tears to promote the health of the ocular surface in the right eye, there was no improvement in the epithelial appearance. Superficial keratectomy was reattempted, and again, there was no significant improvement in central corneal clarity. Because the patient had been stable, we felt that a scleral lens could improve his vision without further disrupting the remaining healthy limbal stem cells.

PROCEDURE: SCLERAL CONTACT LENS TREATMENT

Scleral lenses are large-diameter, rigid, gas-permeable contact lenses that rest on the sclera and vault over the cornea and limbus. The prosthetic replacement of the ocular surface (PROSE; BostonSight, Needham, Massachusetts, USA) lens is the best-studied scleral lens for ocular

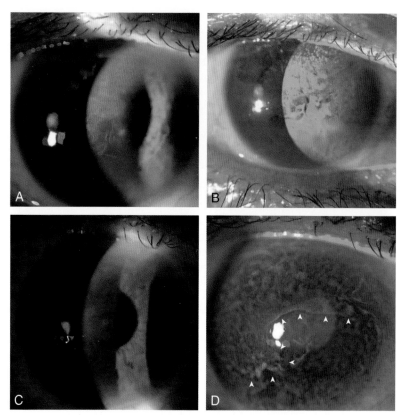

Fig. 21.2 Slit-lamp photos of the right eye from the patient described in case 2. (A–B) Appearance prior to initiating treatment with a scleral contact lens without (A) and with (B) fluorescein. (A) Note the hazy, irregular epithelium extending from the limbus superiorly and covering the central cornea. (B) Superiorly, there is prominent large punctate staining with a wavelike progression of conjunctivalized epithelium that is well visualized with fluorescein. (C–D) Appearance after 2 years of treatment with a scleral lens without (A) and with (B) fluorescein. (C) Central corneal clarity substantially improved with treatment. (B) However, there was still prominent wavelike conjunctivalization that was easily visualized with fluorescein staining (*arrowheads*).

surface disease and LSCD, but other models and manufacturers' lenses can be used.[6,27–29] The lenses are fit using a trial set with customized adjustments to the lens diameter, peripheral curves, base curve, and sagittal depth that allow the best fit for the patient's eye. When fitting scleral lenses in patients with LSCD, we ensure that the lens vaults over the limbus and cornea, as compression in these areas could cause further damage. The depth of vaulting cannot be excessive either, as this could result in corneal hypoxia.[30,31] Also, there is a concern that in patients with poor tear exchange under the lens, a scleral lens could trap inflammatory mediators and, with time, contribute to further epithelial dysfunction. Because of these complexities in fitting scleral contact lenses, especially in patients with ocular surface disease, we refer patients to specialized optometrists to perform these fittings.

For patients with ocular surface disease, we recommend filling the lens bowl with preservative-free 0.9% saline, often supplemented with preservative-free serum/plasma tears.[30] We recommend daily wear of the lenses with removal every evening. However, we occasionally treat patients with persistent epithelial defects with continuous wear in which the lens is removed two to four times during the day to replace the fluid in the bowl. If patients are treated with continuous use for this indication, we add a drop of prophylactic preservative-free fluoroquinolone antibiotic to the bowl and follow the patient every 1–2 days until the epithelial defect heals.[32] If patients have abnormal eyelid function, such as keratinization or the eyelid margin or trichiasis, we often have them insert a bandage soft contact lens after the scleral lens is removed. The scleral lens is cleaned by overnight soaking in a peroxide-based lens cleaning solution.[30]

CASE FOLLOW-UP

The patient has been wearing a scleral contact lens in both eyes for over 5 years with stability of his vision and LSCD during that time. His best-corrected acuity with the scleral lenses is 20/20 in both eyes. The clarity of the central epithelium improved in the right eye, and we did not detect any progression in either eye with scleral lens use (Fig. 21.2). We continue to treat him with cyclosporine 0.05% twice daily (BID) and fluorometholone 0.1% twice weekly.

DISCUSSION

The benefits of scleral contact lenses for LSCD are the result of stabilizing the limbal niche, protection from mechanical trauma, and correcting optical aberrations from the irregular surface.[1,30,31] Kim et al. reported a case series of 31 eyes with LSCD who were treated with scleral lenses. Nearly all patients had improved visual acuity, and approximately 70% gained at least two lines. Most studies evaluating the role of scleral lenses in LSCD include mixed populations of ocular surface disease patients, and they find similar improvements in visual acuity with scleral lens use.[27–29,31] Resolution of persistent epithelial defects, reduction in epithelial defect frequency, and improvement in conjunctivalization have also been reported in LSCD patients treated with scleral lenses.[6,31,33]

We feel that the ideal candidates for scleral contact lenses are patients with mild to moderate partial LSCD, as they have the greatest potential for visual improvement. Prior to utilizing scleral contact lenses, we try to maximize medical management (see Case 1) until improvement has plateaued. This avoids any potential stress to the limbal niche by a contact lens until it has been medically optimized. Additionally, many patients may sufficiently improve with medical therapy alone, precluding the need for a scleral lens. Patients with total LSCD are unlikely to achieve significant gains in visual acuity. However, utilizing a scleral lens to promote healing of a chronic epithelial defect in this subset may be effective.

There are several potential risks in treating LSCD patients with scleral contact lenses. Soft contact lens wear is a well-established cause of LSCD, likely due to hypoxia and mechanical trauma in the setting of a predisposed surface. These factors can certainly be present in an ill-fitting scleral lens and can worsen LSCD.[30,31] Regular monitoring is necessary to evaluate for progression of LSCD while wearing scleral lenses. If progression is detected, patients may need refitting or complete discontinuation of lenses. Infection is also a risk factor, especially if the lenses are being used to treat epithelial defects. Fluoroquinolone antibiotics should be placed in the lens before insertion in such cases to decrease this risk.[6,30,32]

Case 3

A 65-year-old female with a gradual decline in vision in both eyes due to LSCD was referred to our clinic. She had no prior history of contact lens use or chronic drop use. Her best corrected visual acuity was 20/40 in both eyes. She had 2+ papillae on the superior tarsal conjunctiva in both eyes. The right eye demonstrated conjunctivalization, primarily affecting the superior 5 clock hours of the cornea and sparing the visual axis. The left eye had 8 hours of conjunctivalization and a superior Salzmann-like nodule, again sparing the visual axis. She had decreased tear production and a low tear lake. The remainder of the exam was unremarkable. Treatment with preservative-free

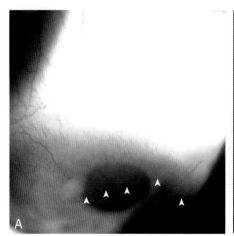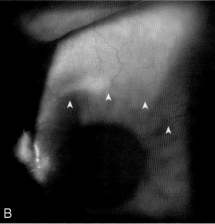

Fig. 21.3 Slit-lamp photos of the right eye from the patient described in Case 3. (A) Appearance prior to superficial keratectomy. Note the presence of conjunctival epithelium with fine vessels extending into the visual axis (*arrowheads*). (B) Improved corneal clarity 6 months after superficial keratectomy. The margin of conjunctivalization (*arrowheads*) remains outside of the visual axis.

tears, cyclosporine 0.05% BID, and intermittent use of topical antihistamines was initiated. Her corneal epithelium stabilized and improved over 4 years of treatment with this regimen, at which point her best corrected acuity was 20/20 in the right eye and 20/25 in the left.

The patient was subsequently lost to follow-up for 7 years, but she returned for declining vision, predominately in the right eye. The best corrected visual acuity had declined to 20/50 in the right eye. Her superior conjunctivalization had progressed into the visual axis, and there was mild subepithelial scarring centrally, consistent with stage II disease (Fig. 21.3). The central cornea remained clear in the left eye (stage I). Medical treatment was reinitiated in both eyes with cyclosporine 0.05% BID, erythromycin ointment every night at bedtime (QHS), and doxycycline 50 mg daily. She was also treated with a taper of loteprednol 0.5% and maintained on daily loteprednol. Despite these measures, the conjunctivalization did not regress in her right eye, and her visual acuity declined to 20/70 after 1 year of treatment. She was also developing an early nuclear sclerotic cataract. We decided to proceed with a superficial keratectomy in the right eye because of the inadequate response to medical management.

PROCEDURE: SUPERFICIAL KERATECTOMY

Supply List

- Topical anesthetic drops (tetracaine or proparacaine)
- Fluoroquinolone antibiotic drops
- Povidone-iodine swab sticks or 5% povidone-iodine solution
- Sterile drape (optional)
- Eyelid speculum
- No. 64 scalpel blade and handle
- Weck-Cel sponges (BVI Medical, Waltham, MA, USA)
- 4-inch × 4-inch gauze
- Sterile 0.9% saline solution or balanced salt solution
- Bandage soft contact lens

A superficial keratectomy can be performed in a minor operating room in clinic or at the slit lamp. Place topical anesthetic in the affected eye, followed by drops of a fluoroquinolone antibiotic. Prep the eye and periocular skin with povidone-iodine swab sticks or 5% povidone-iodine solution. If swab sticks are used, gently dab the inferior palpebral conjunctiva to place some iodine solution on the ocular surface. If the patient is supine for the procedure, a sterile drape can be used. Insert the eyelid speculum. The conjunctival epithelium is more loosely adherent to the cornea than normal corneal epithelium, and we utilize this property to determine the margins of the superficial keratectomy. Gently sweep the affected epithelium with Weck-Cel sponges in a central-to-peripheral direction. The conjunctivalized epithelium should lift while the corneal epithelium remains intact. Continue gently scraping the abnormal epithelium with a Weck-Cel sponge or a no. 64 scalpel blade until the abnormal epithelium is removed all the way to the limbus. Avoid dissecting through the Bowman layer. Rinse the eye with saline or balanced salt solution, instill a drop of fluoroquinolone antibiotic, and place a bandage contact lens.

Postoperatively, we instruct patients to use a fluoroquinolone antibiotic 4 times per day while there is an epithelial defect or while a bandage lens is in place. We ask them to immediately resume their normal medical management. Serum tears may be added to promote epithelialization. We see patients 1 day after the procedure and then weekly until the epithelial defect has resolved.

CASE FOLLOW-UP

Six months after performing a superficial keratectomy on the right eye, the central cornea remains clear. The best corrected visual acuity in the right eye is now 20/40, with a cataract and some residual stromal haze limiting her best corrected visual acuity (Fig. 21.3). She is being maintained on her preoperative medications and has deferred cataract extraction.

DISCUSSION

Superficial keratectomy can effectively restore corneal clarity by allowing normal corneal epithelium to repopulate the conjunctivalized area. However, recurrence is very likely if the health of the limbal niche has not been optimized with medical therapy.[34,35] We recommend continued medical therapy after superficial keratectomy as well in order to prevent regression. Even with an optimized surface, the conjunctival epithelium may repopulate the affected area before the healthy corneal epithelium does.

Amniotic membrane transplantation has been successfully combined with superficial keratectomy to promote growth of the corneal epithelium. For clinic-based procedures, a Prokera (BioTissue, Miami, Florida, USA) can be inserted, or an AmbioDisk (Katena, Parsippany, NJ, USA) can be placed under the bandage contact lens (see Chapter 16). Glued or sutured amniotic membrane transplantation can also be performed in the operating room. If the visually significant conjunctivalization remains after these measures, limbal autografting or allografting should be considered, depending on individual patient circumstances.

Conclusion

LSCD is caused by genetic, developmental, inflammatory, or toxic insults to the limbal niche. Characteristically, patients with LSCD have decreased visual acuity due to growth of conjunctival epithelium onto the corneal surface, and they may later develop complications such as epithelial defects and stromal scarring. Many patients with partial LSCD can be successfully treated with medical management. Here, we have described a series of in-office procedures and advanced techniques that can be used to treat patients who do not respond to initial medical treatment. We feel that these are appropriate interventions for many partial LSCD patients prior to considering more invasive limbal stem cell transplantation techniques.

In Fig. 21.4, we present an algorithm outlining our approach to managing patients with LSCD. Early recognition of LSCD is important so that therapeutic intervention can occur when corneal clarity is still recoverable. For patients in which continued toxic exposure is present, such as preserved drops or contact lens use, strict discontinuation of the exposure is critical. Our approach to management is then contingent on the stage of LSCD. We treat patients in all stages with medical management, even if we feel that surgical intervention will be necessary. However, the intensity and strategy of medical treatment vary based on the underlying

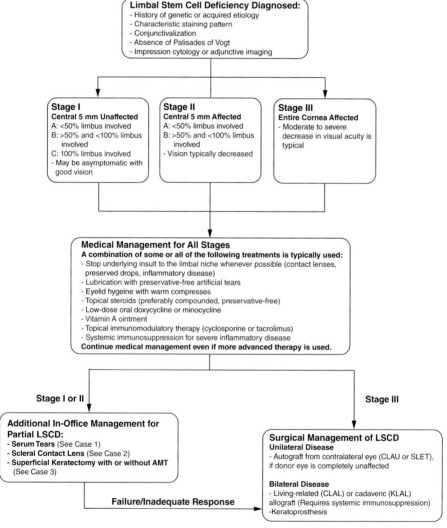

Fig. 21.4 Treatment algorithm for LSCD. *CLAL*, Conjunctival limbal allograft; *CLAU*, conjunctival-limbal autograft; *KLAL*, keratolimbal allograft; *SLET*, simple limbal epithelial transplantation.

etiology and stage of disease. We frequently employ preservative-free serum tears for patients who have an inadequate response to initial medical management, and we often use them early in our treatment approach. For medically optimized stage II patients who have conjunctivalization affecting the visual axis, we will attempt superficial keratectomy with or without amniotic membrane transplantation. We consider scleral contact lenses in stable stage II patients who have improved acuity with the lenses with the caveat that close monitoring is needed to assess for progression. For stage II patients who do not respond to these interventions, we consider advanced limbal stem cell transplantation techniques. The details of these approaches are beyond the scope of this chapter. With timely and appropriate intervention, we can restore vision in patients with partial LSCD and prevent progression to more advanced stages that require limbal stem cell transplantation.

References

1. Yazdanpanah G, Jabbehdari S, Djalilian AR. Limbal and corneal epithelial homeostasis. *Curr Opin Ophthalmol.* 2017;28:348–354.
2. Nubile M, Curcio C, Dua HS, et al. Pathological changes of the anatomical structure and markers of the limbal stem cell niche due to inflammation. *Mol Vis.* 2013;19:516–525.
3. Deng SX, Borderie V, Chan CC, et al. Global consensus on definition, classification, diagnosis, and staging of limbal stem cell deficiency. *Cornea.* 2019;38:364–375.
4. Lekhanont K, Jongkhajornpong P, Anothaisintawee T, Chuckpaiwong V. Undiluted serum eye drops for the treatment of persistent corneal epithelial defects. *Sci Rep.* 2016;6:38143.
5. Tsubota K, Goto E, Shimmura S, Shimazaki J. Treatment of persistent corneal epithelial defect by autologous serum application. *Ophthalmology.* 1999;106:1984–1989.
6. Kojima T, Hasegawa A, Nakamura T, et al. Five-year PROSE treatment for aniridic keratopathy. *Optom Vis Sci.* 2016;93:1328–1332.
7. Puangsricharern V, Tseng SCG. Cytologic evidence of corneal diseases with limbal stem cell deficiency. *Ophthalmology.* 1995;102:1476–1485.
8. Haagdorens M, Behaegel J, Rozema J, et al. A method for quantifying limbal stem cell niches using OCT imaging. *Br J Ophthalmol.* 2017;101:1250–1255.
9. Araújo AL, de, Ricardo JR, Sakai VN, et al. Impression cytology and in vivo confocal microscopy in corneas with total limbal stem cell deficiency. *Arq Bras Oftalmol.* 2013;76:305–308.
10. Yazdanpanah G, Jabbehdari S, Djalilian AR. Emerging approaches for ocular surface regeneration. *Curr Ophthalmol Rep.* 2019;7:1–10.
11. Liu L, Hartwig D, Harloff S, et al. An optimised protocol for the production of autologous serum eyedrops. *Graefes Arch Clin Exp Ophthalmol.* 2005;243:706–714.
12. Semeraro F, Forbice E, Braga O, et al. Evaluation of the efficacy of 50% autologous serum eye drops in different ocular surface pathologies. *Biomed Res Int.* 2014;2014:1–11.
13. Azari AA, Rapuano CJ. Autologous serum eye drops for the treatment of ocular surface disease. *Eye Contact Lens.* 2015;41:133–140.
14. Asbell PA, Potapova N. Effects of topical antiglaucoma medications on the ocular surface. *Ocular Surf.* 2005;3:27–40.
15. Cha S-H, Lee J-S, Oum B-S, Kim C-D. Corneal epithelial cellular dysfunction from benzalkonium chloride (BAC) in vitro. *Clin Exp Ophthalmol.* 2004;32:180–184.
16. Kim BY, Riaz KM, Bakhtiari P, et al. Medically reversible limbal stem cell disease: Clinical features and management strategies. *Ophthalmology.* 2014;121:2053–2058.
17. Giannaccare G, Versura P, Buzzi M, et al. Blood derived eye drops for the treatment of cornea and ocular surface diseases. *Transfus Apher Sci.* 2017;56:595–604.
18. Higuchi A. Autologous serum and serum components. *Invest Ophthalmol Vis Sci.* 2018;59:DES121–DES129.
19. Matsumoto Y, Dogru M, Goto E, et al. Autologous serum application in the treatment of neurotrophic keratopathy. *Ophthalmology.* 2004;111:1115–1120.
20. Lambiase A, Sacchetti M, Bonini S. Nerve growth factor therapy for corneal disease. *Curr Opin Ophthalmol.* 2012;23:296–302.

21. Touhami A, Grueterich M, Tseng SCG. The role of NGF signaling in human limbal epithelium expanded by amniotic membrane culture. *Invest Ophth Vis Sci*. 2002;43:987–994.

22. López-García JS, Rivas L, García-Lozano I, Murube J. Autologous serum eyedrops in the treatment of aniridic keratopathy. *Ophthalmology*. 2008;115:262–267.

23. Akcam HT, Unlu M, Karaca EE, et al. Autologous serum eye-drops and enhanced epithelial healing time after photorefractive keratectomy. *Clin Exp Optom*. 2017;101:34–37.

24. Chen Y-M, Hu F-R, Huang J-Y, et al. The effect of topical autologous serum on graft re-epithelialization after penetrating keratoplasty. *Am J Ophthalmol*. 2010;150:352–359.e2.

25. Celebi ARC, Ulusoy C, Mirza GE. The efficacy of autologous serum eye drops for severe dry eye syndrome: A randomized double-blind crossover study. *Graefe's Archive Clin Exp Ophthalmol*. 2014;252:619–626.

26. Tsubota K, Goto E, Fujita H, et al. Treatment of dry eye by autologous serum application in Sjogren's syndrome. *Brit J Ophthalmol*. 1999;83:390–395.

27. Romero-Rangel T, Stavrou P, Cotter J, et al. Gas-permeable scleral contact lens therapy in ocular surface disease. *Am J Ophthalmol*. 2000;130:25–32.

28. Parra AS, Roth BM, Nguyen TM, et al. Assessment of the prosthetic replacement of ocular surface ecosystem (PROSE) scleral lens on visual acuity for corneal irregularity and ocular surface disease. *Ocular Surf*. 2018;16:254–258.

29. Nguyen MTB, Thakrar V, Chan CC. EyePrintPRO therapeutic scleral contact lens: Indications and outcomes. *Can J Ophthalmol*. 2018;53:66–70.

30. Harthan JS, Shorter E. Therapeutic uses of scleral contact lenses for ocular surface disease: Patient selection and special considerations. *Clin Optom (Auckl)*. 2018;10:65–74.

31. Kim KH, Deloss KS, Hood CT. Prosthetic replacement of the ocular surface ecosystem (PROSE) for visual rehabilitation in limbal stem cell deficiency. *Eye Contact Lens*. 2020;1.

32. Lim P, Ridges R, Jacobs DS, Rosenthal P. Treatment of persistent corneal epithelial defect with overnight wear of a prosthetic device for the ocular surface. *Am J Ophthalmol*. 2013;156:1095–1101.

33. Schornack MM. Limbal stem cell disease: Management with scleral lenses. *Clin Exp Optom*. 2011; 94:592–594.

34. Jeng BH, Halfpenny CP, Meisler DM, Stock EL. Management of focal limbal stem cell deficiency associated with soft contact lens wear. *Cornea*. 2011;30:18–23.

35. Rossen J, Amram A, Milani B, et al. Contact lens-induced limbal stem cell deficiency. *Ocular Surf*. 2016;14:419–434.

CHAPTER 22

Corneal Suturing and Adjusting at the Slit Lamp

Marjan Farid ■ Alexander Knezevic

Introduction

Corneal suturing and adjusting at the slit lamp present many advantages but also unique challenges. When possible, it is faster and easier for patients without the added hassles of emergency room visits or going to the operating room. Identifying the cooperative patient and appropriate pathology to be repaired in an in-office setting is key. For a busy practice where penetrating keratoplasty (PKP) is frequently performed, efficient management of postoperative wound leak or suture adjustment is instrumental. While many practices may have a minor room, setting up equipment and patient transportation can present added challenges. This chapter is intended as a guide for in-office suturing of appropriate corneal pathology.

Patient selection is an important factor in pursuing corneal suturing and adjustment at the slit lamp. A host of patient factors, including underlying medical conditions that could affect positioning, psychiatric conditions, or patient temperament, may impact performing the procedure. As no anesthesia provider is present, the surgeon must have confidence in the patient's cooperation.

Case 1 Corneal Laceration

A 50-year-old male presents to the emergency room with severe foreign body sensation after a work-related eye injury. The cornea is found to have a radial laceration that is full thickness. The wound is Seidel positive on examination. No foreign bodies are found.

PROCEDURE: CORNEAL SUTURING OF CORNEAL LACERATION

Supplies: Box 22.1

A topical anesthetic drop and a drop of broad-spectrum antibiotic are placed in the conjunctival fornix. The lids and lashes are prepped with betadine in typical fashion for an ocular procedure.[1-3] An eyelid speculum is placed, and the patient is brought forward to the slit lamp (Fig. 22.1).

The primary goal of corneal suturing in the setting of laceration or a leaking wound is to balance sealing the cornea while minimizing scarring and astigmatism. Monofilament 10-0 nylon suture material on a fine spatula microsurgical needle is used. Corneal sutures should be 90% of stromal depth and equal depth on both sides of the wound. Shallow sutures may be structurally weak and difficult to rotate. Long sutures may cause unnecessary astigmatism or scarring. Full-thickness sutures may lead to suture track leaks and subsequent microbial invasion or endophthalmitis.

Corneal sutures should be passed with the tip of the needle perpendicular to the corneal surface with the needle rotated along the curve of the needle exiting along the cut surface. If the wound is well approximated, the needle can be passed through the opposite side of the wound.

BOX 22.1 ■ Supplies

- Barraquer eye speculum
- 0.12-mm forceps
- Povidone-iodine 5%
- Ofloxacin ophthalmic solution 0.3% (or equivalent antibiotic eye drop)
- Proparacaine hydrochloride 0.5% (or equivalent anesthetic eye drop)
- Suture scissors
- Needle driver
- Monofilament 10-0 nylon suture on a spatula-designed microsurgical needle
- Tying forceps (straight and bent)

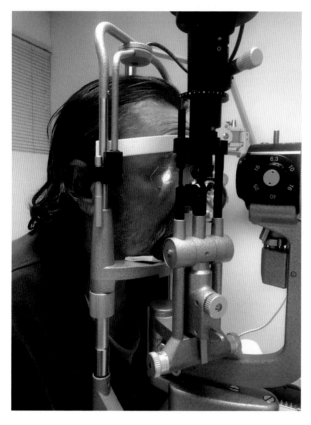

Fig. 22.1 Positioning the patient at the slit-lamp microscope with a speculum to hold the eyelids. (Courtesy M. Farid and A. Knezevic).

If the wound is too superficial or too deep, an adjustment can be made at this time to properly approximate the anterior surface. Prior to passing the needle, the suture length can be trimmed so there are no long ends that will drag over the face and cheek area. A slipknot allows for maximal control in a setting where patient movement can be a complicating factor. Tying the suture at the slit lamp can be challenging and will require the use of tying forceps or, alternatively, two jeweler forceps with thin grasping tips to maneuver vertically. After trimming the suture ends with a corneal scissor, the knot is rotated with tying forceps without burying the knot in the wound to prevent wound gape[4] (Fig. 22.2).

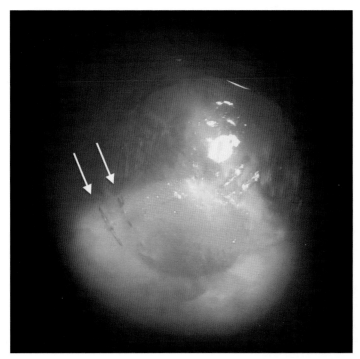

Fig. 22.2   Sutures placed through corneal laceration with no evidence of further leak with Seidel testing.

Different laceration morphologies may require various angles of suture placement. These can be individualized based on type and location of laceration.

DISCUSSION

In the setting of trauma where other facial or bodily injuries may have occurred, prompt referral to an emergency room with ophthalmic coverage may be appropriate. Past ocular and medical history, including prior ophthalmic surgeries, should be obtained. If a new injury has occurred, documentation should reflect how the injury occurred and the events that followed.[5] Foreign body should always be suspected. In particular, vegetable matter has a high risk of contamination.[6]

External examination of the face and eyelids should document any lacerations or bony step-offs. Baseline visual acuity and a pinhole should be assessed, as they are an important prognostic indicator. Pupillary examination will help assess whether there is a ruptured globe or involvement of the optic nerve. This includes documentation for the presence or absence of a relative afferent papillary defect. Extraocular movement restriction can tip off orbital pathology.

With slit-lamp examination, the presence and extent of subconjunctival hemorrhage should be documented. Any visible corneal laceration, including depth, length, limbal, or scleral involvement, should be noted. Seidel testing should be used to evaluate any suspicious areas.[7] In the setting of prior PKP, areas of graft-host junction (GHJ) step-off or bulging may be the site of a leak. Any tight sutures causing corneal flattening or loose sutures causing staining should be identified. The anterior chamber may be shallow in a penetrating or perforating injury or, conversely, deep if there is lens dislocation. Evaluation of the anterior segment is completed with documentation of the iris, lens, and lens capsule and the presence of vitreous or foreign bodies.

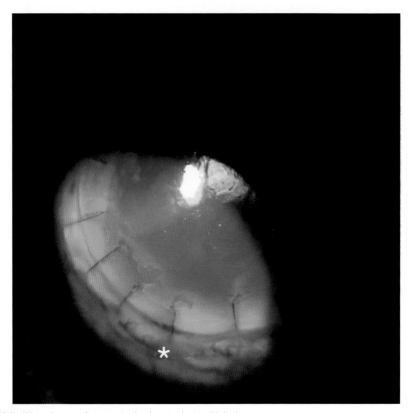

Fig. 22.3 Wound gape after penetrating keratoplasty with leak.

In settings of acute trauma, examination of the vitreous and retina should be performed on both eyes. A Shafer sign should be identified as red blood cells or pigment in the vitreous, as it may indicate retinal tears. Retinal or choroidal detachment or choroidal rupture may all be identified on the initial examination, which impact both management and predict outcomes.

Advanced corneal trauma where the limbus and sclera are involved or shallow anterior chamber with uveal prolapse should alert the examiner that a more serious injury has occurred. In the case of a suspected foreign body, computed tomography scanning of the eye and orbit is indicated.[8] These cases should be repaired in a more controlled setting of the operating room.

Case 2 PKP Wound Leak

A 72-year-old male presents to clinic for a postoperative-week-1 examination after penetrating keratoplasty (PKP). A slow leak is detected at the GHJ at 7 o'clock (Fig. 22.3)

PROCEDURE: CORNEAL SUTURING OF A PKP WOUND

Supplies: Box 22.2

The eye is prepped similar to case 1. Taking care to turn the wrist so that the needle enters the tissue perpendicular to the wound and follows the curve to exit will allow a smooth equidistant pass

> **BOX 22.2 ■ Supplies**
>
> - Barraquer eye speculum
> - 0.12-mm forceps
> - Povidone-iodine 5%
> - Ofloxacin ophthalmic solution 0.3% (or equivalent antibiotic eye drop)
> - Proparacaine hydrochloride 0.5% (or equivalent anesthetic eye drop)
> - Suture scissors
> - Needle driver
> - Monofilament 10-0 nylon suture on a spatula-designed microsurgical needle
> - Tying forceps (straight and bent)

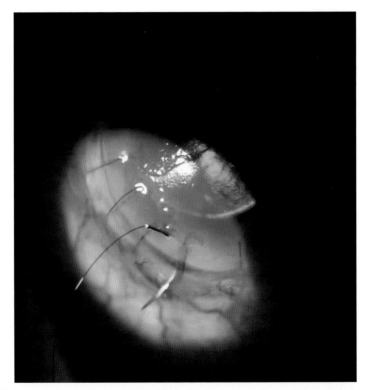

Fig. 22.4 Suture needle passed (at the slit lamp) through wound edge with even bite through donor and host tissue.

between donor and host tissue (Fig. 22.4). Now, a cross stitch is placed across the leak (Fig. 22.5). The knot is buried. Care should be taken to approximate the graft-host anterior edge to create a smooth transition without step-offs. Additionally, the tension of the newly placed stitch cannot be more than the neighboring sutures, as this can cause not only significant striae and astigmatism but also can create loosening of the neighboring areas. The wound is confirmed to be Seidel negative with fluorescein staining (Fig. 22.6). An additional drop of antibiotic is placed on the eye, and the speculum is removed.

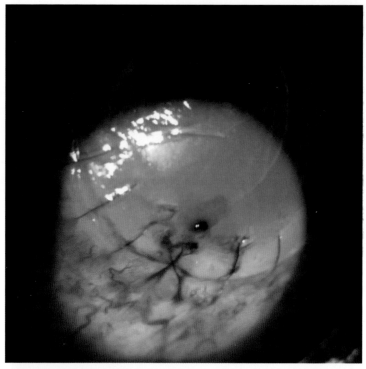

Fig. 22.5   A mattress suture X stitch is placed to close the wound gape and seal the leak.

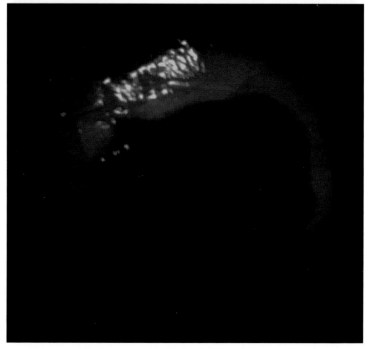

Fig. 22.6   Seidel testing at the slit lamp confirms no further wound leak.

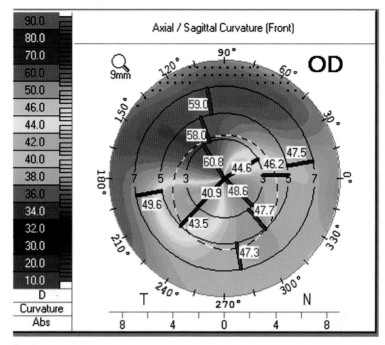

Fig. 22.7 Postkeratoplasty topography showing steepness at the 128-degree axis and flatness at the 210-degree axis.

Case 3 Post-PKP High Astigmatism With a Running Suture

A 36-year-old female who is 3-months post-PKP for keratoconus presents for her postoperative visit. Her uncorrected visual acuity is 20/150. Her topography reveals 8.3 D of irregular cylinder at 128 degrees (Fig. 22.7), and the manifest refraction also reveals that with 7.5 D of cylinder at 120 degrees, the visual acuity improves rapidly to 20/25. Since she has a 24-bite running suture, a suture adjustment to redistribute the tension of the running suture can dramatically decrease the effective cylinder within the graft and improve the visual acuity.

PROCEDURE: ADJUSTMENT OF A RUNNING PKP SUTURE

Supplies: Box 22.3

A topical anesthetic drop and a drop of broad-spectrum antibiotic are placed in the conjunctival fornix. An eyelid speculum is placed, and the patient is brought forward to the slit lamp. The topography is analyzed with a plan to start with the suture loops in the flatter areas of the topography. Those suture loops are tightened, and suture slack is redistributed to the steeper axis of the topography. The first loop must be gently grabbed by flat- and larger-tip jeweler forceps and pulled forward. The next loop does not need to be grabbed, but, rather, one prong of the jeweler forceps is passed beneath it, and the loop is pulled out. This is done consecutively from the area of loose loops, and these are redistributed to the areas of tighter loops. For this case, the first loop that is tightened would start at 210 degrees, and the loose loops are fed into the 120-degree axis. As the

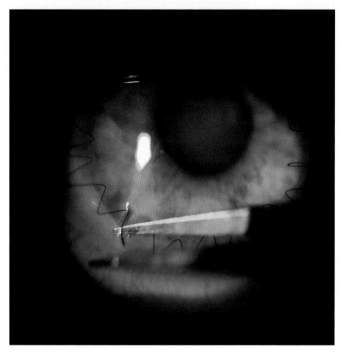

Fig. 22.8 A jeweler forceps is used to redistribute suture tension on a running suture postkeratoplasty (at the slit lamp).

knot at 90 degrees is a hard stop and cannot be adjusted through, a second readjustment of suture tension from the 30-degree axis to the 300-degree axis is performed. Care should be taken that the jeweler prong is kept flat so that the suture does not slide along the edge of the medal, which can risk suture breakage (Fig. 22.8). See Video 22.1.

If the running suture breaks, an interrupted suture can be passed in the area of break, and the two ends are tied to the two broken ends of the running suture. As this would create two additional knots, these can either be gently buried or a bandage contact lens can be used for 1–2 months until the entire suture can be removed safely.

Conclusion

Corneal suturing at the slit lamp is a useful skill for the corneal or anterior segment surgeon to maximize efficiency and convenience for both the patient and physician. Patient selection and appropriate pathology are important concerns. Small corneal lacerations, PKP wound leak, and PKP running suture adjustment, as described in this chapter, are ideal cases for slit-lamp suturing.

References

1. Carrim ZI, Mackie G, Gallacher G, Wykes WN. The efficacy of 5% povidone-iodine for 3 minutes prior to cataract surgery. *Eur J Ophthalmol.* 2009;19:560–564. https://doi.org/10.1177/11206721090190 0407.
2. Halachmi-Eyal O, Lang Y, Keness Y, Miron D. Preoperative topical moxifloxacin 0.5% and povidone-iodine 5.0% versus povidone-iodine 5.0% alone to reduce bacterial colonization in the conjunctival sac. *J Cataract Refract Surg.* 2009;35:2109–2114. https://doi.org/10.1016/j.jcrs.2009.06.038.
3. Speaker MG, Menikoff JA. Prophylaxis of endophthalmitis with topical povidone-iodine. *Ophthalmology.* 1991;98:1769–1775. https://doi.org/10.1016/s0161-6420(91)32052-9.
4. Macsai M. *Ophthalmic Microsurgical Suturing Techniques.* Springer Verlag, 2007.
5. Aslam SA, Sheth HG, Vaughan AJ. Emergency management of corneal injuries. *Injury.* 2007;38:594–597. https://doi.org/10.1016/j.injury.2006.04.122.
6. Greven CM, Engelbrecht NE, Slusher MM, Nagy SS. Intraocular foreign bodies: Management, prognostic factors, and visual outcomes. *Ophthalmology.* 2000;107:608–612. https://doi.org/10.1016/s0161-6420(99)00134-7.
7. Madhusudhana KC. Corneal abrasion or corneal penetration? *J Trauma.* 2006;60:687. https://doi.org/10.1097/01.ta.0000205801.38299.6e.
8. Arey ML, Mootha VV, Whittemore AR, Chason DP, Blomquist PH. Computed tomography in the diagnosis of occult open-globe injuries. *Ophthalmology.* 2007;114:1448–1452. https://doi.org/10.1016/j.ophtha.2006.10.051.

CHAPTER 23

Corneal Transplant Complications

Kendall E. Donaldson

As corneal specialists, we are fortunate to be able to provide our patients with an expanding array of options that allow them to improve their vision despite potentially sight-threatening conditions. Over the past two decades, we have seen significant advancements in lamellar kerato-plasty and the correction of astigmatism. This has allowed us to provide our patients with faster visual recovery, better visual potential, and the means to adjust their vision postoperatively without returning to the operating room. While our techniques have advanced, we use several minor pro-cedures to facilitate visual recovery.

Case 1

The patient is a 67-year-old male with a history of bilateral chronic anterior keratouveitis associ-ated with herpetic uveitic glaucoma (Fig. 23.1) The patient had undergone bilateral Baerveldt glaucoma implants and had previously undergone a penetrating keratoplasty (PKP) twice in the right eye, as well as an endothelial keratoplasty followed by a PKP in the left eye. The left eye was his primary functional eye, as the right eye was cupped with a cloudy, failed graft. The graft in the left eye had remained clear following his second corneal surgery. The patient presented to clinic with a 2-day decline in vision in the left eye. New Descemet folds and a mild anterior chamber reaction were observed. The patient was started on hourly prednisolone acetate 1% ophthalmic drops and cyclosporin 0.5% drops 4 times a day and was advised to return in 1 week for consid-eration of a sub-Tenon Kenalog injection if no improvement. Upon his return in 1 week, he con-tinued to struggle with his vision, and his corneal exam remained unchanged; thus, a sub-Tenon Kenalog injection (40 mg/ml) was administered in the inferior fornix (Box 23.1).

PROCEDURE: MANAGEMENT OF GRAFT REJECTION WITH TRAIMCINOLONE ACETONIDE (SUB-TENON KENALOG-40) INJECTION

These injections can be performed in the examining chair in a semisupine position. Preservative-free 4% lidocaine solution on a sterile cotton swab is used as a pledget in the inferotemporal fornix following a 5% povidone-iodine prep of the lids with a drop of povidone-iodine on the surface of the eye along with a drop of antibiotic. Either lidocaine 4% drops or viscous lidocaine can be used for anesthesia. However, if viscous lidocaine is used, it is essential to place povidone-iodine before the gel to ensure appropriate povidone-iodine penetration for the semisterile procedure. The Kenalog is drawn out of the vial with a 25-gauge needle. Once in the syringe, the needle is switched from a 25-gauge to a 27-gauge needle in the interest of patient comfort. However, a 30-gauge needle is notably too thin to manage viscous Kenalog. Kenalog also separates into its components, so it is very important to roll the syringe between your hands (or shake the syringe) to resuspend the 2 components before injection. As my assistant gently pulls the lower lid inferior, I have the patient look up and insert the needle into the temporal tarsal fornix, injecting 0.5 cc of Kenalog-40. Patients find this procedure very comfortable and tolerable, avoiding the use of a lid speculum. An antibiotic drop is then applied.

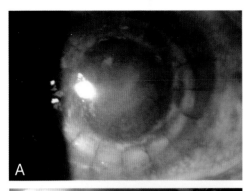

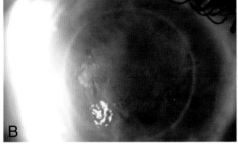

Fig. 23.1 (A–B) Graft rejection unresponsive to topical agents. Appropriate for sub-Tenon Kenalog injection.

BOX 23.1 ■ Supplies for Sub-Tenon Triamcinolone Injection

- Triamcinolone (Kenalog-40)
- 0.5% Tetracaine or lidocaine 4% drops, preservative free
- Topical antibiotic drop
- 5% Povidone-iodine prep/swabs
- 27-gauge needle
- 3-cc syringe
- Wire-lid speculum
- Cotton-tip applicators (pack of 2)

DISCUSSION

Graft rejection is always a disappointment to both the surgeon and the patient, but it is even more challenging when the cause is unknown and the patient is compliant with medical management and follow-up appointments. Of course, great surgical technique and appropriate medical management are the mainstays of rapid recovery; however, at times, we need to move forward with procedural options. With initial rejection, steroids are increased to an hourly dosing regimen, and compounded cyclosporin 0.5% is often added to suppress the inflammatory/immune response. Any underlying condition causing inflammation should be treated (such as systemic rheumatoid disease, herpetic infection, retained lens material, or poorly positioned glaucoma implant). If there is no improvement within a week, consider a sub-Tenon Kenalog injection in the office. Both subconjunctival and sub-Tenon injection of triamcinolone have been shown to decrease anterior segment inflammation in patients after corneal transplantation.[1] Although either an inferior or superior approach can be taken, an inferior approach may be easier and safer, avoiding any risk of globe penetration. In some cases of aggressive rejection, an additional superior subconjunctival injection of dexamethasone can also be given at the same time as the Kenalog to facilitate a more rapid response.

Case 2

The patient is a 79-year-old female with a history of bilateral cataract surgery with Baerveldt glaucoma implants for severe open-angle glaucoma. The patient had done well for several years after her glaucoma surgery; however, she then began to experience a progressive decline in the vision of the left eye associated with the onset of corneal edema. The tube in the left eye extended approximately 4 mm into the anterior chamber and was noted to be near the corneal endothelium in the superotemporal quadrant of the cornea. Over a period of 3–4 months, the visual decline was dramatic, resulting in unstable, fluctuating 20/400 vision. There appeared to be significant endothelial decompensation and corneal edema. It was decided that the patient would undergo a Descemet stripping with endothelial transplantation (DSEK) procedure in addition to repositioning the tube into the sulcus. On postoperative day 1, the DSEK graft had detached and was found to be sitting at the inferior angle. The patient was suffering from hand motion vision. The patient was immediately prepared for rebubbling and repositioning of the DSEK graft in the minor procedure room (since the graft was fully detached) (Box 23.2).

PROCEDURE: REBUBBING AND REPOSITIONING OF THE DSEK GRAFT

DSEK rebubbling can be performed either at the slit lamp in a sitting position or supine on a bed under an operating microscope in a minor procedure room (in office) or the operating room. If the detachment is partial and the tissue is still centered in a good position, the procedure can be approached at the slit lamp. However, if the graft is fully detached, the rebubbling and repositioning are best approached in the supine position in a minor procedure room (or laser suite) with the availability of an operating microscope in the office. Before the procedure is approached, the lids and lashes should be cleaned with povidone-iodine in the usual sterile ophthalmic fashion, and sterile lid drapes (similar to laser-assisted in situ keratomileusis drapes) should be positioned over the lids to retract the lashes and avoid contamination. When performed with the patient in the supine position, the surgeon is seated superiorly. The surgeon may be able to reopen the original superior paracentesis for passage of instruments if the rebubbling occurs within the first 3 postoperative days. However, if necessary, a superior paracentesis can be formed with a no. 75 blade or supersharp paracentesis blade. It is a good idea to keep a syringe of balanced salt solution (BSS) and a syringe of filtered air available on the mayo stand throughout the procedure. A reverse Sinsky

---

BOX 23.2 ■ Supplies

- Topical antibiotic drop
- 0.5% Tetracaine or 4% lidocaine drops (preservative free)
- 5% Povidone-iodine prep
- Metal lid speculum
- 27-gauge needle
- 3-cc syringe × 2 (1 for air and 1 for balanced salt solution)
- Reverse Sinsky hook
- Balanced salt solution
- No. 75 blade or supersharp blade (to create paracentesis for repositioning; not necessary if only rebubbling)
- 27-gauge cannula
- Air filter

hook can be used to grab the superior edge of the graft and lift it out of the inferior angle, using BSS to maintain the stability of the anterior chamber as needed. Once the graft is well centered, a cannula of filtered air is placed beneath the tissue and extended to the central anterior chamber over the intraocular lens but above the iris (to avoid pupillary block). If the graft is not centered or needs to be repositioned periodically, one may need to reinflate the anterior chamber with BSS and then replace the bubble. Once a partial bubble of reasonable size has been formed (enough to keep the tissue in place), refocus on adding air through the paracentesis. Instead of placing the cannula through the paracentesis, it can be gently placed at the mouth of the paracentesis to create a 100% anterior chamber fill. This can be achieved through a slow but forceful injection of air without fully opening the paracentesis. The aim is to leave a full bubble for 1 hour while the patient remains supine in the office and intraocular pressure can be monitored. One must ensure that the intraocular pressure is not excessive and the patient is not in pain during the observation time. If the patient has a glaucoma tube shunt, a full air fill is reasonable, as loss of air through the tube can happen more rapidly. If the patient does not have a tube shunt, a small amount of BSS is injected into the anterior chamber while allowing some air to escape to leave approximately an 80% fill. A drop of antibiotic 0.5% is placed at the conclusion of the case, and the patient continues an antibiotic drop for 1 week following the procedure. Usually, this is performed within the first postoperative week, so the patient is already taking an antibiotic drop which can be continued just a few days longer in the case of rebubbling. If the graft detachment is partial and the DSEK lenticule is still centered, an air bubble can be slowly injected through a previously or newly made paracentesis port via a cannula on an air-filled syringe while the patient is at the slit lamp.

Case 3

The patient is an 84-year-old female with a history of Fuchs dystrophy, anterior basement membrane dystrophy, and mild, dry, age-related macular degeneration. She had previously undergone uncomplicated cataract surgery in both eyes and a successful DSEK surgery in the left eye. Since the time of her original surgery, the standard of care had evolved to indicate that a Descemet membrane endothelial keratoplasty (DMEK) graft could potentially offer the patient better vision, higher long-term endothelial cell counts, and a more rapid recovery relative to surgery in the other eye.[2] She underwent DMEK surgery in the right. On postoperative day 1, she was noted to have an attached DMEK graft with a central 3-mm Descemet detachment diagnosed on anterior segment optical coherence tomography (OCT) (Fig. 23.2).[3] Since this area accounted for less than 1/3 of the total graft area, a decision was made to observe, and the patient returned in 1 week. The area overlying the graft detachment remained edematous and developed a corneal epithelial defect. Given the area of decompensation overlying the localized graft detachment, the patient was rebubbled with filtered air in the office. Early on in the DMEK learning curve, we would observe an area less than 1/3 of the total graft area; however, we now rebubble much more quickly, even with small areas of central detachment, avoiding potential overlying corneal decompensation and continued corneal edema associated with poor visual acuity. We realize that the complications of leaving an area detached are more significant than the inconvenience of performing a minor in-office procedure. We also realize the visual recovery is much faster if the graft is reattached sooner, and it is much easier to place a bubble when much of the graft is still attached as opposed to waiting until the graft is detached and then requires a new graft and a trip back to the operating room to obtain visual recovery (Box 23.3).

PROCEDURE: DMEK REBUBBLING AT THE SLIT LAMP

DMEK rebubbling can also be approached either at the slit lamp or in a supine position in a minor procedure room. (Figs. 23.2–23.6) Although DSEK tissue can easily be repositioned in

BOX 23.3 ■ Supplies

- Topical antibiotic drop
- 0.5% Tetracaine or 4% lidocaine drops (preservative free)
- 5% Povidone-iodine prep
- Metal lid speculum
- 27-gauge needle
- 1-cc or 3-cc syringe (tuberculin syringe)
- Air filter

Alternative Technique – Additional Tools[2]

- Sulfur hexafluoride 20% dilution (optional)
- Intravenous tubing (optional)

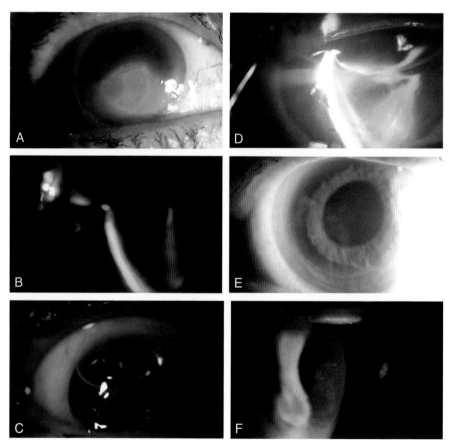

Fig. 23.2 Patient 1. Descemet membrane endothelial keratoplasty (DMEK) rebubbling. (A–B) Before rebubbling: epithelial defect with rolled borders in the area of Descemet detachment. (C–D) Immediately after rebubbling. (E–F) One month after DMEK rebubbling.

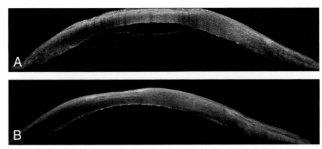

Fig. 23.3 (A–B) Patient 1. Anterior segment optical coherence tomography (OCT) before and after Descemet membrane endothelial keratoplasty (DMEK) rebubbling. (A) Patient 1 before DMEK rebubbling. (B) Patient 1 after DMEK rebubbling.

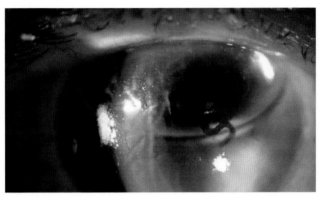

Fig. 23.4 Descemet membrane endothelial keratoplasty (DMEK) rebubbling. Patient 2 postop day 1 with central detachment, attached peripherally, and 50% sulfur hexafluoride (SF6) bubble, resulting in significant corneal edema. Air added with 30-gauge needle at slit lamp.

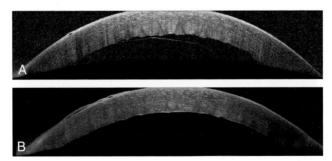

Fig. 23.5 (A–B) Patient 2. Anterior segment optical coherence tomography (OCT) before and after Descemet membrane endothelial keratoplasty (DMEK) rebubbling. Fig. 23.5 (A) Before Descemet membrane endothelial keratoplasty (DMEK) rebubbling at slit lamp. (B) After DMEK rebubbling.

the office with a reverse Sinsky hook, DMEK tissue cannot easily be repositioned in the office, and for this reason, it is best to intervene as early as possible if there is potential incomplete graft attachment. A povidone-iodine prep of the lids is performed following application of 1% tetracaine or 4% lidocaine anesthetic drops. Air injection can often be performed with a 30-gauge needle through a preexisting paracentesis. Generally, the detachment is inferior if the patient

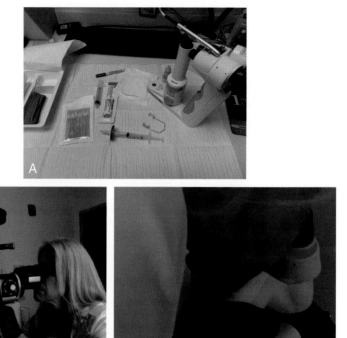

Fig. 23.6 (A–C) Descemet membrane endothelial keratoplasty (DMEK) rebubbling at the slit lamp. (A) Tools for DMEK rebubbling. (B) Injection of air at the slit lamp through the inferior paracentesis on postoperative day 3. (C) Evaluation of the DMEK graft after rebubbling in the supine position. One hour after rebubbling, the patient was examined with an anterior segment optical coherence tomography (OCT) to ensure full graft attachment with no interface fluid.

is at the slit lamp and looks upward; one can place the needle through the inferior paracentesis and extend the needle into the anterior chamber superior to the area of detachment, injecting slowly to flatten out the detached area of the graft (Fig. 23.6). Once the graft is flattened, a little additional air at the mouth of the paracentesis is added to ensure full adhesion. The patient is instructed to lie on their back for 1 hour after the procedure before going home to ensure the best success. One must ensure that the intraocular pressure is not excessive and that the patient is not in pain during this time of full air fill. At the end of the hour, the patient is sat upright at the slit lamp to ensure the inferior peripheral iridotomy is not covered by the bubble and there is no risk of pupillary block. If needed, a small amount of air can be removed by gently compressing the outer lip of the paracentesis or by slowly inserting the 30-gauge needle with the stopper of the syringe removed. One must be careful not to remove too much air, leaving an adequate bubble, as the air can exit rapidly in the early postoperative period when the paracentesis is fresh. An anterior segment OCT at this time can be very helpful to ensure full graft adhesion with resolution of any interface fluid (Fig. 23.3 and Fig. 23.5). Antibiotic drops are placed both before and after the procedure.

An alternative procedure for DMEK rebubbling has been published by Sales et al.[4]

The rebubbling apparatus was composed of a standard 43-inch intravenous extension tube, a 5-cc syringe, and a 27-gauge cannula. The cannula was screwed onto one end of the extension tubing, and a 5-cc syringe that has been filled with air was screwed onto the opposite end. With the patient seated at the slit lamp, the cannula was positioned in the anterior chamber by the surgeon with one hand while the other hand operates the syringe and the joystick. In this particular publication, the authors found this technique to be ergonomically preferable to the traditional technique described earlier.

Case 4

The patient is a 67-year-old male with a history of PKP following a contact lens–related penetrating ulcer (Fig. 23.7A–C). The patient achieved a clear graft and underwent successive suture removal over a period of approximately 15 months.[5] After complete suture removal, the patient was left with significant residual regular astigmatism (Fig. 23.7B). Due to a history of rheumatoid arthritis (limiting his manual dexterity) and a history of contact lens intolerance, the patient was highly motivated to pursue procedural options for alleviation of his residual astigmatism. The pros

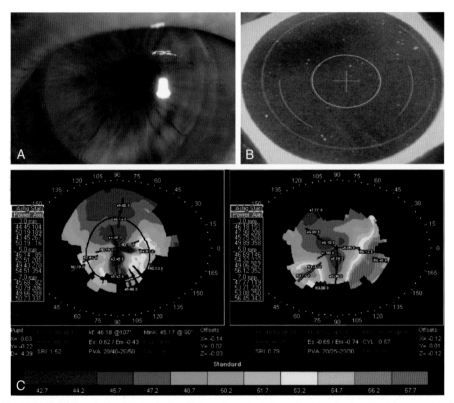

Fig. 23.7 (A–D) Penetrating keratoplasty with irregular astigmatism. Awaiting femtosecond laser–assisted astigmatic keratectomy. Representative image courtesy of Sonia Yoo, MD. (A) Post–penetrating keratoplasty with irregular astigmatism. Now post–femtosecond laser–assisted astigmatic keratectomy. (B) Laser pattern with 6.5-mm optical zone (8-mm corneal graft). (C) Topography before and after femtosecond astigmatic keratotomy (AK) with reduction in astigmatism from 4.4 D to 0.67 D. Uncorrected vision improved from 20/60 to 20/50, and best corrected visual acuity (BCVA) improved from 20/50 to 20/32.

TABLE 23.1 ■ Supplies for Astigmatic Keratotomy

Supplies for Slit-Lamp Astigmatic Keratotomy	Supplies for Femtosecond Laser–Assisted Astigmatic Keratotomy
Topical antibiotic drop	Topical antibiotic drop
0.5% Tetracaine or 4% lidocaine drops	0.5% Tetracaine or 4% lidocaine drops
5% Povidone-iodine prep	5% Povidone-iodine prep
Adjustable-depth astigmatic keratotomy blade (Moria)	Sinsky hook
Sinsky hook	Itralase iFS laser (Johnson and Johnson)
Bandage contact lens (optional, for comfort)	Bandage contact lens (optional, for comfort)

and cons of surgical versus manual limbal relaxing incisions were discussed. Given the mild asymmetry in his pattern of astigmatism, it was decided to use the femtosecond laser, as it would help us design and apply a precise pattern of asymmetric astigmatism correction at a specific optical zone (within the graft)[5] (Table 23.1).

PROCEDURE: MANAGING ASTIGMATISM AFTER PENETRATING KERATOPLASTY–ASTIGMATIC KERATOTOMY

Astigmatic keratotomy (AK) should only be performed after all sutures have been removed from a PKP or deep anterior lamellar keratoplasty. Once all sutures have been removed, a refraction and topography/tomography should be performed. Two to three serial refractions and topographies should be performed at 4- to 6-week intervals to ensure stability and prior to final procedure planning. At this point, astigmatism can be differentiated into regular astigmatism and irregular astigmatism. Irregular astigmatism is very difficult to treat and may be due to a combination of ocular surface disease and asymmetry of graft scar formation and secondary to suture removal. Regular astigmatism may be treatable with AK incisions created manually or with the use of a femtosecond laser.[5–8] One must keep in mind that long AK incisions may temporarily or permanently worsen ocular surface disease. In addition, more centrally placed incisions can induce or worsen irregular astigmatism. The incisions are made approximately 1 mm or more within the graft-host junction and are aligned with the steep corneal axis based on corneal topography.[8] The treatment pattern is usually designed in a symmetric pattern according to the steep axis, and the depth is calculated based on 80% of the corneal thickness as measured by anterior segment OCT in the areas of planned treatment. However, the treatment can also be applied in an asymmetric pattern designed to match the topographic map.

Given the typical prolonged period of suture removal (generally greater than 1 year), a topographically designed treatment pattern can be determined and applied only after suture removal has been completed and the refraction and topographic maps are stable. The AK incisions should be placed at least 1 mm within the graft-host junction (which is generally at approximately a 6.5- to 7.0 -mm optical zone).[8] The incisions are made at approximately 65%–80% corneal depth, which can be assessed by anterior segment OCT or by tomography (not as precise, and cannot target the particular location for incision placement). Nomograms vary according to whether the incisions are made manually versus with the use of the femtosecond laser (Table 23.2A and B).[8] For best effect, the AK incisions can be opened at the time of surgery (with a Sinsky hook), or they may be opened during the postoperative period as determined by topography. Generally, AK incisions in a PKP tend to have a greater effect than AK incisions in a native cornea; therefore, a conservative approach is advocated.

TABLE 23.2 ■ A. Nomogram for Manual Astigmatic Keratotomy Incisions: Hanna Nomogram for Astigmatic Keratotomy for Correction of Post–Keratoplasty Astigmatism[8]

Refractive Astigmatism (D)	Optical Zone Diameter (mm)	Incision Depth (% of Corneal Thickness)	Angular Length of Incision (Degrees)
2.50–3.75	6.75	75	60
4.00–5.00	6.50	75	60
5.00–6.25	6.50	75	70
6.50–7.50	6.25	75	70
7.75–8.75	6.25	75	80
9.00–15.00	6.00	75	80

*Older than or younger than age 30 years: increase or decrease efficacy by 0.05 diopters (D) per year.

TABLE 23.2 ■ B. Nomogram for Femtosecond Laser–Created Astigmatic Keratotomy Incisions[8]

Preop DK	Incision Magnitude	Correction (%)	Incision Depth (% Corneal Thickness)	Arc Length (Degrees)	Optical Zone Diameter (mm)
2	1.311	0.87	85	60	7.0
3	1.784	0.82	85	75	6.8
4	2.176	0.78	85	85	6.7
5	2.508	0.72	85	90	6.6
6	2.791	0.98	90	90	6.6
7	3.036	0.91	90	90	6.5
8	3.249	0.87	90	90	6.4
9	3.438	0.83	90	90	6.3
10	3.605	0.81	90	90	6.2

DK, Delta K (difference between the steepest and flattest keratometry values).

Conclusion

All of these techniques are useful postsurgical adjuncts to help us achieve the very best results for our patients. Patients are much more amenable to in-office procedures relative to additional surgery, as these procedures are perceived by the patient as an "enhancement" or "adjustment" following surgery rather than a repeat surgery after a "failed procedure." Additionally, these procedures are typically lower risk, require less recovery, and are lower cost compared to a return to the operating room. Mastering these simple techniques is a key component to providing our patients with the very best care.

References

1. Yannis A, Michael T, Anant S, Parwez H. Subconjunctival triamcinolone acetonide in the management of ocular inflammatory disease. *Ocul Pharmacol Ther.* Jul-Aug 2013;29(6):516–522.
2. Feng MT, Price M, Miller JM, Price FW. Air reinjection and endothelial cell density in DMEK: 5-year follow-up. *J Cataract Refract Surg.* 2014;40:1116–1121.

3. Yoh RY, Quilendrino R, Musa FU, Liarakos VS, Dapena I, Melles GRJ. Predictive value of OCT in graft attachment after DMEK. *Ophthalmology*. 2013;120:240–245.
4. Sales C, Straiko M, Terry M. Novel technique for rebubbling DMEK grafts at the slit lamp using intravenous extension tubing. *Cornea*. 2016;35(4):582–585.
5. Chang JSM. Femtosecond laser-assisted astigmatic keratotomy: A review. *Eye Vis (Lond)*. 2018;5:6.
6. Yoo S, Hurmeric V. Femtosecond laser-assisted keratoplasty. *Am J Ophthalmol*. Feb 2011;151(2):189–191.
7. Kymionis GD, Yoo S, Ide T. Culbertson WW Femtosecond-assisted astigmatism keratotomy for post-keratoplasty irregular astigmatism. *J Cataract Refract Surg*. 35 (1): 11–13.
8. Ryan M St Clair, Anushree Sharma, David Huang, et al. Development of a nomogram for femtosecond laser astigmatic keratotomy for astigmatism after keratoplasty. *Cataract Refract Surg*. Apr 2016;42(4):556–562.

INDEX

Note: Page numbers followed by *f* indicate figures; *t*, tables; *b*, boxes